AF441802

PAIN MECHANISMS AND MANAGEMENT

Pain Mechanisms and Management

Edited by

S.N. Ayrapetyan

Biophysics Center, Armenian National Academy of Sciences
Yerevan, Armenia

and

A.V. Apkarian

Department of Neurosurgery, SUNY Health Science Center
Syracuse, NY, USA

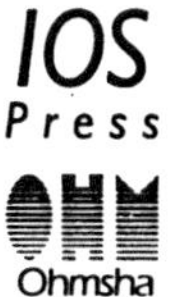

IOS Press

Ohmsha

Amsterdam • Berlin • Oxford • Tokyo • Washington, DC

ISBN 90 5199 306 4 (IOS Press)
ISBN 4 274 90135 1 C3047 (Ohmsha)

Publisher
IOS Press
Van Diemenstraat 94
1013 CN Amsterdam
Netherlands

Distributor in the UK and Ireland
IOS Press/Lavis Marketing
73 Lime Walk
Headington
Oxford OX3 7AD
England

Distributor in Germany
IOS Press
Spandauer Strasse 2
D-10178 Berlin
Germany

Distributor in the USA and Canada
IOS Press, Inc.
P.O. Box 10558
Burke, VA 22009-0558
USA

Distributor in Japan
Ohmsha, Ltd.
3-1 Kanda Nishiki-cho
Chiyoda-ku
Tokyo 101
Japan

LEGAL NOTICE
The publisher is not responsible for the use which might be made of the following information.

v

Contents

1. Metabolic Regulation of the Neuron

2. Peripheral and Spinal Cord Physiology

3. Supraspinal Physiology

4. Pharmacology

5. Pain Management (Social Issues)

6. Pain Management (Clinical Issues)

Foreword

Is the pain more dangerous than the medicine we use to cure it?
Who can answer this simple flat question?
What fool?
And who can argue with pain?
What fool?
Arguing with pain is like the sea arguing with the salt.

From "The world's old wounds" by Barooyr Sevag, 1971,
Translation by Peter Balakian.

This book is the result of a symposium held from 22 to 28 September 1996, in Stepanakert and Yerevan in the Nagorno Karabagh Republic (NKR) and the Republic of Armenia. For 6 days, forty-five participants enjoyed the good will and hospitality of the Armenians in both lands. Given the remoteness of the meeting site, participation had to be limited. Several of the chapters are written by scientists who could not attend the meeting. However, we were fortunate enough to attract a group of eminent scientists, and enjoyed intense discussions on the topical presentations. These plenary discussions are included with the corresponding essays.

The scope of current pain research is vast, and this book--and the symposium--could not adequately portray the field. Instead it presents some important issues in pain research, including molecular biology, pharmacology, central physiology and functional brain imaging, and portrays the most recent directions that pain research is branching into. The book is the reflection of an effort to expand the scope of discussion in pain research and therapy by cross-fertilization between western and Former Soviet Union (mainly Armenian) scientists. The special circumstances of the country of meeting prompted due consideration of pain issues largely ignored in current thinking, namely the impact of war and natural disasters on pain perception and pain management, particularly in circumstances where resources are limited. These considerations acquire great significance when we bear in mind that, at any one time, about one third of the world's nations are at war.

The topics of the papers largely represent the particular interests of the Armenian scientists, such as the mechanisms of metabolic regulation of the neuron, the role of the hypothalamus in pain, and the biochemistry of opiate drugs. Armenian scientists conducted special field studies and presented the results on biologically active substances unique to the Armenian lands that may be used for development of new pain drugs.

It is worth mentioning, in this context, that our meeting was the first international scientific meeting to be held in NKR. Many colleagues asked why we decided to conduct the meeting in such a remote place. I believe that most of the participants came to understand the scientific, political, and personal motivations underlying the effort. Unfortunately, the reader can only partake of the scientific discourse. In this space, I thought it worthwhile to share a few of the experiences of the symposium.

The amphitheater in Stepanakert where the meeting was held was renovated weeks before the meeting started. Our conference was the first event hosted there. During the war, this building had been hit by more than 700 aerial bombs. To us it was just another beautifully lit structure with facilities for seating more than 500 people. On behalf of all the participants I thank the government of NKR and the people of NKR who presented to us a large number of such miracles.

While discussions regarding the mechanisms of Halothane anesthesia and receptor binding properties of opiates were ongoing, a small group of the participants visited Stepanakert's hospital, the main health care center of NKR. We arrived just in time to witness a surgical procedure performed on a child while the mother was restraining her because the surgery had to be done without anesthesia since the hospital had run out of the necessary drugs.

Credit for the success of the meeting is primarily due to all the participants. I want to thank all those who attended, as well as those who contributed essays despite their inability to attend the meeting. Particular thanks go to the numerous individuals that contributed variously to the success of the meeting. Many thanks go to Catherine Porter, president of the Human Rights Alliance, who dedicated her office and staff to help us procure the funds necessary for the symposium; she was unfortunately unable to attend the meeting because of health problems. We also thank Carolyn Mugar and Prof. J.M. Besson for financial assistance. We wish to acknowledge the scientific and government institutions that provided funds for the meeting, or for particular scientists, including the US NIH, Naval Research Office, the Gulbenkian Foundation in Portugal, the British MRC, the International Pharmacological Society, the International Biophysical Society, the National Academy of Science in Armenia, the International Association for the Study of Pain, the International Brain Research Organization, Monsanto Company and the Lebanese government. Personal thanks go to the organizing committees in Armenia and NKR, and to Narine Khatchatrian and Heike Newman for helping with the manuscript and the meeting. Thanks also to my sister, Gassia Apkarian, and brother, Prof. V. Ara Apkarian, for their support in this endeavor.

A.V.A.

Preface

This volume represents the materials of the International Symposium on the Application of the Theory of Metabolic Regulation to Pain, held in Stepanakert, Nagorno-Karabagh Republic and Yerevan, Republic of Armenia on the 22-28th of September, 1996. The lectures (with their discussions) of the participants from different countries, who are working on molecular, cellular, physiological, pharmacological and therapeutic aspects of pain are presented here.

The purpose of this symposium was to bring together basic researchers and clinicians to discuss mechanisms of nociception and pain. Strategies for adequate management of pain in developing countries were a major topic of discussion. The book is divided into six sections. The first section deals with the fundamental properties of the neuron, its metabolic regulation both in normal and ischemic states, and its molecular properties regarding axoplasmic transport and neurotransmission. Here, Ayrapetian introduces the notion that metabolic pathways underlying abnormal discharges of neurons may explain nociceptive transmission. The second section examines peripheral and spinal cord mechanisms of pain, with a strong emphasis on receptor dynamics, neuro-immune modulation, and cellular and metabolic pathways underlying nociceptive physiology. The third section is composed of chapters regarding the supraspinal physiology of nociception and pain. This section includes animal physiology and brain imaging and transcranial stimulation studies in humans, and a broad discussion of the correspondence between animal and human studies. The section also reflects the recent expansion in supraspinal pathways thought to be involved in pain perception and pain modulation. Chapters in section expound on the pharmacology of pain, and studies regarding molecular modeling and the use of natural resources for developing new drugs are presented. Section five deals with social issues regarding pain management, especially in disaster areas in countries with limited resources. Chapters in the sixth section are by Austrian pain researchers and clinicians who have conducted multi-centered studies regarding various approaches for clinical management of pain.

S.N.A. and A.V.A.

Salutatory Address

Arthur B. Tovmasian
Speaker of the House of Representatives of Nagorno-Karabagh Republic

Dear participants, chairmen, ladies and gentlemen,

I am privileged to greet you on behalf of the President of Nagorno-Karabagh Republic, Robert Kocharian, the National Congress and the Government of our republic.

The government and the people of our republic consider it to be a great honor for our newly independent republic that such authoritative international organizations as the International Brain Research Organization (IBRO), International Association for the Study of Pain (IASP), International Union of Pure and Applied Biophysics (IUPAB), International Pharmacological Society and Human Rights Alliance have decided to hold this important meeting in the capital of NKR - Stepanakert.

The problem of pain has for years been the most important one for our people. Thousands of young people have been wounded and killed during the years of the independence of our republic. I am mentioning this fact just for you to imagine what a psychological factor in pain relief the organization of this meeting can be. Taking this fact into consideration, the government of NKR, even not having convenient living conditions, met the request of our scientists halfway to hold this meeting in NKR. We hope that our guests will be indulgent to our inconvenient living conditions and we hope that we will meet you in the future as well and that we will have the possibility to provide you with more convenient living and working conditions. I hope it becomes possible for the scientists of NKR to succeed in organizing a Center for Pain Research, which would be of regional importance, and it would be possible to use it in future as a good factor for the promotion of and establishing and strengthening of friendly ties between regional countries.

I wish you great success in your work and I hope you will enjoy yourselves in Karabagh and Armenia to your hearts content.

Thank you for your attention.

Opening Address

Sinerik N. Ayrapetyan
Director of Biophysics Center
Armenian National Academy of Sciences
Yerevan, Armenia

I am happy to greet all of you in my motherland, in the capital of five years old independent Nagorno-Karabagh Republic (NKR), Stepanakert. NKR was one of the first administrative units in Former Soviet Union that declared independence on the basis of the right to self-determination of nations. That's why it was involved in the war against Soviet and Azerbeijan armies. During this war thousands of Karabaghtsi patriots and FSU and Azerbeijani soldiers were killed.

Before opening this meeting let us for a minute rise in memory of these young people. Thank you. Now our symposium is declared open.

The present symposium is patronized and sponsored by seven famous international organizations. Leading scientists from more than 17 different countries working in the medical and biological sciences take part in this symposium. I hope that during the next five days discussions we can move far in understanding the cellular mechanism of pain signal generation and find rational ways for pain relief and pain management.

Besides the research program you will also have the opportunity to get informed about two old Armenian republics. We hope that we will be able to compensate our inconvenient living conditions by warm Karabaghtsi hospitality.

Armenians are proud of being the first nation in the world who adopted Christianity as a state religion in 301, and the Armenian Apostolic Church played a very important role in science and education. Historically even in very tragic situations Armenians did not forget the importance of science and education in the survival of our nation. The State University of NKR was founded five years ago when the nation was involved in war.

Following this tradition NKR leaders are trying to make this small land a peaceful country. The organization of this symposium is the proof of it. We hope that this symposium will be the starting point of international collaboration between life scientists and will serve as an appeal to reject uncivilized relationships between different nations and religions. To promote this friendship, especially between regional countries, and make it more effective, Biophysics Center in collaboration with the School of Public Health of SUNY at Albany (dean - Prof. David O. Carpenter) is organizing the Life Science International Higher Education School (LSIHES). We will appreciate those scientists and organizations who will help us in our efforts

I'd like to explain the meaning of an Armenian expression "Tsavet Danem" that you can hear in Karabagh and in Armenia and which means: let me take your pain away (see book cover).

I hope your work in our meeting will be fruitful and enjoyable. Thank you for your attention and good luck to everyone.

Metabolic Regulation of the Neuron

Pain Mechanisms and Management
S.N. Ayrapetyan and A.V. Apkarian (Eds.)
IOS Press, 1998

The Application of the Theory of Metabolic Regulation to Pain

Sinerik N. Ayrapetyan
Biophysics Center, Armenian National Academy of Sciences
Yerevan, Armenia

Abstract. Pain is considered abnormal cell membrane excitability of nerve endings. It has been shown that cell membrane protein molecules, determining membrane function, are in functionally active and inactive states, and that the ratio of active and inactive molecules is changed depending on the size of the active surface membrane area. Cell swelling leads to the increase, while shrinking to the decrease, of the number of functional active molecules in the membrane. It has been suggested that abnormal hydration leads to abnormal excitation. Therefore, the cell hydration is considered as a second messenger for transformation of external and internal signals to pain signals. Na-K pump and Na:Ca exchange are the main mechanisms through which metabolism regulates cell hydration. As Na-K pump is more sensitive to the metabolic activity of the cell than Na:Ca exchange, in pathology first Na-K pump is damaged and as a compensatory mechanism it switches on Na:Ca exchange in reversal mode (Na efflux, Ca influx). It is suggested that in pathology Na:Ca exchange is a universal extrasensitive sensor for different extraweak chemical, physical and metabolic signals by which the modulation of cell membrane excitation takes place.
In oocyte, Na:Ca exchange and its sensitivity towards extraweak signals are absent. The nicotinic ACh, GABA and Glutamate receptors in oocyte membrane, which are expressed by preliminary injection of mRNA from mouse brain are insensitive to low concentrations of transmitters. The injection of total RNA from mammalian brain activates Na:Ca exchange in oocyte membrane, but it is insensitive to transmitters. Thus, the transmitter sensitive Na:Ca exchange in neuronal membrane can be considered a universal and extrasensitive sensor through which the external extraweak signals could modulate the abnormal excitation in the nociceptive region.

Introduction

As with other senses, pain also has its own signal, which from a biophysical point of view can be considered as abnormal membrane excitability (AME) of nerve ending. As pain can be generated by different phenomena, starting from mechanical damage to the breakdowns of different metabolic pathways, it must be a universal target (or a common second messenger) for various physical, chemical and metabolic factors which could develop abnormal membrane excitation. At the same time, it is well known that pain signals can be generated or modulated by extraweak chemical and physical stimuli, the intensity of which is far from the threshold of ionic channels in the membrane. Therefore, the mechanism responsible for pain signal generation must be a common cellular mechanism, which has properties to receive extra- and intracellular signals by extrasensitive sensors and transfer them to AME.

During the last two decades, the problem of metabolic regulation of membrane excitability was the subject of investigation of Biophysics Center of Armenia NAS. The obtained data allow us to develop a theory of metabolic regulation of membrane excitability, according to which cell volume is a fundamental cell parameter through which the interaction between membrane excitation and cell metabolism takes place; cell hydration can serve as a common "second" messenger through which the effects of external and internal signals on membrane excitability are realized. From this point of view, abnormal cell hydration could produce abnormal cell membrane excitation, which is interpreted in the CNS network as pain (nociceptive) signal. Below are briefly presented the data proving this suggestion.

It is well known that cell swelling takes place in any cell pathology. Cell swelling precedes cell death irrespective of the reason (apoptosis or necrosis) (Bennett & Huxlin, 1996). Although from clinical observations we know that pain is accompanied with swelling of nerve endings, the physiological meaning of cell hydration in the regulation of membrane excitability is not clear yet. To understand this issue it was necessary to study the following two questions:
1. the dependence of neuromembrane functional activity on cell volume;
2. the metabolic regulation of cell volume.

The Dependence of Neuromembrane Functional Activity on Cell Volume

It is known that the cell swells in hypotonic or shrinks in hypertonic solutions, by taking in or giving out water through the cell membrane. The dependence of membrane I-V characteristics (Ayrapetyan, 1980), excitability and chemosensitivity (Ayrapetyan & Arvanov, 1979) on external tonicity, in snail and Aplysia neurons, as well as in squid and crawfish axons, was studied. It was shown that there is a certain correlation between cell volume (membrane surface) and functional membrane activity. Cell swelling leads to the increase of membrane permeability, excitability (Ayrapetyan, 1980, Kojima et al., 1984), chemosensitivity (Ayrapetyan & Arvanov, 1978), and Na-K pump activity (Ayrapetyan et al., 1984), while cell shrinkage has the opposite effect.

Through a more detailed investigation of the mechanism of correlation between functional membrane activity and cell surface, it was shown that membrane proteins which have enzymatic, chemoreceptive and ionophoretic properties are in functionally active and inactive (reserved) states, and that the number of functionally active molecules in the membrane is determined by the membrane surface. Cell swelling leads to the increase, while its shrinking--to the decrease of the number of functionally active protein molecules in the membrane (Ayrapetyan et al., 1984).

This fact can be clearly seen on Table 1, where the dependence of the number of ouabain receptors (Na^+K-ATPase molecules) in cell membrane on external solution tonicity is presented.

It is apparent that all concentrations of ouabain binding sites are higher in hypotonic solutions than in iso- and hypertonic solutions. In order to change the tonicity without altering the ionic strength, the NaCl content of standard solution was reduced by 50%, and sucrose was used to obtain media of different tonicities (T): hypotonic (T=0.5) contains 0 mM and hypertonic (T=2)--189 mM sucrose. 1 Mol of NaCl was taken as osmotic equivalent to 1.57 Mol of sucrose.

Table 1. Binding of [³H] ouabain to Helix pomatia cell membrane as a function of concentration of glycoside in solutions with different tonicities (x10^8 molecules/mg dry weight)

Ouabain content	Incubation medium		
(Mol)	Hypotonic	Isotonic	Hypertonic
1x10^{-10}	4.59 ± 0.32	3.23 ± 0.24	2.03 ± 0.16
3x10^{-10}	18.3 ± 1.4	11.7 ± 0.87	6.29 ± 0.41
6x10^{-10}	28.9 ± 2.0	17.9 ± 1.2	10.0 ± 0.67
1x10^{-9}	32.0 ± 2.2	21.1 ± 1.4	12.2 ± 0.9
3x10^{-9}	144 ± 29.4	90.5 ± 5.7	53.8 ± 3.1
6x10^{-9}	431 ± 29.4	266 ± 15.8	147 ± 9.7
1x10^{-8}	793 ± 45.6	508 ± 30.1	283 ± 19.4

To elucidate whether the number of functioning pump units is changed under normal conditions in response to increased passive membrane permeability, the binding of [³H] ouabain to the membrane was studied in the presence of synaptic transmitters. From Table 2 it can clearly be seen that ACh and GABA increased ouabain binding significantly. Therefore, we suggest that the increased membrane permeability brought about by exposure to synaptic transmitters is accompanied by corresponding alteration in the number of functioning pump units in the membrane.

Table 2. The effects of ACh and GABA on [³H] ouabain binding to neuronal membrane

Ouabain content in the medium (mol)	Normal Ringer	Normal Ringer containing 10^{-4} M ACh	Normal Ringer containing 10^{-4}M GABA
1x10^{-10}	3.16 ± 0.48	5.13 ± 0.62	4.24 ± 0.21
1x10^{-9}	20.56 ± 0.55	30.54 ± 1.55	27.63 ± 3.17
5x10^{-9}	109.40 ± 10.47	170.29 ± 13.36	139.62 ± 11.43
1x10^{-8}	143.54 ± 8.91	270.93 ± 28.53	174.48 ± 13.54
1x10^{-7}	3254.47 ± 74.20	3944.33 ± 107.23	-
1x10^{-6}	23938.20 ± 852.44	28686.96 ± 963.47	-

Thus, these data allow us to conclude that any abnormal cell swelling will cause hyperfunctional activity (hyperexcitability) as a result of transferring all reserved protein molecules (receptors, channels and enzymes) to a functionally active state.
At present it is known that any channel (receptor binding and potential dependent) activation leads to cell swelling (Ayrapetyan, 1980, Tasaki et al., 1982). Through experiments by Tasaki and coworkers, it was shown that even during the rising phase of a single action potential the neuronal hydration increases, while in its hyperpolarization phases the cell shrinks (Tasaki et al., 1982). Therefore the depolarization-induced cell swelling is a potentiation factor for further cell excitation as a result of increasing the number of functionally active molecules in the membrane. It was shown also that water uptake has direct activation effect on inward ionic currents (Ayrapetyan et al., 1991).
Thus, in excitation-induced hydration, the number of functionally active ionic channels in the membrane increases by a positive feed-back mechanism. If the metabolic mechanisms responsible for regulation of cell hydration are unable to contract to the excitation-induced hydration, the cytoskeleton stretching could lead to long lasting depolarization (LLP), which could serve as a pain signal. Therefore it is suggested that finding out the metabolic mechanisms which are regulating cell hydration allows us to understand the mechanism of metabolic regulation of pain signal generation.

Metabolic regulation of cell volume

Previously it was shown that electrogenic Na-K pump, which is operated by a ratio of 3Na:2K, is a powerful mechanism through which metabolism regulates cell volume: the inhibition of the pump causes an increase in cell volume, while the activation of the pump leads to cell shrinking (Ayrapetyan & Sulejmanian, 1979). Therefore, the pump-dependent cell volume regulation has physiological significance in metabolic regulation of functional membrane activity (Ayrapetyan, 1980).

The next mechanism controlling cell volume is the phosphorylation and dephosphorylation of cytoskeleton. The latter consists of contractile proteins, such as actomyosin (Minkoff L. and Damadian R., 1976). The phosphorylation of cytoskeleton leads to the shrinking of the cell while the dephosphorylation has a swelling effect on it.

Previously, in our laboratory the close correlation between Na-K pump activity and the level of intracellular cAMP and Na:Ca exchange (Azatian et al., 1993) was shown. Those factors which have an inhibitory effect on Na-K pump activity increase the intracellular level of cAMP and Na:Ca exchange. The latter, through a cAMP-dependent mechanism, regulates the intracellular Ca^{2+} ion concentration (Saghyan, 1991). As Na:Ca exchange also operates an electrogenic regime (3Na out 1 Ca), its activation has a strong dehydration effect on the cell.

These data allowed us to conclude that the negative correlation between Na-K pump and Na:Ca exchange has a protective reaction for the cell. Pump inactivation leads to cell swelling (MHE), and at the same time the elevation of intracellular cAMP stimulates Na:Ca exchange and shrinks the cell. As in the normal state, the activity of Na-K pump is much higher than that of Na:Ca exchange, the contribution of Na-K pump in the regulation of cell hydration is much higher than in Na:Ca exchange, while in cell pathology pump activity depresses the major role in cell hydration which is played by electrogenic reversal Na:Ca exchange.

As the small elevation of intracellular Ca^{2+} ions concentration leads to dramatic activation of enzymatic systems which participate in phospholipid turnover, which is supplying additional substrate for ATP production, it can serve as another metabolic pathway through which cell dehydration is realized.

The next negative feed-back mechanism between membrane excitation and cell hydration is the cell swelling-induced activation of reserved pump units in the membrane, which could activate the pump and dehydrate the cell (see table 2).

Thus, cell volume (membrane surface) is a very dynamic and highly metabolic dependent structure, the regulation of which is presented in figure 1.

From this scheme, it can be seen that any activating receptor and potential dependent channels and depression of Na-K pump cause cell swelling and initiate MHE. The latter through the increase of internal Na and Ca content switches on metabolic cascades through which the protective reaction of the cell is realized. One of these metabolic pathways is Ca-dependent activation of lipid turnover, which switches on the cascade of metabolic messenger systems regulating membrane sensitivity for external signal and stimulates the ATP production through their oxidation. The second pathway, through which the protective reaction of the cell is realized, is Ca-activated calmodulin-dependent NO synthase (NOS). Our recent data have shown that NO stimulates cGMP - dependent Na:Ca exchange as a result of which the realization of intracellular Ca and the reactivation of Na-K pump takes place (Azatian et al., 1996). There are a number of positive and negative feed-back mechanisms between AME and cell swelling.

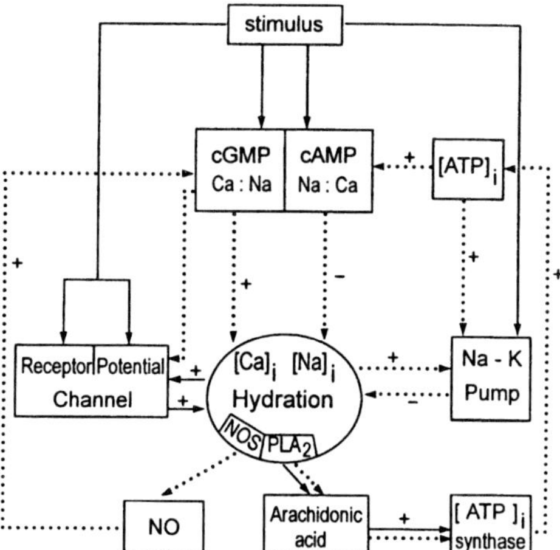

Figure 1. The schema of metabolic regulation of membrane excitation.
(Non-metabolic pathways are shown as solid lines, metabolic pathways as dotted lines.)

It is clear that if the positive feed-back mechanisms have passive, thermodynamically irreversible characters, the negative feed-back mechanisms have a metabolic nature. Therefore the capacity of negative feed-back mechanisms will depend on the reversibility of cell abnormal hydration and AME (nociceptive) state.

It is well known that, in AME state, very weak physical and chemical stimulation could elevate or depress the painful signal. The study of the nature of these universal extrasensitive sensors was the subject of our investigation during the last few years.

The aim of the next series of experiments was to find an extrasensitive and universal sensor, which could receive extraweak signals, and transform it through cell hydration to membrane excitation. Figure 2 shows the effect of ACh and GABA on ^{22}Na efflux from the cells in K-free, 10^{-4} M ouabain-containing solution.

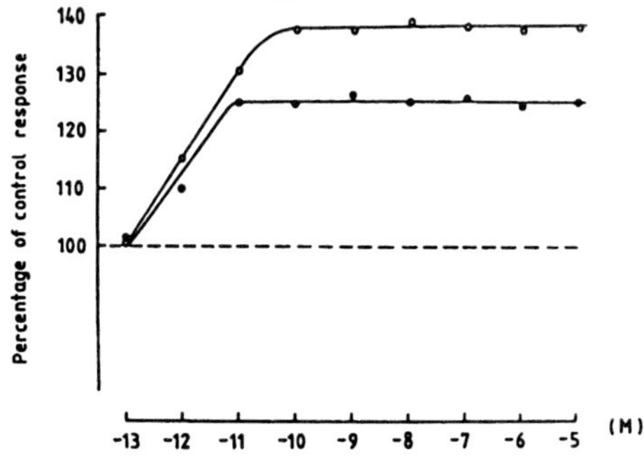

Figure 2. Effect of ACh (•) and GABA (o) on ^{22}Na efflux from the cells in K-free, 10^{-4}M ouabain containing solution. Abscissa: log concentration of transmitters, Ordinate: ACh and GABA - induced changes of ^{22}Na efflux from the cells as compared with the efflux in K-free, 10^{-4} M Ouabain containing solution.

It can be seen that these transmitters in very low concentrations of ACh and GABA, which are far from the threshold of activation for receptor binding ionic channels (higher than 10^{-7} M), have an activation effect on Na efflux. Previously it was shown that in this medium Na efflux in neuronal membrane is realized through the Na:Ca exchange mechanism (Saghyan ,1991).

It is well known that intracellular injection of cAMP leads to the generation of abnormal discharge in the neuron (Kononenko and Scherbatko, 1985). It has also been shown that the epileptogenic drug induced abnormal discharge is accompanied with significant elevation of intracellular cAMP level (Sugaya et al., 1973). On the basis of these data, it was suggested that weak signal induced modulation of pain signal can be realized by elevation of intracellular cAMP. The study of the effect of low concentration of transmitters on intracellular cAMP proved this suggestion (Ayrapetyan et al., 1992). As it can be seen in figure 3, low doses of ACh elevate intracellular cAMP concentration.

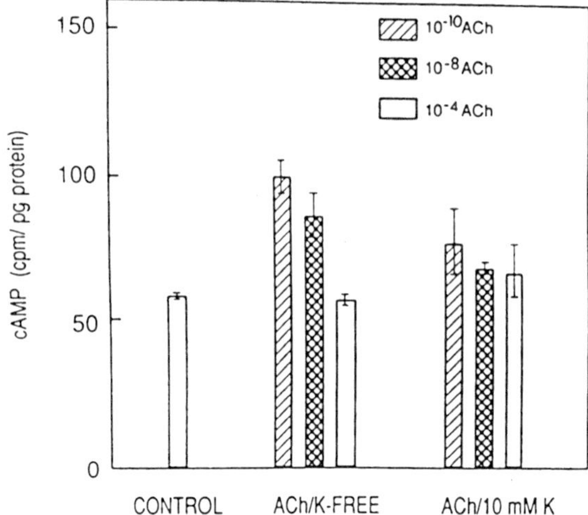

Figure 3. The effect of ACh on intracellular level of cAMP in Aplysia neurons in K-free and normal physiological solutions.

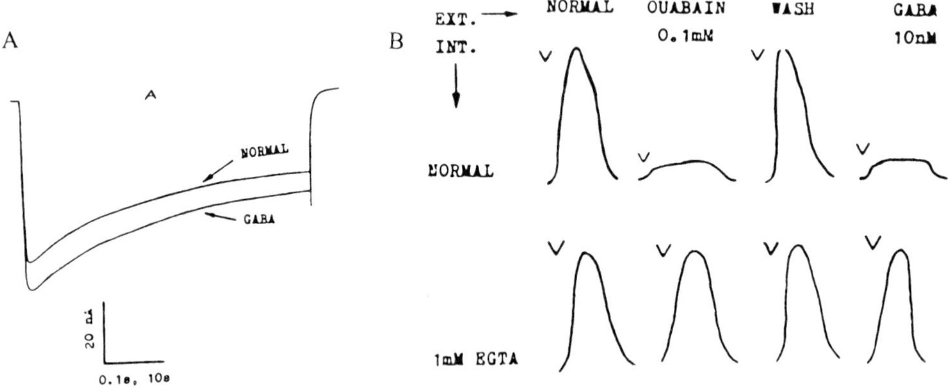

Figure 4. Enhancement of Ca-inward current (A) and depression ACh-induced responses of snail neuronal membrane by 10 nM GABA (B). The ouabain and GABA-induced inhibition of ACh responses was absent when the neuron was internally perfused by 1mM EGTA.

As can be seen in figure 4, a low concentration of GABA could effectively modulate the potential dependent Ca inward current and ACh-induced ionic current in internal dialyzed snail neurons. Earlier it was shown that ouabain depressed Cl-dependent ACh-induced current is reversed by Na:Ca exchange, as a result the intracellular Na concentration increases (Arvanov et al., 1992). The fact that low concentration of GABA-induced ACh responses were absent in the presence of intracellular EGTA showed that this inhibition is caused by elevation of intracellular Ca concentration.

The low concentration of ACh leads to the depression of GABA-induced outward current in Aplysia neurons (fig 5).

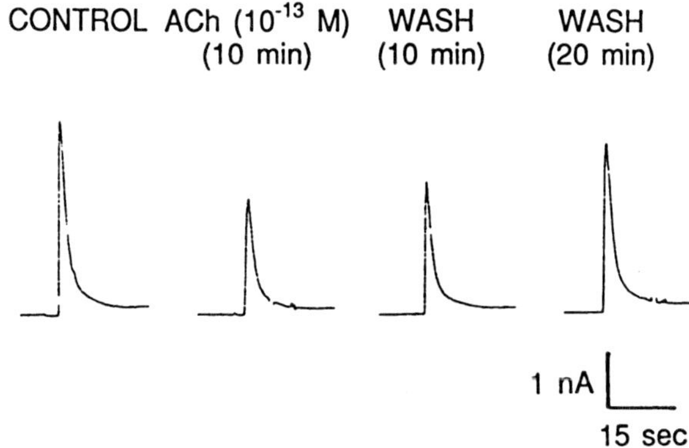

Figure 5. Effect of 10^{-13}M ACh on GABA responses of medial plural neuron.

More detailed investigation of this question showed that low dose (LD) ACh induced inhibition of GABA responses is also induced by cAMP-dependent reversion of Na:Ca exchange (Ayrapetyan and Carpenter, 1991).

It is interesting to note that in neurons the electrogenic Na pump-induced outward membrane current is also sensitive to low concentration of transmitters.

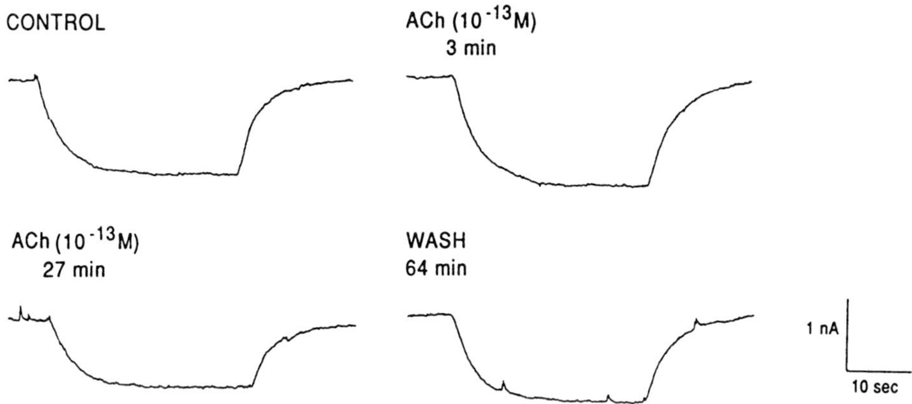

Figure 6. The effect of prolonged microperfusion of a solution containing 10^{-13} M ACh on K-free solution-induced inward (pump inhibition) currents in Aplysia neuron. The neuron was perfused by normal sea water before 1 minute exposure in K-free solution.

As can be seen in figure 6, after long incubation in 10^{-13} M ACh containing medium, the amplitude of pump current is reversible to depressing. To understand the underlying mechanism of the effect of LD neurotransmitters, it is necessary to answer the following two questions:

1. whether the sensors for weak signals have different structure than channel binding receptors;

2. whether Na-K pump and Na:Ca exchange are responsible for membrane sensitivity to LD neurotransmitters (NT).

For this purpose, the next series of experiments were carried out on xenopus oocyte injected with different mRNA from rat brain. These experiments have shown that in oocyte membrane Na-K pump induced current is insensitive to transmitters and Na:Ca exchange is absent.

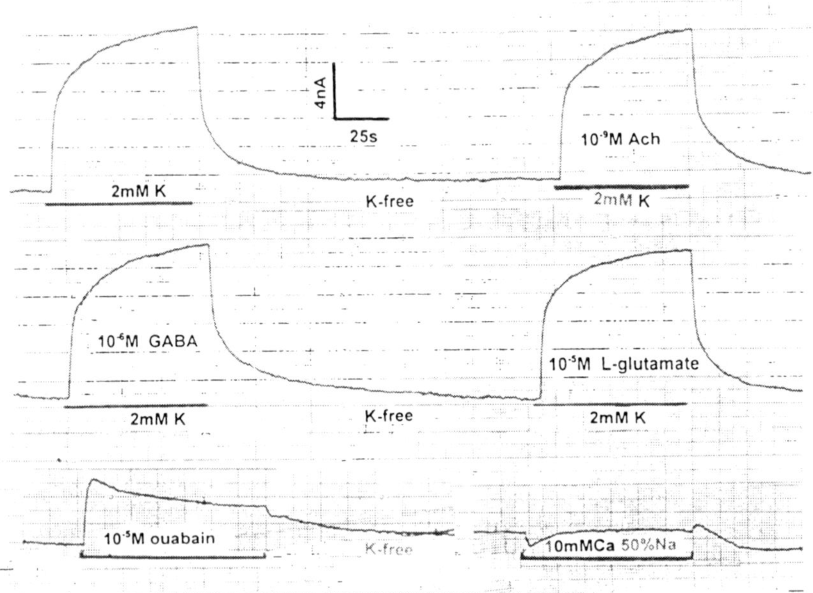

Figure 7. The insensitivity 2mM-induced outward (pump) currents to transmitters.
Fresh isolated oocytes, which were continuously perfused by K-free per 2 minutes, for one minute it was exposed 2mM K containing medium with different transmitters. In the bottom ouabain depressed the pump current while 10mM Ca and 50% Na containing medium has no significant changing of study level of membrane current.

Figure 7 shows that 2 mM K-induced outward currents are insensitive to ACh, GABA, and glutamate, while they are depressed by ouabain 10^{-5} M. In the neuronal membrane decreasing the extracellular concentration of Na ions generates an outward current which is due to the activation of Na:Ca exchange in a reversible mode (Saghyan, 1991). As it can be seen from these data, a similar decrease of external Na did not produce any change of membrane current. By measuring the ^{45}Ca uptake it was shown that Na:Ca exchange is absent in defoliculated oocytes.

In the study of sensitivity of specific rat brain mRNA-expressed receptors in oocytes it was shown that transmitter-induced responses are insensitive to LD of NT (figures 8 and 9).

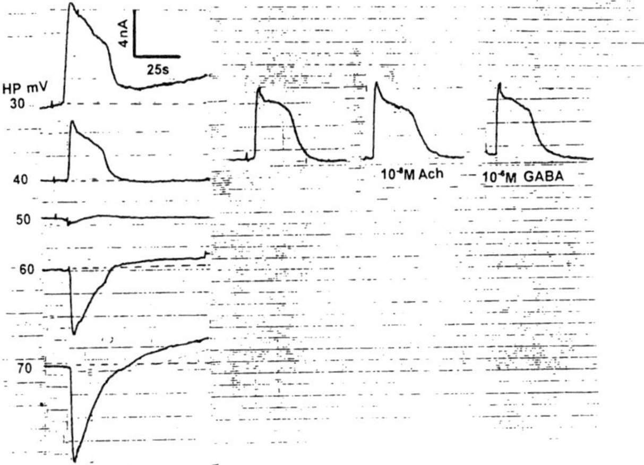

Figure 8. The insensitivity of nicotinic ACh responses of oocytes to low concentration of ACh and GABA.

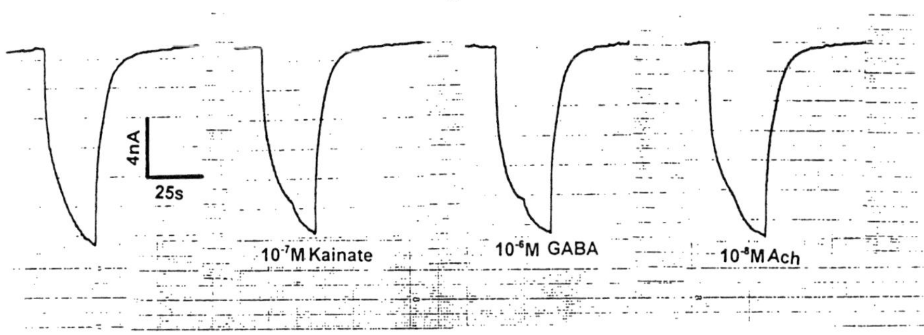

Figure 9. The insensitivity of kinate (10^{-4}M) responses of oocytes to 10^{-7}M kinate, 10^{-6}M GABA and 10^{-8}M ACh. Holding potential was 50mV.

If in neuronal membrane there are high affinity receptors for low concentrations of ouabain, in oocyte membrane these receptors are absent (Ayrapetyan et al., 1994). Our recent data shows that the function of these receptors correlates with that of Na:Ca exchanger (Saghyan et al., 1996). All these data showed that extrasensitive sensors as well as Na:Ca exchanger are specific for neurons and are absent in oocyte membrane.

Thus, our observation suggests that the degree of cellular hydration represents a new, not yet fully recognized, signal for control of membrane excitability which acts as a missing link (i.e. like a second or third messenger) mediating the effects of different external and internal signals on cellular metabolism and excitability. From this point of view, we suggest that the abnormal membrane excitation (pain signal) is an abnormal activation of all protein molecules (enzymes, receptors and channels) in the membrane as a result of abnormal cell hydration, while the cAMP dependent Na:Ca exchange in neuronal membrane is an extrasensitive and universal sensor through which the weak stimuli-induced modulation of nociception is realized.

Plenary discussion

Wall P.: When you speak of pain do you mean nociception?

Ayrapetyan S.: I am speaking about pain signal generation. I don't use the term "nociception," because, from the point of view of fundamental neuroscience, I don't consider it an adequate category.

Wall P.: The behavior of isolated neurons differs from their behavior in situ.

Ayrapetyan S.: Yes, of course it differs. I am speaking about the fundamental mechanism responsible for membrane excitability both in vitro and in situ. I think that in this case pain signal generation is equivalent to the abnormal discharge of neurons. My theory explains the cellular mechanism of abnormal discharge generation in isolated neurons and neurons in situ.

Wall P.: Does membrane excitability differ from cytoskeletal excitability?

Ayrapetyan S.: As you know, under the membrane there are molecular layers of actin-like proteins, phosphorylation and dephosphorylation of which play an important role in the regulation of cell surface as well as membrane excitability. I suggest that the abnormal stretching of the cytoskeleton could serve as an additional mechanism through which cell hydration could generate abnormal discharges (pain signals) in the membrane.

Reeh W.: What is the relationship between Helix pomatia with nociceptive nerve ending?

Ayrapetyan S.: According to my suggestion there are no special nociceptive nerve endings. Therefore, membrane mechanisms responsible for nociception in mammalian nerve endings are the same as those in mollusk neurons.

Besson J.-M.: It is difficult to accept your theory (swelling-shrinkage) when considering clinical findings related to the activation of specific nociceptors and to the activation of large (non-nociceptive) primary afferent fibers.

Ayrapetyan S.: There are abundant clinical data showing that nociception is accompanied with nerve ending swelling, which according to our data could produce abnormal excitation of nerve membrane. I suggest that there are no specific nociceptive and non-nociceptive pathways. These two pathways differ only in the threshold for generating an action potential.

Amassian V.: Regarding your interesting hypothesis on hydration, I think we need to distinguish what occurs in the receptor as distinguished from the axon. Concerning the axon, there is the question of the importance of the Na+-K+ in resisting pathological effects. For example, a small weight dropped on cat spinal cord that is followed by complete recovery of long tract function within 30 min. is irreversible if the spinal cord has been topically pretreated with Strophanthidin, a pump poison. It would be of interest to your hypothesis to see the effect of locally injected Strophanthidin on nociceptor sensitivity to trauma. (The dose would have to be very low to avoid nerve fiber block). Mining from your schema we find a reference to loss of Na inactivation, a powerful influence promoting ionic imbalance in the cell and loss of function.

Ayrapetyan S.: Thank you very much for your interesting question and advice. According to our data, Na^+-K^+ pump could modulate membrane excitability by a number of potential independent mechanisms, by transmembrane water efflux and by changing the number of functionally active ionic channels in the membrane. These properties of the Na^+-K^+ pump correlate with its electrogenicity; the latter, as you know, strongly depends on membrane resistance. As nerve endings have incomparably higher resistance than the axon, the mentioned modulation effect of the Na^+-K^+ pump in nerve ending is much higher than in axon.

Regarding the local injection of Srophanthidin in nociceptive regions, as you have suggested, Srophanthidin must potentiate membrane excitation. However, I will definitely check this experimentally.

References

Arvanov VL, Ovakimyan KS, Stepanian AS, Ayrapetyan SN (1992) The effect of cAMP, Ca +2 and phorbol ester TPA on ouabain induced depression of neuron responses induced by rapid ACh application. Cell Molec Neurobiol 12,153-161.

Arvanov VL, Tsai M-Ch, Walker RJ (1993) Interaction of concanavalin A and wheat germ agglutinin with Helix acetylcholine receptors. Brain Research Elsev Sci Publishers 615, 252-258.

Ayrapetyan SN (1980) On the physiological significance of pump-induced cell volume changes. Adv Physiol Sci 23, 3, 67-82, Budapest.

Ayrapetyan SN, Carpenter DO, Azatian KV, Dadalian SS, Martyrosian DM, Saghian AA, Mndalian VG (1992) Extralow neurotransmitter dozes-induced triggering of neuronal intracellular messenger systems. In: Cellular Signalization (PG Kostyuk and MA Ostrovskii eds) "Nauka" Moscow p. 89-96.

Ayrapetyan SN, Arvanov VL (1979) On the mechanism of the electrogenic sodium pump dependence of membrane chemosensitivity. Comp Biochem physiol 64A, 601-604.

Ayrapetyan SN, Suleymanyan MA, Sagian AA, Dadalyan SS (1984) Autoregulation of electrogenic sodium pump. Cell Mol Neurobiol 4, 367-384.

Ayrapetyan SN and Arvanov VL (1988) The metabolic regulation of membrane chemosensitivity. In: Neurobiology of Invertebrates (J Salanki ed) Budapest 669-684.

Ayrapetyan SN, Carpenter DO (1991) Synaptic transmitters for membrane functional activity (in Russian). Evol Biochem and Physiol 26, 513-528.

Ayrapetyan SN and Carpenter DO (1991) Very low concentration of acetylcholine and GABA modulate transmitter responses. Membrane and Cellular Biophysics and Biochemistry NeuroReport 2, 563-565.

Azatian KV, Ayrapetian SN, Carpenter DO (1996) The metabotropic effect of low doses of GABA. J Physiol (in press).

Azatian KV, Karapetian ITz, Ayrapetian SN (1993) Effect of low dose acetylcholine on Ca ions influx into Helix Pomatia neurons. Biological membranes 10, 317-320.

Bennett MR and Huxlin KR (1996) Neuronal Cell death in the Mammalian Nervous System: The Calmortin Hypothesis Gen Pharmac 27, 407-419.

Kojima K, Ayrapetyan SN, Koketsu K (1984) On the mechanism of the sodium pump-induced inhibition of spontaneous electrical activity of Japanese land snail neurons. Comp Biochem Physiol 77A, 577-583.

Kononenko NI, Scherbatko AL (1985) The Effect of Elevation of Intracellular cAMP on Electrical Characteristics of Identified Neurons of Snails. Neurophysiology v. 17, N1, 78-84.

Minkoff L, Damadian R (1976) Biological ion exchanger resins. The cytotonus hypothesis Physiol Chem Phys 8, 349-382.

Saghyan AA (1991) The ouabain-insensitive fraction of sodium efflux from Helix pomatia neurons. Biol Membr 8, 711-718.

Saghyan AA, Ayrapetyan SN, Carpenter DO (1996) Low dose of ouabain stimulates the Na:Ca exchange in Helix neurons. Cell Mol Neurobiol 16, 180-192.

Sugaya A, Sugaya E, and Tsujitani M (1973) Pentilentetrazol-induced intracellular potential changes of the neuron of the Japanese land snail,Jap. J Physiol 23, 261-274.

Tasaki I, Iwasa K (1982) Rapid pressure changes and surface displacements in the squid giant axon associated with production of action potentials. Jpn J Physiol 32, 69-81.

Pain Mechanisms and Management
S.N. Ayrapetyan and A.V. Apkarian (Eds.)
IOS Press, 1998

Effects of Metabolic Disruption on Neuronal Excitability

D.O. Carpenter*, M.W. Riepe[#] and N. Hori[+]
Wadsworth Center for Laboratories and Research
New York State Department of Health and School of Public Health
State University of New York, Albany, NY, USA
[#] *Department of Neurology, University of Ulm*
Ulm, Germany
[+] *Department of Pharmacology, Faculty of Dentistry*
Kyushu University, Fukuoka, Japan

Abstract. We have utilized transient ischemia, inhibition of oxidative phosphorylation, and inhibition of sodium-potassium transport as tools with which to determine the metabolic dependence of neuronal excitability. Transient cerebral ischemia in both animals and man often results in a period of unconsciousness followed by recovery of function, but with secondary loss of function after a period of hours to days. In the hippocampus, area CA1 is particularly susceptible to this delayed loss of function, and pyramidal neurons die and disappear 3-7 days after global cerebral ischemia. Using electrophysiological recordings from brain slices of animals subjected to global ischemias, or slices from control animals subjected to ischemic damage, we find that there is a prolonged hyperexcitability after a transient ischemic episode. Responses to synaptic activation become prolonged and induce repetitive discharge. The hyperexcitability is blocked by antagonists of NMDA receptors, while such antagonists have almost no effect in controls. Thus, the hyperexcitability appears to be due to the appearance of NMDA responses not present in controls. When NMDA is applied ionophoretically to control and ischemic slices, the transient ischemia appears to have altered the ability of Mg^{2+} to block the NMDA channel, which we believe to be the cause of the hyperexcitability. In contrast, metabolic blockade applied to brain slices by inhibition of oxidative phosphorylation or Na-K-ATPase results in neuronal death as a result of loss of ion exchange and concentration gradients, not mediated via excitatory amino acid transmitters.

Introduction

Like all cells, neurons are dependent upon metabolic processes for normal function, and will die if denied adequate oxygen and/or glucose, or if metabolically poisoned so as to be unable to utilize oxygen and glucose. However, not all neurons are equally vulnerable to ischemic damage for reasons that have not been understood. Moreover, the sequence of events leading to irreversible loss of cell excitability and viability have also not been identified. A variety of processes are known to be involved, including cell swelling, loss of ability to maintain concentration gradient because of failure of ion transport systems, and release of excitatory neurotransmitters from presynaptic terminals which causes excessive postsynaptic activation and triggering the process of apoptosis, leading to a programed cell death. While all of these processes undoubtedly contribute to cellular damage in severe ischemia or metabolic poisoning, the sequence and identification of the process which first results in irreversible damage is important clinically in that this information would suggest targets of appropriate intervention in humans subjected to cerebral vascular accidents and other forms of metabolic injury.

Degenerative neurologic diseases in humans are characterized by selective neuronal loss, but the reasons for loss of some neurons but not others are poorly understood. For example, in amyotrophic lateral sclerosis upper and lower motor neurons die, but other neurons are relatively spared. In addition, the extraocular motor neurons are spared for unknown reasons. In Alzheimer's Disease there is massive cell loss of hippocampus and other forebrain areas, but little loss in hindbrain cortical areas such as visual cortex. Several investigators have speculated on roles of specific transmitters (Jansen et al., 1990; Palmer and Gershon, 1990) and specific metabolic or transport deficits (Colvin et al., 1991; Deng et al., 1993; Rothstein et al., 1992) as the explanation for the selective patterns seen in these diseases, but in fact the origin of the patterns of cell loss are still uncertain.

Ischemic brain damage may result either from a global (such as prolonged hypoglycemia or transient cardiac failure) or local (cerebral vascular occlusion) insults, but both circumstances result in selective cell loss when the injury is transient. The goal of the present experiments is to identify factors that may explain why some neurons are more sensitive than others to cell death, what cellular mechanisms cause this increased vulnerability, and which factors are most important in leading to irreversible cell damage. We have focused our studies on the hippocampal brain slice, and have applied cellular insults both directly to the isolated slices and to the intact animal prior to preparation of the brain slice.

Methods

Male rats (150-200 gms) were used for all studies, and the methods have been described in detail in previous publications (Carpenter and Gregg, 1984; Hori et al., 1991; Hori and Carpenter, 1994a and b; Riepe et al., 1992; 1995; 1996; Riepe and Carpenter, 1995). After cervical dislocation the brain was rapidly removed, blocked and slices of hippocampus cut on a vibrating microtome. After a prolonged preincubation to allow for recovery of the injury of preparation, the slices were mounted in a submersion chamber and perfused with oxygenated Krebs-Ringer solution to which drugs were added as appropriate. The perfusion solution was normally equilibrated with 95% O_2/5% CO_2. When ischemia was applied to the isolated slice, the perfusion solution was changed to one lacking glucose and equilibrated with 95% N2/ 5% CO_2. A monopolar stimulating electrode was placed on the Schaffer collateral pathway in order to monosynaptically activate pyramidal neurons in the CA1 region. Depending upon the specific experiment to be done, the recordings were either made with large extracellular microelectrodes for recording the population response of a large number of neurons, or with fine, sharp intracellular microelectrodes for recordings from a single neuron.

Transient global cerebral ischemia was applied to rats in some experiments, utilizing the protocol of Pulsinelli and Brierley (1979), in which after coagulation of the vertebral arteries, ligatures placed on both carotids were tightened for a period of about 10 min after which the animal was allowed to recover and survive for several days before preparation of brain slices as above. In some experiments animals were given an IP injection of 3-nitroproprionic acid (20 mg/kg) one hour prior to preparation of brain slices.

Results

Mechanisms of Delayed Neuronal Death Following Transient Ischemia: Figure 1 illustrates the selective neuronal cell death seen in area CA1 after a transient global ischemic challenge to a rat 7 days earlier.

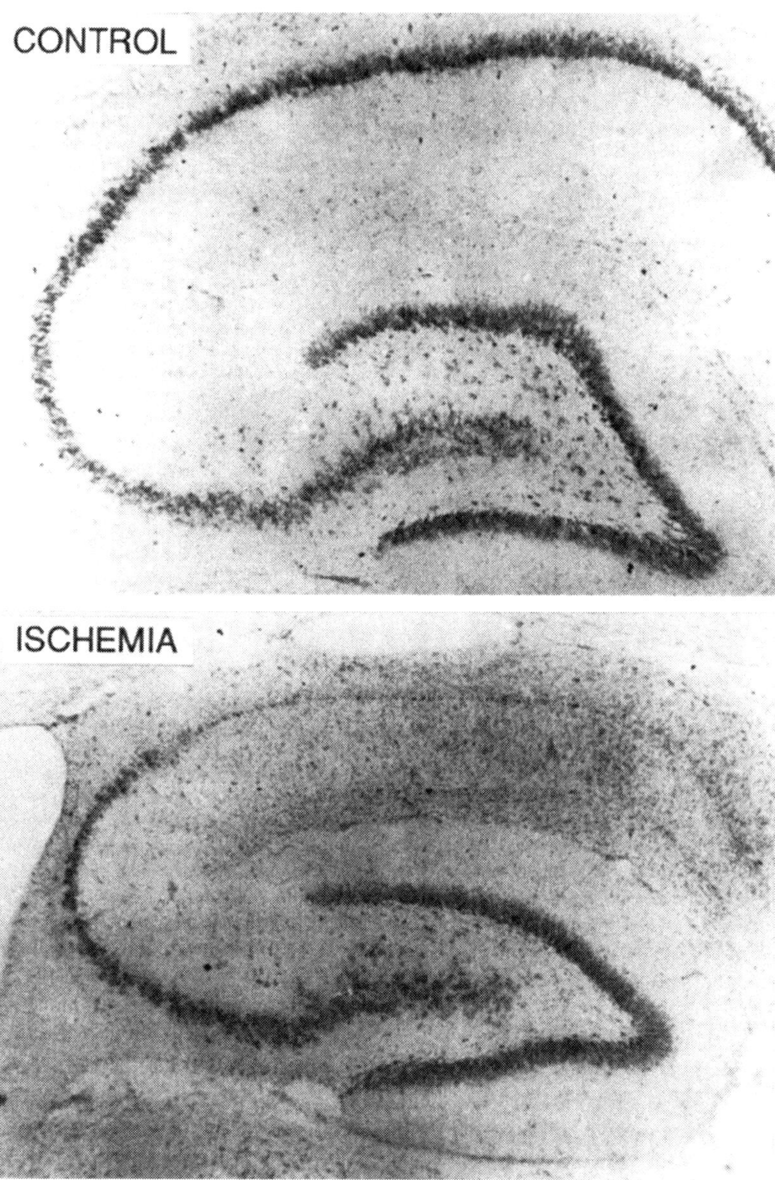

Figure 1. Histological sections of hippocampi of control animals and animals subjected to four vessel occlusion for a period of 10 min 7 days prior to removal from the animal and fixation. The brain was removed and fixed in 2.5% glutaraldehyde in Krebs-Ringer overnight and frozen sections were cut at 10 mm and stained with cresyl violet. Note the loss of neurons in CA1 in the hippocampus subjected to ischemia (indicated by arrows). (From Hori et al., 1991, reproduced with permission).

Pyramidal neurons in CA1 have almost totally disappeared in the ischemic animal as compared to control, while there is little, if any, change in cell density in CA3 or in the dentate. When the electrical activity of slices of these animals exposed to transient ischemia are recorded, population responses show a striking hyperexcitability in both areas CA1 and CA3 after two days (Figure 2). However, while almost all activity in CA1 has disappeared by 7 days, due to loss of neurons, that in CA3 remains hyperexcitable. Although not illustrated, the electrical response in the dentate was similar to that in control animals, not showing any hyperexcitability. These observations pose three clear questions: 1. What are the mechanisms responsible for the hyperexcitability? 2. Why does this appear only in CA1 and CA3? 3. Why does this hyperexcitability result in cell death in CA1 but not in CA3?

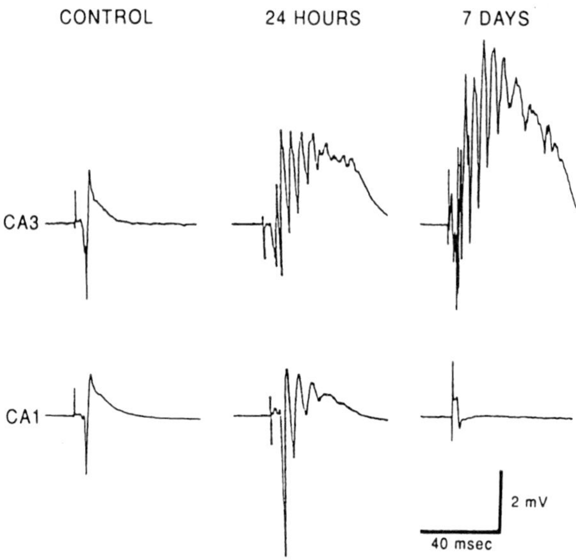

Figure 2. Population EPSP recordings from CA1 and CA3 from three different animals. The control responses are from slices prepared from normal animals. The response consists of a sharp negative wave, reflecting the population discharge of the postsynaptic neurons, followed by a positive wave which reflects the slower EPSP. In all control slices there is little or no indication of additional population discharges on the falling phase of the slow wave. The other slices were prepared from animals subjected to bilateral four vessel occlusion for 10 min applied 24 h and 7 d, respectively, before slice preparation. In all preparations the stimulus strength was 10 V and 50 ms duration. Note the multiple discharge spikes in both slices at 24 h and 7 d. No postsynaptic response was obtained from CA1 at 7 d. (From Hori et al. 1991, used with permission).

Figure 3 shows intracellular recordings from a CA1 pyramidal neuron in a control slice and a slice from an animal subjected to 10 min global ischemia 28 h earlier. Resting membrane potential of the two neurons is similar. Upon a comparison of membrane potential and input resistance, measured by application of constant current pulses, in eight control and eight cells following ischemia, we found no significant difference in either parameter. Figure 3 shows, however, that there was a significant difference in the synaptic response resulting from monosynaptic excitation of the Schaffer collateral input to these neurons. While in the control a half maximal stimulation gives a synaptic depolarization and single action potential which then rapidly decays back to the baseline, in the post-ischemic slice the underlying synaptic response is very prolonged. This would appear to be the basis for the hyperexcitability. In order to determine what the origin of this prolonged synaptic response was, a series of pharmacologic studies were performed. As illustrated in the middle traces, application of the specific inhibitor of responses mediated by the N-methyl-D-aspartate (NMDA) type of excitatory amino acid receptor, amino phosphonovaleric acid (APV), had very little effect in the control slice, but blocked the prolonged synaptic potential in the post-ischemic cell. This observation indicates that after transient ischemia there is the appearance of NMDA responses not present in control, and suggests that this is the origin of the hyperexcitability.

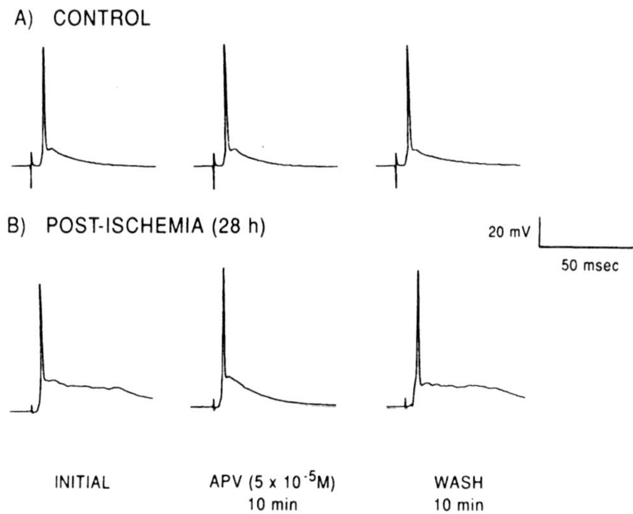

Figure 3. Intracellular recordings from two CA1 pyramidal neurons from slices from a control animal and an animal subjected to four-vessel occlusion 28 h prior to slice preparation, and effects of amino-phosphonovaleric acid (APV, $5{\times}10^{-5}$M), an antagonist of NMDA receptors. While resting potential and spike amplitude are similar in the two neurons, that after ischemia has a prolonged synaptic response which is APV sensitive. There is little or no APV sensitive component in the control. (In part from Hori et al., 1991; used with permission.)

The appearance of new NMDA responses could reflect either new receptors, or some alteration in the receptor/channel complex which makes activation more efficient. NMDA responses are known to be blocked by physiological concentrations of Mg^{2+} at most sites where they have been studied, and this channel blockade has been shown to impart a voltage dependence to the NMDA response which does not occur with other excitatory amino acid responses. In order to evaluate whether there was some change in the ability of Mg^{2+} to block NMDA responses after ischemia, we performed experiments with ionophoresis of NMDA and quisqualate onto single pyramidal neurons, and recorded responses at different membrane potentials in slices from control and post-ischemic animals. Since these were current clamp recordings, and the membrane potential was altered via a bridge circuit which results in some uncertainty of actual membrane potential, results were expressed on the basis of the current applied. Figure 4 shows that as expected the quisqualate responses were larger when membrane potential was increased in both control and post-ischemic slices, reflecting a lack of voltage dependence of this response which is known to result from a increase in conductance of monovalent cations (Mayer and Westbrook, 1987). In contrast, in the control neurons the NMDA response is reduced in amplitude by an applied hyperpolarization, reflecting Mg^{2+} blockade. However, this potential dependence is abolished after ischemia, and now the NMDA responses are not different from those to quisqualate with regard to voltage dependence. These observations suggest that the hyperexcitability preceding cell death in CA1 results from a loss of the ability of Mg^{2+} to block NMDA responses.

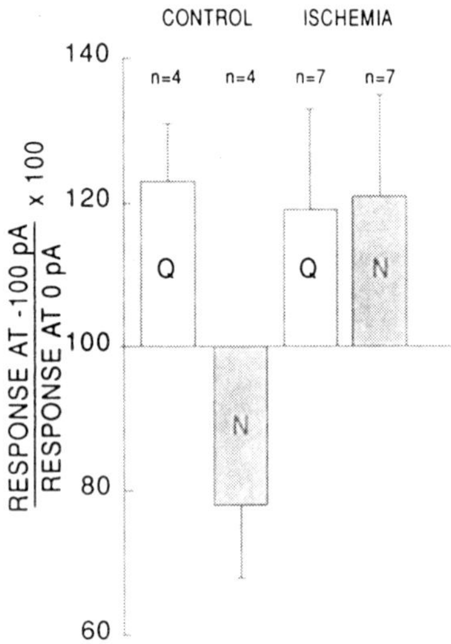

Figure 4. NMDA (N) but not quisqualate (Q) responses change after ischemia. Histogram of ratios of Q and N response amplitudes with 100 pA hyperpolarizing currents as compared with resting membrane potential in control animals and animals subjected to a transient 10 min ischemic episode 24-48 h earlier. The voltage dependence of Q and N responses in the control are significantly different at the P = 0.05 level in the control, and the voltage dependence of the N responses in the control and post-ischemia are also significantly different at the P = 0.05 level by the Student's t-test (from Hori and Carpenter, 1994; used with permission).

Mechanisms of Cell Death Following Acute Ischemia or Metabolic Inhibition: Figure 5 shows the effect of changing the perfusion solution of a hippocampal slice from one with normal oxygenation and glucose concentration, to one lacking both for a period of 10 min on the synaptic response recorded intracellularly from a CA1 pyramidal neuron upon stimulation of the Schaffer collateral pathway. There was no significant loss of membrane potential during this transient ischemic episode, but the size of the synaptic potential was dramatically reduced to the point that the cell no longer discharged after 10 min of ischemia. In addition, there was only a small reduction of input resistance, as measured by application of constant current hyperpolarizing pulses. The change in input resistance was too small to explain the reduced excitability. If the ischemia were continued there was ultimately an irreversible loss of membrane potential. However, after reperfusion with oxygenated solution containing normal glucose concentration soon after the loss of synaptic excitation, excitability returns and, as in the in vivo ischemic experiments, the slices show hyperexcitability. There were no significant effects of inhibitors of NMDA responses on the loss of synaptic excitability (see Figure 6 in Hori et al., 1991). In separate experiments in which ouabain, an inhibitor of Na-K-ATPase was applied to brain slices, we found that there was little, if any, effect on the population synaptic response for the first 10 min, but thereafter the population response decayed and excitability was totally lost after about 20 min (Carpenter and Gregg, 1984).

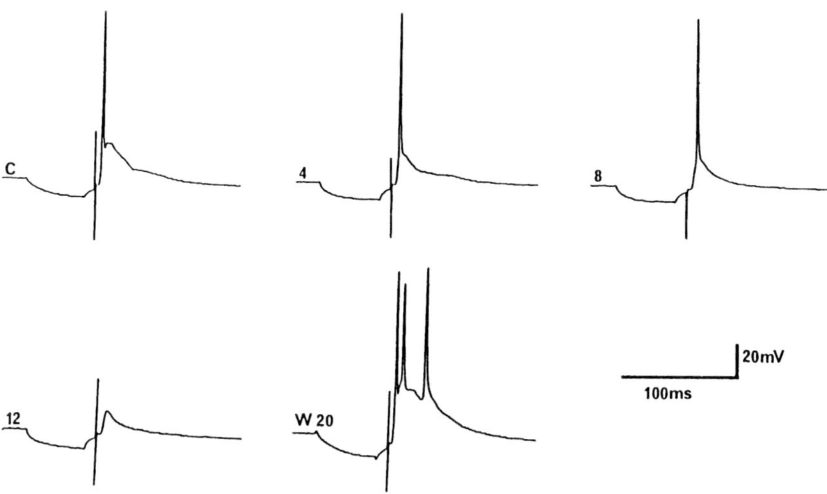

Figure 5. Intracellular recordings from a pyramidal neuron during ischemia application. Each trace shows the voltage change caused by a constant current pulse of 0.2 nA and the response elicited by activation of the Schaffer collateral pathway. The ischemic condition was applied for 10 min. The times of recording are indicated. Synaptic transmission was lost without significant loss of membrane potential or resistance. After a 20 min wash the same stimulation gave a prolonged response. (From Hori et al., 1991; used with permission).

We have used the fungal toxin, 3-nitroproprionic acid (3-NP), a selective inhibitor of succinic dehydrogenase and thus uncouples oxidative phosphorylation, as a tool to follow the electrical events that occur when cell metabolism is shut down. Figure 6 shows the series of events found when recording intracellularly from hippocampal pyramidal neurons in CA1 upon perfusion of 1 mM 3-NP. Under conditions of normal glucose concentration, 3-NP caused a small transient depolarization in some neurons (3 of 12), followed by a rather large hyperpolarization which after a prolonged period decayed to an irreversible depolarization. In 12 neurons the average hyperpolarization was 12 mV at 30-60 min following onset of perfusion of 3-NP. The hyperpolarization is accompanied by a significant increase in membrane conductance. The hyperpolarization was blocked by application of glibenclamide, a specific antagonist of ATP-sensitive potassium channels. Figure 7 shows that glibenclamide induces a depolarization and discharge in control neurons, and that diazoxide, an activator of ATP-sensitive potassium channels, causes a hyperpolarization of these neurons. Thus, cellular ATP concentration has a direct effect in regulation of membrane potential and conductance of hippocampal neurons. The late depolarization began after 65 to 140 min, and was relatively rapid (3-7 mV/min). As seen in Figure 6, application of antagonist of the excitatory amino acids has no effect on the late depolarization, indicating that this is not due to activation of these receptors. The presence of glibenclamide did not influence the time course of the irreversible depolarization, but totally blocked the transient hyperpolarization.

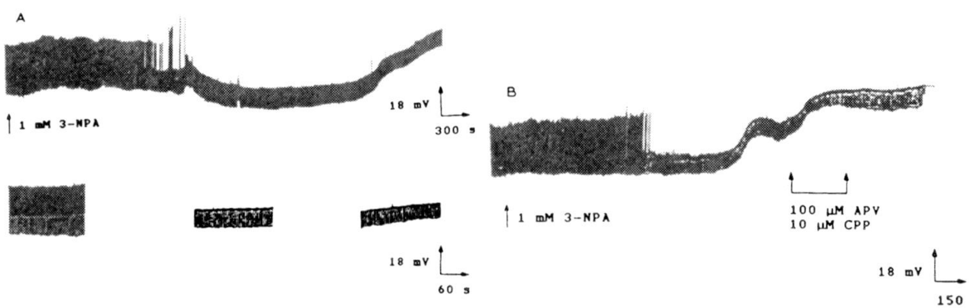

Figure 6. A: Intracellular recording in a CA1 pyramidal neuron under continued perfusion of 3-NPA in normal Krebs-Ringer containing 10 mM glucose. Hyperpolarizing constant current pulses, 0.5 nA, 50 ms duration, 0.3 Hz, were applied to monitor input resistance. The lower records are expanded traces. In B the same conditions were applied but with glucose concentration reduced to 4 mM. (From Riepe et al., 1992; used with permission).

It has widely been speculated that the depolarization following ischemia is secondary to excessive release of glutamate from presynaptic terminals. Since excitatory amino acid antagonists had no effect on the terminal depolarization following 3-NP, we performed some additional investigations of the effects of 3-NP on membrane potential and responses to application of ionophoretic excitatory amino acids (Figure 8). These studies show that the responses to application of the excitatory amino acid agonist is decreased, not increased, following inhibition of oxidative phosphorylation.

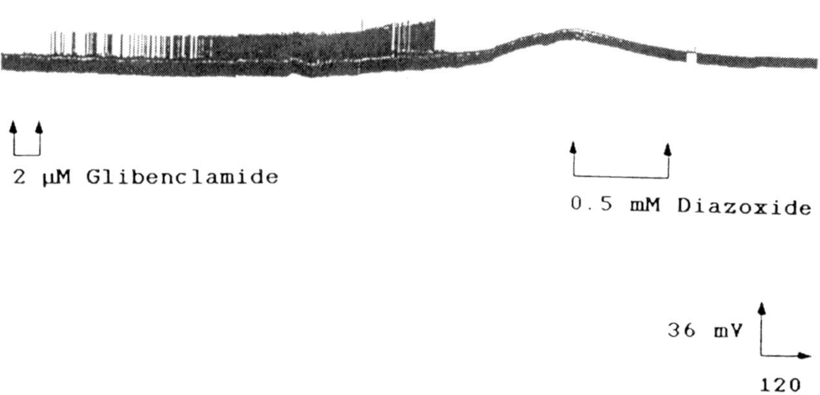

Figure 7. Diazoxide (0.5 mM) reverses depolarization induced by glibenclamide (2 mM) under conditions of continued application of 1 mM 3-NPA. Resistance was monitored by application of 0.5 nA hyperpolarizing current pulses as in Figure 6. (From Riepe et al., 1992; used with permission.)

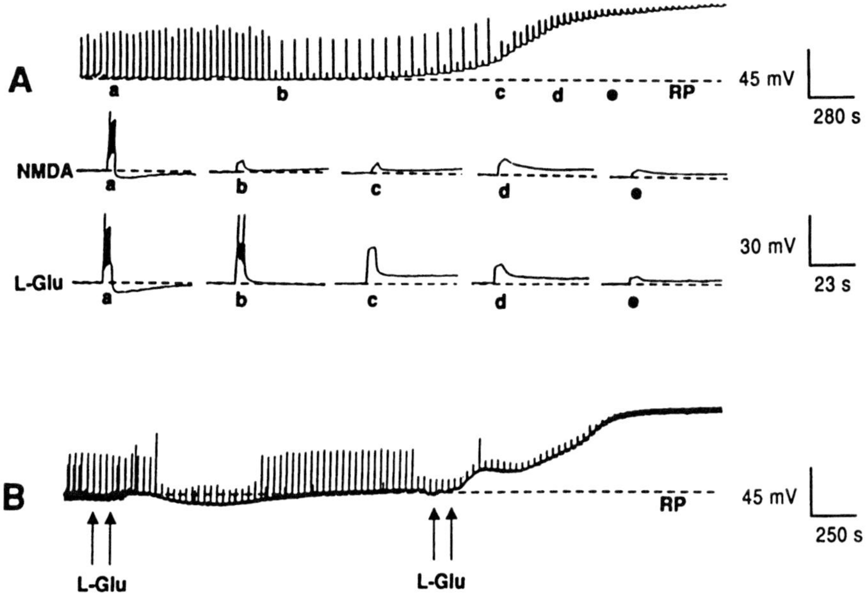

Figure 8. Ionophoretic application of glutamate (L-Glu) and NMDA on a pyramidal neuron in CA1. A: The upper row shows recordings at a slow time base where the upward deflections are responses alternating to NMDA (50 mM in 150 mM NaCl, 24 nA) and glutamate (150 mM, 23 nA), while the second and third rows show expanded traces at times indicated. Note action potential generation upon application of glutamate and NMDA initially and incomplete repolarization after prolonged inhibition, although the induced depolarization decreased. B: Ionophoretic and superimposed bath application (5 mM, arrows) of glutamate at the beginning of inhibition of energy metabolism and after decrease in ionophoretic responses. (From Riepe et al., 1995; used with permission).

Prior to metabolic inhibition, there is a prominent hyperpolarization following the response to ionophoretic glutamate or NMDA. As shown in Figure 9, this hyperpolarization is blocked within a few minutes by application of ouabain, an inhibitor of sodium-potassium transport, indicating that the hyperpolarization results from activation of electrogenic sodium transport. However, the electrogenic component is totally blocked without any massive depolarization of resting potential. These observations are consistent with our demonstration some years ago (Carpenter and Gregg, 1984) that the time course of loss of cellular excitability after ouabain is over a period of 20 to 45 min, which is very similar to that seen with 3-NP. Together these observations indicate that it is inhibition of maintenance of ionic concentration gradients, not excessive action of glutamate triggered by release from presynaptic terminals, that causes the terminal depolarization.

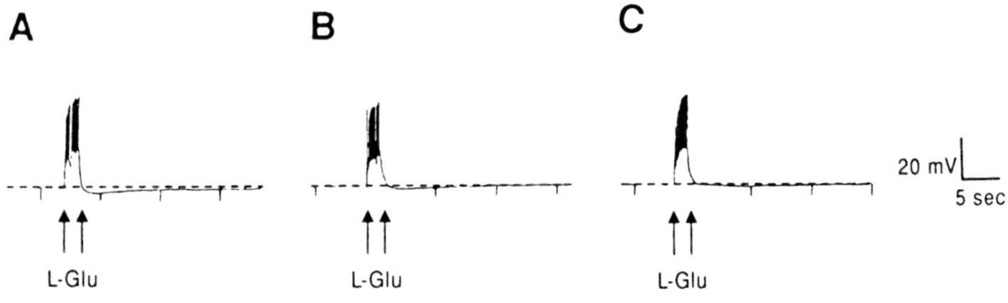

Figure 9. Ionophoretic application of glutamate on a pyramidal neuron and the effect of a bathing solution containing 10 mM ouabain. A: Control. B: Ouabain, 3 min. C: Ouabain, 6 min. (From Riepe et al., 1995; used with permission).

Discussion

All cells require metabolic energy for survival. For neurons that energy is derived from glucose, which is utilized to generate ATP via the process of oxidative phosphorylation. ATP supports a variety of metabolic functions, but one of the most significant is the maintenance of the ionic concentration gradients to critical ions such as Na^+, K^+ and Ca^{2+}.

Our results, together with studies from a number of other laboratories, suggest the following sequence of events following metabolic challenge to a neuron. Prolonged ischemia, inhibition of sodium transport or metabolic inhibition results in cell death after a period of time during which cellular energy stores of ATP are depleted. Our results with 3-NP suggest that this irreversible depolarization is a result primarily of loss of ionic concentration gradients, and does not suggest any particular role for increased release of excitatory amino acid transmitters. This conclusion is in general agreement with that of Zeevalk and Nicklas (1991), who demonstrated that both cyanide and iodoacetate elicited effects beyond those attributable to excitatory amino acids.

There is no question but that if glutamate were released, it would have such effects, although we have identified several mechanisms which would tend to reduce such release. One of these is the ATP-dependent K^+ channels. The relatively large hyperpolarization activated by 3-NP or diazoxide and blocked by glibenclamide reflects the functional contribution of this channel. Since this channel is opened when ATP levels are reduced, and since when the channel is opened the membrane potential and membrane conductance are both increased, the ATP-dependent K^+ channel serves as a protective factor against rapid depolarization under circumstances when ATP levels are reduced. We have been, in fact, surprised that the hyperpolarization appears to be due to ATP-dependent K^+ channels, and not Ca^{2+}-dependent K^+ channels. However, these Ca^{2+}-dependent K^+ channels could also serve a similar function, responding to damaging rises in intracellular Ca^{2+} concentration by reducing excitability (Leblond and Krnjevic, 1989). It is likely that these Ca^{2+}-dependent K^+ channels also play a role in protecting neurons, at least to a degree, from metabolic challenges, but at least in CA1 pyramidal neurons it appears that the ATP-dependent K^+ channels are of greater significance.

Another protective mechanism is probably responsible for the loss of synaptic transmission at a time during ischemia when membrane potential and resistance are more or less maintained. While we have not studied the mechanism of this effect ourselves, it is almost certainly a result of release of adenosine, which blocks presynaptic release of glutamate (Sciotti et al., 1992; Simpson et al., 1992). This is a rapid effect, and is probably the major mechanism which prevents excessive actions of the excitatory amino acids.

In cell culture systems, there is good evidence that excitatory amino acid release is not only an important source of rapid cellular damage, but also is associated with significant cell swelling. However, our experiments provide little evidence for either excessive glutamate release or significant cell swelling early in the process of cell death. Certainly our investigations do not rule out there being a contribution from either cause, but they suggest that other factors are more significant. By use of the confocal microscope we have been able to visualize CA1 pyramidal neurons during perfusion of kainate, and found that the cell volume increased only during relatively late periods, long after total loss of membrane potential (Riepe and Carpenter, 1995). In total our results in brain slices contrast with results from isolated neurons, and suggest that these various regulatory mechanisms are more intact in in vivo preparations and isolated brain slices, and together they serve to reduce the cell swelling and excitatory amino acid release which is so clear in cell culture systems (Rothman, 1985).

The regulatory mechanisms brought into play during ischemia appear to be somewhat more varied than those available during metabolic inhibition or inhibition of sodium transport. The very rapid inhibition of synaptic transmission upon acute ischemia, probably mediated via presynaptic adenosine receptors, does not occur with either application of 3-NP or ouabain. The evolution of this control mechanism is probably a reflection of the fact that transient ischemia is a relatively frequent event, for which protective actions are required.

Accumulation of intracellular calcium is usually considered to be a critical event in cell death, and it is somewhat surprising that our experiments have not indicated this to be as important a factor as we expected. This is not to say that calcium accumulation is unimportant, of course, since it is well documented to occur both upon application of excitatory amino acid agonists (Hajos et al., 1986; MacDermott et al., 1986) and during ischemia (Kass et al., 1989; Kass and Lipton, 1986). It is also clear that calcium accumulation can kill neurons (Choi , 1986) and can trigger a sequence of events such as proteolysis (Mallgren, 1987) and alteration of other ionic conductances (Zucker, 1992). However, our studies suggest strongly that cellular ATP levels and maintenance of ionic concentration gradients via operation of the sodium pump are of greater importance, at least in acute cell death.

The delayed neuronal death seen in CA1 is a quite different phenomenon, and here it may be that calcium accumulation is the critical event. Delayed neuronal death appears to follow the hyperexcitability that occurs after a transient ischemic episode. Our results show this hyperexcitability to be due to the loss of voltage dependence of NMDA channels, consistent with the independent observations of Zeevalk and Nicklas (1992) in retina. While we have not determined the mechanism whereby voltage dependence is lost, it is presumably a result of some change in the structure of NMDA channels, probably induced through activation of some intracellular kinase or phosphatase. There is accumulating evidence that delayed neuronal death is, in fact, apoptosis or genetically programed cell death (Gwag et al., 1995). Furthermore, there is evidence from a variety of studies that apoptosis can be triggered by increases in intracellular calcium concentration (Richter, 1993).

In summary, metabolic insult to neurons results in activation of a variety of counter measures which tend to delay and prevent cell damage. These include activation of ATP-

and calcium-dependent K^+ channels and adenosine release. While many factors contribute to cell damage leading to cell death, our observations indicate the importance of loss of ionic concentration gradients as being of primary importance. Delayed neuronal death following ischemic damage, on the other hand, appears to result from apoptosis, probably triggered by the increase in intracellular calcium resulting from activity of NMDA activated ion channels, and the loss of the normal voltage dependent blockade of these channels which occurs following a transient ischemic episode.

Acknowledgements

This study was supported by NINDS NS2380709 to DOC.

Plenary discussion

Wall P.: Irreversible changes and cell death are not related to clinical pain states.

Carpenter D.: I totally agree with your comment, and in no way did I imply that they were related. What is relevant to pain from these studies is the variety of compensatory events that can be triggered by ischemia or metabolic inhibition--including activation of ATP-dependent or Ca^{++}-dependent K^+ channels, alternation of electrogenic Na^+-K^+ pump or Na^+-Ca^{++} exchange, depression of transmitter release by adenosine and others. These are events that can possibly be involved in generator potential mechanisms at nociceptive receptor terminals. Obviously my studies are not of pain but rather of compensatory events resulting from harmful stimuli.

Reeh W.: You seem to imply that depolarization is deleterious to the survival of ischemically injured nerve cells. Could it not be the other way around? Depolarization may reduce metabolic turnover and actually improve ischemia tolerance, as is the case in diabetic neuropathy when axons are depolarized, propagating impulses slower and with smaller amplitude than normal, but with increased tolerance against pressure and ischemia (and hypoxia).

Carpenter D.: In the case of ischemia, my view is that the terminal depolarization, resulting from loss of ionic concentration gradients, is harmful to the cell, and that mechanisms endogenous to the cell protect against it. However, this is not to imply that cell depolarization is harmful. In part, one of our primary conclusions is that there are several compensatory measures that may be different with different insults but often have important roles in maintaining functions. Your example of the depolarization with diabetic neuropathy may well be one such example. We have for example found that 3-NP applied at sub-lethal doses to animals prior to acute administration to the isolated brain slice has resulted in some presently unknown compensatory mechanism which results in an improved tolerance to the acute metabolic inhibition.

Eaton S.: What are the time course and the subcellular mechanism responsible for the loss of the unusual voltage dependency of the NMDA-receptor mediated EPSP component following anoxia?

Carpenter D.: We see hyperexcitability after in vitro ischemia almost as soon as excitability occurs, which is within 20 min. We do not yet know the mechanism. The hypothesis we are presently testing is that there is some phosphorylation or dephosphorylation of the NMDA channel which is responsible for the hyperexcitability.

Eaton S.: What changes in inhibition occur following anoxia?

Carpenter D.: There is a decrease of GABA inhibition as well as an increase in NMDA-mediated excitation, but our present evidence suggests that the change in excitability predominates in explaining the hyperexcitability.

References

Carpenter DO and Gregg RA (1984) Functional significance of electrogenic pumps in neurons. In: Electrogenic Transport: Fundamental Principals and Physiological Implications (MP Blaustein and M Lieberman eds) Raven Press, NY pp 253-270.

Choi DW (1986) Calcium-mediated neurotoxicity: Relationship to specific channel types and role in ischemic damage. Trends Neurosci 11: 465-469.

Colvin RA, Bennett JW, Colvin SL, Allen RA, Martinez J and Miner GD (1991) Na^+/Ca^{2+} exchange activity is increased in Alzheimer's disease brain tissues. Brain Res 543: 139-147.

Deng H-X, Hentati A, Tainer JA, Iqbal Z, Cayabyab A, Hung W-Y, Getzoff ED et al. (1993) Amyotrophic lateral sclerosis and structural defects in Cu,Zn superoxide dismutase. Science 261: 1047-1050.

Gwag BJ, Lobner D, Koh JY, Wie MB and Choi DW (1995) Blockade of glutamate receptors unmasks neuronal apoptosis after oxygen-glucose deprivation in vitro. Neuroscience 68: 615-619.

Hajos F, Garthwaite C and Garthwaite J (1986) Reversible and irreversible neuronal damage caused by excitatory amino acid analogues in rat cerebellar slices. Neuroscience 18: 417-436.

Hori N and Carpenter DO (1994a) Transient ischemia causes a reduction of Mg^{2+} blockade of NMDA receptors. Neurosci Letts 173:75-78.

Hori N and Carpenter DO (1994b) Functional and morphological changes induced by transient in vivo ischemia. Exp Neurol 129: 279-289.

Hori N, Doi N, Miyahara S, Shinoda Y and Carpenter DO (1991) Appearance of NMDA receptors triggered by anoxia independent of voltage in vivo and in vitro. Expt Neurol 112:304-311.

Jansen KLR, Faull RLM, Dragunow M and Synek BL (1990) Alzheimer's disease: Changes in hippocampal N-methyl-D-aspartate, quisqualate, neurotensin, adenosine, benzodiazepine, serotonin and opioid receptors-an autoradiographic study. Neuroscience 39: 613-627.

Kass IS, Chambers G and Cottrell JE (1989) The N-methyl-D-aspartate antagonists aminophosphonovaleric acid and MK-801 reduce anoxic damage to dentate granule and CA1 pyramidal cells in the rat hippocampal slice. Exp Neurol 103: 116-122.

Kass IS and Lipton P (1986) Calcium and long-term transmission damage following anoxia in dentate gyrus and CA1 regions of the hippocampal slice. J Physiol Lond 378: 313-334.

Leblond J and Krnjevic K (1989) Hypoxic changes in hippocampal neurons. J Neurophysiol 62: 427-438.

MacDermott AB, Mayer ML, Westbrook GL, Smith SJ and Barker JL (1986) NMDA-receptor activation increases cytoplasmic calcium concentration in cultured spinal cord neurones. Nature 321: 519-522.

Mallgren RL (1987) Calcium-dependent proteases: An enzyme system active at cellular membranes? FASEB J. 1: 110-115.

Mayer ML and Westbrook GL (1987) The physiology of excitatory amino acids in the vertebrate central nervous system. Prog Neurobiol 28: 197-276.

Palmer AM and Gershon S (1990) Is the neuronal basis of Alzheimer's disease cholinergic or glutamatergic? FASEB J 4: 2745-2752.

Pulsinelli WA and Brierley JB (1979) A new method of bilateral hemispheric ischemia in the unanesthetized rat. Stroke 307: 462-465.

Richter C (1993) Pro-oxidants and mitochondrial Ca2+: Their relationship to apoptosis and oncogenesis. FEBS Letts 325: 104-107.

Riepe M and Carpenter DO (1995) Delayed increase of cell volume of single pyramidal cells in live rat hippocampal slices upon kainate application. Neurosci Letts 191: 35-38.

Riepe M and Carpenter DO (1995) Delayed increase of cell volume of single pyramidal cells in live rat hippocampal slices upon kainate application. Neurosci Letts 191: 35-38.

Riepe MW, Hori N, Ludolph AC and Carpenter DO (1995) Failure of neuronal ion exchange, not potentiated excitation, causes excitotoxicity after inhibition of oxidative phosphorylation. Neuroscience 64: 91-97.

Riepe M, Hori N, Ludolph AC, Carpenter DO, Spencer PS and Allen CN (1992) Inhibition of energy metabolism by 3-nitropropionic acid activates ATP-sensitive potassium channels. Brain Res 586: 61-66.

Riepe MW, Niemi WN, Megow D, Ludolph AC and Carpenter DO (1996) Mitochondrial oxidation in rat hippocampus can be preconditioned by selective chemical inhibition of succinic dehydrogenase. Exp Neurol 128: 15-21.

Rothman SM (1985) The neurotoxicity of excitatory amino acids is produced by passive chloride influx. J Neurosci 5: 1483-1489.

Rothstein JD, Martin LJ and Kungl RW (1992) Decreased glutamate transport by the brain and spinal cord in amyotrophic lateral sclerosis. N Engl J Med 326: 1464-1468.

Sciotti VM, Roche FM, Grabb MC and Van Wylen GL (1992) Adenosine receptor blockade augments interstitial fluid levels of excitatory amino acids during cerebral ischemia. J Cereb Blood Flow Metab 12: 646-655.

Simpson RE, O'Regan MH, Perkins LM and Phillis JW (1992) Excitatory transmitter amino acid release from the ischemic rat cerebral cortex: Effects of adenosine receptor agonists and antagonists. J Neurochem 58: 1683-1690.

Zeevalk GD and Nicklas WJ (1992) Evidence that the loss of the voltage-dependent Mg^{2+} block at the N-methyl-D-aspartate receptor underlines receptor activation during inhibition of neuronal metabolism. J Neurochem 59: 1211-1220.

Zeevalk GD and Nicklas WJ (1991) Mechanisms underlying initiation of excitotoxicity associated with metabolic inhibition. J Pharmacol Exp Therap 257: 870-878.

Zucker RS (1992) Calcium regulation of ion channels in neurons. In: Intracellular Regulation of Ion Channels (M Morad and Z Agus eds) Springer-Verlag, Berlin Heidelberg, pp. 191-201.

Signal Transduction Mechanism and Metabolic Regulation of Axoplasmic Transport in Superior Cervical Ganglion Cells

T. Takenaka, T. Kawakami, H. Hori, Y. Hashimoto and T. Kusakabe*
*Department of Physiology and Anatomy**
Yokohama City University, Yokohama, Japan

Neuronal and hormonal systems are the main control system in our physiological activity (Ochs, 1982). The functional activity of the neuronal system is also controlled by the neurotransmitters and hormones. Axoplasmic transport is thought to supply neuron materials and to be related to physiological activity like a feedback system. If the axoplasmic transport reflects the nerve cell activity, the increase or decrease of axoplasmic transport expresses the nerve cell condition. We have found that treatment with neurotransmitters dramatically alters the organelle transport in superior cervical ganglion (SCG) cells. Treatment with acetylcholine depresses axoplasmic transport and adrenaline enhances axoplasmic transport in SCG cells (Kawakami et al. 1995, Takenaka et al. 1992, Takenaka et al. 1993 and Takenaka et al. 1994). This increase or decrease of axoplasmic transport relates to the nerve cell activity, especially transmitter release. For example, treatment of the SCG cells with adrenaline results in long term potentiation. This paper discusses the transduction mechanism responsible for the change in axoplasmic transport induced by neurotransmitters.

Modulation of axoplasmic transport by neurotransmitters

SCG cells from 3-month-old C57BL mice were cultured on 50 mm thick polylysine-coated cover glasses for 3 days. Movements of individual particles were observed with differential interference contrast optics and video enhanced microscopic techniques (Allen et al. 1981, Takenaka et al. 1990, and Takenaka et al. 1992). The number of particles passing through one region of a neurite was 20-60 per minute in both anterograde and retrograde directions, which mainly depends upon the diameter of the fiber. The velocity distribution of these particles was 0.2-3.0 mm /sec in both directions. There are faster moving small particles, up to 6.0 mm /sec, but these particles were not taken into account because of measurement inaccuracies. The transported particles reported here were generally longer than 0.1 mm and were mainly lysosomes and mitchondria which moved in linear fashion along microtubules.

The number of the transported particles in neurites decreased to 30-60% within 5 min after application of ACh 1×10^{-3}-1×10^{-7} M in both anterograde and retrograde directions. These changes were completely reversed by washing out the ACh solution (Takenaka et al. 1992). The velocity of the transported particles is also decreased by about 25% in ACh application. This modulatory action of neurotransmitter on axoplasmic transport is not a specific phenomenon observed only in sympathetic ganglion cells. Transported particles are also suppressed in a similar fashion in dorsal root ganglion neurons by the application of g-aminobutyric acid. These modulations of axoplasmic transport by neurotransmitters are a physiological phenomenon in nerve cells, and the suppression of axoplasmic transport might be one common aspect of neural regulation.

In contrast, adrenaline (1×10^{-5}-1×10^{-7} M) increased the number of the transported particles to 150-200% in SCG cells (Takenaka et al. 1994). The application of 0.1 mM adrenaline increased the particle flow within 5 minutes. The peak increase occurred about 10 minutes after application in both anterograde and retrograde directions. The increase was about twice the control value and completely reversible. Desensitization was also observed. The velocity of the transported particles are also increased to about 150% in both retrograde and anterograde directions.

Transduction mechanism of neurotransmitters in axoplasmic transport

Pharmacological experiments were performed to determine which type of ACh receptors is involved in the suppression of the transport. Arecoline, a muscarinic agonist, decreased the transport reversibly, but nicotine had no effect (Kumamoto and Kuba, 1986). Thus, muscarinic receptors mediate the suppression of the axoplasmic transport by ACh. There are five muscarinic receptor subtypes, m_1, m_2, m_3, m_4, m_5 which have been identified by molecular biological techniques. Stimulation of both m_1 and m_3 muscarinic receptor subtypes evoked outward K current dependent on calcium ion mediated phosphoinositide hydrolysis. m_2, m_4 evoked the suppression of adenylyl cyclase and decreased cAMP which does not depend on calcium ion. m_1, m_3, m_5 also activate phospholipase C mediated GTP-binding protein (G-protein) which is insensitive to islet activating protein (IAP). In contrast, stimulation of m_2, m_4 receptors inhibits the adenylyl cyclase and decreases cAMP mediated G_i-protein which is sensitive to IAP. IAP, a specific inhibitor of inhibitory GTP-binding protein (G_i-protein), blocked the ACh effect on axoplasmic transport, so G_i-protein related with these effects (Takenaka et al. 1992). In addition, we found that there was no increase of calcium during the suppression of axoplasmic transport by arecoline (Takenaka et al. 1992). These data suggest that muscarinic Ach receptor m_2 or m_4 is to be considered. This suggests that inhibitory effect of ACh on axoplasmic transport was mediated by decreased cAMP production as a result of either m_2 or m_4 receptor activation. We carried out in situ hybridization studies in order to determine which muscarinic receptor subtypes are present on SCG cells (Takenaka et al. 1993). Labeling with cDNA indicated that m_1 and m_2, but not m_3 or m_4 subtypes were present. Immunoreactivity of m_2 was also detected in the cultured SCG neuron. Thus, we concluded that the muscarinic ACh receptor is m_2 and not m_4 (Takenaka et al. 1993). These results suggest that ACh via ACh receptor m_2 decreases the rate of fast axoplasmic transport through the activation of G_i-protein.

Adrenaline increased the number of transported particles in both anterograde and retrograde directions. These effects were antagonized by a b_2-antagonist, butoxamine, but not by b1- or a-antagonists, atenolol or phentolamine. The b_2-agonist, albuterol, mimicked the adrenaline effect on the axoplasmic transport, but b_1, a_1, and a_2-agonists did not. Thus, the effects of adrenaline may involve stimulation of the b_2-receptors (Takenaka et al. 1994).

An activator of adenylyl cyclase, forskolin, increased the axoplasmic transport. Similarly, application of dibutyryl cAMP mimicked the stimulatory effect of adrenaline. 300 nM KT5720, specific inhibitor of cAMP dependent protein kinase (protein kinase A,

PKA) decreased axoplasmic transport to about 50%. Another PKA inhibitor, H89, also decreased the axoplasmic transport. This suggests that PKA mediates the effect of adrenaline. Thus it appears that adrenaline binding to b_2-adrenergic receptors activates adenylyl cyclase through a stimulatory GTP-binding protein, Gs. The resultant rise in endogeneous cAMP initiates a sequence of metabolic processes which presumably includes the phosphorylation of specific proteins by PKA. This phosphorylation modulates the axoplasmic transport. In contrast, acetylcholine presumably suppresses axoplasmic transport via decreased of cAMP and then decreased PKA.

Adrenaline and ACh control axoplasmic transport

Our conclusion on how adrenaline and ACh control axoplasmic transport in SCG cells are as follows (Fig.1). Acetylcholine suppresses axoplasmic transport by lowering the basal concentration of cAMP and adrenaline increases it by raising cAMP. The changes in cAMP are mediated via Gi and Gs effects on adenylyl cyclase. Increases in cAMP activate PKA which in turn phosphorylates another enzyme, phosphorylase kinase. Activation of this enzyme leads to phosphorylation of motor proteins like kinesin and dynein that are involved in axoplasmic transport.

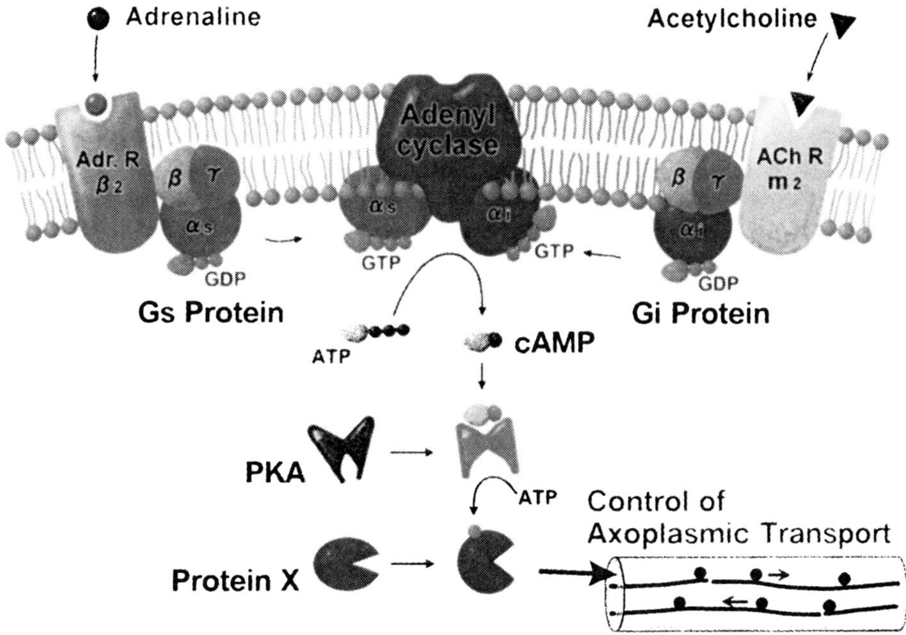

Figure 1. Schematic diagram of how adrenaline and acetylcholine modulate axoplasmic transport. G-proteins linking ACh or adrenaline receptors activate or inactivate adenylyl cyclase, thereby altering the intracellular concentration of the intracellular messenger cAMP. The cAMP in turn activates PKA, which phosphorylates another enzyme, phosphorylase kinase. It in turn phosphorylates motor proteins like kinesin or dynein involved in the axoplasmic transport. Under normal conditions cAMP level stays at a normal level. Adrenaline increases cAMP activity, thereby increasing the axoplasmic transport. On the other hand ACh suppresses axoplasmic transport by decreasing the concentration of cAMP. Ad-R b_2: b_2-adrenergic receptor, ACh-R m_2: m_2 acetylcholine receptor, Gs-prot.: stimulatory GTP-binding protein, G_i-prot.: inhibitory GTP-binding protein, AC: adenylyl cyclase, cAMP: cyclic AMP, PKA: cyclic-AMP-dependent protein kinase.

We can hypothesize as follows. The SCG cells contain a basal quantity of cAMP in a quasi-stable state. Acetylcholine suppresses axoplasmic transport by lowering the concentration of cAMP and adrenaline increases it by raising the concentration of cAMP. The concentration of cAMP in the cell controls the nervous activity. For example, Kuba and Kuramoto showed that the quantal content of the first excitatory post-synaptic potentials was potentiated for more than several hours after treatment with adrenaline, which causes increased transmitter release (Kuba and Kumamoto, 1986 and Kumamoto and Kuba, 1986). Azderian et al. reported that cAMP stimulates axoplasmic transport in the neurites of Aplysia bag cell neurons (Azderian et al. 1991). Forscher et al. also reported that cAMP induced regulation of organelle transport in bag cell growth cones of aplysia (Forsher et al. 1987).

This modulatory action is not a specific phenomenon observed only in sympathetic ganglion cells. Axoplasmic flow in dorsal root ganglion cells is also suppressed in a similar fashion by the application of g-aminobutyric acid (unpublished data). Thus, modulation of axoplasmic transport by neurotransmitters is a physiological phenomenon in neurons which could work synergistically with presynaptic release in the regulation of neuronal information.

The relation between physiological neural activity and modulatory action of axoplasmic transport

The enhancement of axoplasmic transport means that many substances are transported, which in turn increases transmitter release. The quantal content of the excitatory post-synaptic potential was potentiated after treatment with adrenaline, which causes increased transmitter release (Kuba and Kumamoto, 1986 and Kumamoto and Kuba, 1986). Forsher et al. also reported that cAMP induced changes in distribution and transport of organelles within growth cones of aplysia bag cell neurons (Forsher et al. 1987). On the other hand, the decrease of axoplasmic transport causes changes in neural architecture and plasticity. When the axoplasmic transport is depressed, the transported materials accumulate in certain places in the neurite. Membranous lamellipodia have been observed in these areas. New branches were forming where the particles were accumulated (Takenaka et al. 1991). The substances which are transported by the axoplasmic transport have to be dropped off from the microtubules acting as tracks. Using these accumulated materials, the neurite produces new branches. This phenomenon is a kind of plasticity. The results demonstrate that neurotransmitters play an important role in regulating neuronal activity.

Plenary discussion

Basbaum A.: Is there any effect of adrenalectomy on transport mechanisms in vivo?

Takenaka T.: Our experimental materials are tissue cultured SCG cells, but we do the same experiment using tissue cultured hypocampal cells, and we have found that cAMP does increase the axoplasmic transport.

Basbaum A.: Where is the muscarinic receptor m_2 subtype located? Is it on the presynaptic terminal or the postganglionic fiber?

Takenaka T.: In tissue cultured SCG cells, the m_2 receptor exists in the cell body, neurite, and growth cone.

Basbaum A.: What might be the in vivo source of acetylcholine that acts on the transport mechanisms?

Takenaka T.: We did not do in vivo experiments.

Eaton S.: If cAMP levels are increased, can you see increased velocity of neuronal tracer transportation?

Takenaka T.: Yes, if cAMP levels are increased the increased velocity is also observed in SCG cells.

References

Allen RD, Allen NS and Travis JL (1981) Video-enhanced contrast, differential interference contrast (AVEC-DIC) microscopy: a new method capable of analyzing microtubule-related motility in the reticulopodial network of Allogromia laticollaris. Cell Motil 1: 291-302.

Azderian E, Lin CH, Hefner D, Forsher P and Kaczmarek LK (1991) Cyclic AMP increases the quantity of ELH-containing proteins in the neurites of Aplysia bag cell neurons. 21st Ann Meet Soc for Neurosci Abstr. p59.

Forscher P, Kaczmarek LK, Buchanan JA and Smith SJ (1987) Cyclic AMP induces changes in distribution and transport of organelles within growth cones of Aplysia bag cells neurons. J Neurosci 7: 3600-3611.

Kawakami T, Takenaka T, Hori H and Hashimoto Y (1995) Effects of acetylcholine and adrenaline on axoplasmic transport at different regions of mouse superior cervical ganglion cells in culture. Brain Res 683: 88-92.

Kuba K and Kumamoto E (1986) Long-term potentiation of transmitter release induced by adrenaline in bull-frog sympathetic ganglia. J Physiol 374: 515-530.

Kumamoto E and Kuba K (1986) Mechanism of long-term potentiation of transmitter release induced by adrenaline in bullfrog sympathetic ganglia. J Gen Physiol 87: 775-793.

Ochs S (1982) Axoplasmic transport and its relation to other nerve functions. John Wiley & Sons.

Takenaka T, Kawakami K, Hikawa N and Gotoh H (1990) Axoplasmic transport of mitochondria in cultured dorsal root ganglion cells. Brain Res 528: 285-290.

Takenaka T, Kawakami T, Hikawa N, Gotoh H and Bandou Y (1991) Neurotransmitter regulation of axoplasmic transport and neuronal growth. Biomedic Res Supp 1.2: 171-172.

Takenaka T, Kawakami K, Hikawa N, Bandou Y and Gotoh H (1992) Effect of neurotransmitters on axoplasmic transport: acetylcholine effect on superior cervical ganglion cells. Brain Res 588: 212-216.

Takenaka T, Kawakami T, Bandou Y, Hikawa N and Gotoh H (1993) How neurotransmitters affect axoplasmic transport. Jap J Physiol 43: Suppl.1, 205-207.

Takenaka T, Kawakami T, Hori H and Bandou Y (1994) Effect of neurotransmitters on axoplasmic transport: how adrenaline affects superior cervical ganglion cells. Brain Res 643: 81-85.

Takenaka T and Kawakami T (1996) Signal transduction mechanism responsible for change in axoplasmic transport caused by neurotransmitters. Neurochem Res 21: 553-556.

Pain Mechanisms and Management
S.N. Ayrapetyan and A.V. Apkarian (Eds.)
IOS Press, 1998

Molecular and Cellular Mechanisms in Neurotransmitter Release

J.-M. Trifaró, L. Zhang and M.G. Marcu
Secretory Process Research Program
Department of Pharmacology, University of Ottawa
Ottawa, Canada

Abstract. Secretory vesicle exocytosis is the mechanism of release of neurotransmitters and neuropeptides. Secretory vesicles are localized in at least two morphologically and functionally distinct compartments: the reserve pool and the release-ready vesicle pool. Filamentous actin networks play an important role in this compartmentalization and in the traffic of vesicles between these compartments. The cortical F-actin network constitutes a barrier (negative clamp) to the movement of secretory vesicles to release sites and it must be locally disassembled to allow translocation of secretory vesicles in preparation for exocytosis. The disassembly of the cortical F-actin network is produced by scinderin (a Ca^{2+}-dependent F-actin severing protein) upon activation by Ca^{2+} entering the cells during stimulation. There are several factors that regulate scinderin activation (i.e. Ca^{2+} levels, PIP_2, etc.). The results suggest that scinderin and the cortical F-actin network are components of the exocytotic machinery.

Introduction

Neurons as well as other neurosecretory cells store classical neurotransmitters, nucleotides and peptides in membrane-bound organelles: the secretory vesicles (Trifaró, 1977). Upon stimulation, the soluble contents of the vesicles are released to the cell exterior by exocytosis (Trifaró, 1977 and Trifaró and Poisner, 1982). Secretory vesicles are present in these cells in at least two compartments: a) the release-ready vesicle pool and b) the reserve pool (Heinemann et al. 1993, Neher and Zucker, 1993 and Vitale et al. 1995). The traffic of vesicles between these compartments is subject to a fine regulation. Experimental evidence has suggested that an F-actin microfilament network plays an important role in this regulation (Vitale et al. 1991 and Vitale et al. 1995). This is evident in chromaffin cells where F-actin forms a cortical network which excludes the large majority of the secretory vesicles from plasma membrane docking (Burgoyne et al 1982 and Vitale et al. 1995). Therefore, the F-actin network acts as a barrier (negative clamp) blocking the access of secretory vesicles to exocytotic sites at the plasma membrane. Disassembly of cortical F-actin in response to stimulation is thought to allow the movement of vesicles from the reserve compartment into the release-ready pool (Vitale et al. 1991 and Vitale et al. 1995). Vesicles in this pool seem to be in two stages of releasability (i.e. non-prime and prime or fusion competent and fusion incompetent vesicles). It seems that Mg^{2+}-ATP is required in order to make the secretory vesicles fully competent (Parsons et al. 1995). Thus the release reaction has been divided into two sequential steps, priming (Mg^{2+}-ATP-dependent) and triggering (Mg^{2+}-ATP-independent, Ca^{2+}-dependent step) (Bittner and Holz, 1992). Interaction of vesicles with the plasma membrane is brought about by the intervention of the SNARE complex (the fusion machinery), a series of vesicle membrane and plasma membrane proteins (synaptobrevin, syntaxin, SNAP25, etc.) which interact in the presence of cytosolic factors (NSF) (Sudhof and Jahn, 1991). The SNARE complex interaction promotes the docking and fusion of secretory vesicles. Synaptotagmin (p65, $65K_d$-CMBP) is a second negative clamp preventing vesicle fusion, and only in the presence of Ca^{2+} is the inhibitory effect of synaptotagmin removed (Bommert et al. 1993 and Popov and Poo, 1993). Following vesicle-plasma membrane fusion there is a formation of the fusion pore followed by the subsequent expansion of the pore to give rise to a full exocytotic event (Alvarez de Toledo et al. 1993).

In recent years, we have been interested in the role of cytoskeleton dynamics in exocytosis (Trifaró and Vitale, 1993), and the model we have used in our studies is the chromaffin cell (Trifaró, 1982). This cell has shown itself to be one of the most useful systems for the study of cellular and molecular mechanisms in neurotransmitter release (Trifaró, 1977). Chromaffin cells derive embryologically from the neural crest, sharing a common origin with neurons (Trifaró, 1977 and Trifaró, 1984). Moreover, early observations of this secretory cell have been the starting point of many important observations on the mechanisms of neurosecretion (Douglas, 1968). Regulated secretion is triggered by an increase in intracellular Ca^{2+} (Douglas, 1968 and Trifaró, 1977). However, despite the fact that the role of Ca^{2+} in neurosecretion was observed many years ago (Douglas and Rubin, 1961, Harvey and MacIntoch, 1940 and Houssay and Molinelli, 1928), the mechanisms in which Ca^{2+} is involved in this process are still poorly understood. An attractive hypothesis is that one of the sites of action for Ca^{2+} in secretion is in the control of actin networks (Trifaró and Vitale, 1993). The actin cytoskeleton network interacts not only with plasma membranes but also with different organelles, including secretory vesicles (Jockush et al. 1977 and Trifaró et al. 1985). The cytoskeleton is a dynamic structure which changes according to different stages of cell function. In the following pages the dynamic changes observed in the cytoskeleton during release from chromaffin cells, are discussed.

Cortical actin microfilament network during cell stimulation

Chromaffin cells are among neurosecretory cells that have subplasmalemmal areas largely devoid of secretory vesicles (Cheek and Burgoyne, 1991 and Vitale et al. 1995). This cortical area is occupied by a network of actin filaments (Fig.1,A; Fig.2,A) as indicated in earlier immunohistochemical studies from our laboratory (Lee and Trifaró, 1981). Indeed, the cortical actin cytoskeleton has been considered to be a physical barrier to secretory vesicles, excluding them from releasing sites on the plasma membrane (Vitale et al. 1991). Most chromaffin vesicles are apparently retained within the cortical actin network and they associate with actin bundles through short filaments (Nakata and Hirokawa, 1992). The interaction of chromaffin vesicles with cytoskeletal elements suggests the presence of anchorage proteins in chromaffin cells. a-Actinin was found to be associated with chromaffin vesicles (Jockush et al. 1977 and Trifaró, 1984). The dependence of the binding of actin filaments to chromaffin vesicles on Ca^{2+} may be due to a-actinin. Fluorescent microscopy studies using actin antibodies or rhodamine-labelled phalloidin (a probe from filamentous actin), have demonstrated that catecholamine secretion is accompanied by focal and transient disruption of the cortical actin network (Fig.1,B,C; Fig.2,B) (Vitale et al.

1991). A decrease in chromaffin cell F-actin and a concomitant increase in G-actin, as evaluated by the DNase I inhibitory assay (Cheek and Burgoyne, 1986 and Trifaró et al. 1989), and a reduction in the amount of actin associated with the cytoskeleton, also occur upon nicotinic receptor stimulation or membrane depolarization (Burgoyne et al. 1989 and Trifaró, 1989). Moreover, in intact or permeabilized cells, the presence of substances that destabilize actin networks, such as cytochalasin D or DNase I, enhance stimulation-induced catecholamine release. The above observations suggest that the cortical actin network must be locally removed for secretion to occur. F-actin network disassembly has also been observed in depolarized synaptosomes (Bernstein and Bamburg, 1985). Removal of the stimulus (i.e. nicotine, high K$^+$) restores the cortical actin networks through an increased actin polymerization in the areas showing F-actin disassembly during stimulation (Fig.3,B) (Vitale et al. 1991). Therefore, F-actin disassembly/assembly is a dynamic and cyclic event occurring during cell depolarization.

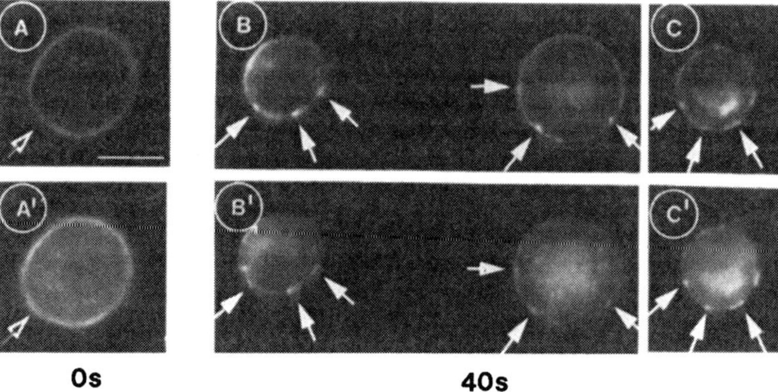

Figure 1. Localization of actin and scinderin by double-staining fluorescence microscopy. Chromaffin cells were incubated with Locke's solution for 40 s in the absence (control) or presence (stimulated) of 10 mM nicotine. Cells were sequentially stained with rhodamine-labelled phalloidin followed by scinderin antibody and FITC-anti-rabbit IgG. A control cell in (A,A') shows continuous and intense rings of fluorescence for F-actin (A) and scinderin (A') colocalized at the sub-plasmalemmal region (open arrows). Stimulated cells display a disrupted cortical fluorescent pattern either for F-actin (B,C,D) or scinderin (B',C'.D'). There is a correspondence between the patched distribution of both actin and scinderin in each cell (compare B and B', and C and C', D and D'). Some patches are indicated by arrows (Vitale et al. 1991).

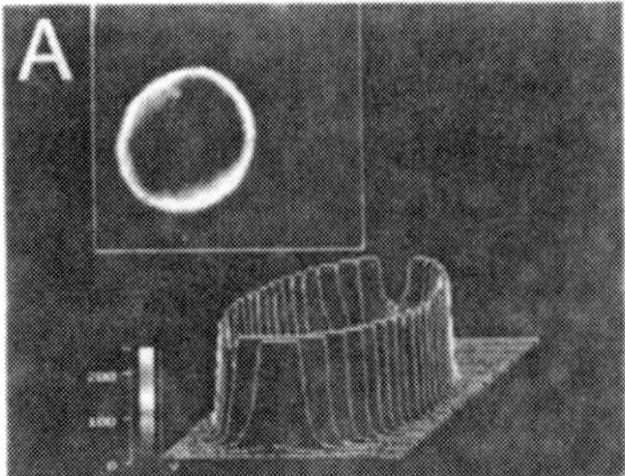 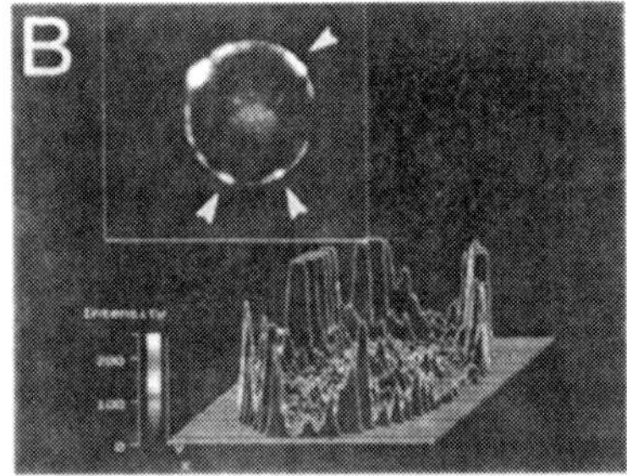

Figure 2. Effect of nicotine on cortical F-actin:video-enhanced image analysis of F-actin fluorescent profiles in single chromaffin cells. Cultured chromaffin cells were incubated with Locke's solution alone (A) or 10^{-5}M nicotine (B) for 40 s, and preparations were then immediately processed for fluorescence microscopy. Cells incubated with Locke's solution alone showed a continuous and bright cortical fluorescence ring (A). Nicotine stimulation caused the disruption of the cortical fluorescence ring. Some fluorescent patches are shown by arrowheads. Three-dimensional image analysis of the cells is shown at the bottom of (A) and (B). In control cells (A) there is a uniform cortical fluorescent pattern. In cells stimulated by nicotine (B), the cortical fluorescence intensity pattern shows irregularities such as valleys and peaks. The peaks correspond to the fluorescent patches observed in the cell shown in (A). The intensity of the fluorescent peaks was 250 arbitrary units. This value is similar to the intensity of the cortical fluorescence pattern observed in control cells.

The cortical actin networks control the size of the release-ready vesicle pool and the initial rate of exocytosis

It has been proposed that chromaffin vesicles may be in various stages of releasability depending upon, in part, the proximity to the plasma membrane (Neher and Zucker, 1993). Vesicles that are relatively close to the membrane constitute the release-ready vesicle pool and those vesicles retained by the actin cytoskeleton constitute the reserve vesicle pool (Neher and Zucker, 1993 and Vitale et al. 1995). Until very recently, there was no morphological evidence for either the existence of these functionally distinctive vesicle pools in chromaffin cells or the cellular structure that controls the delivery of vesicles to exocytotic sites. Morphological, biochemical and membrane capacitance studies carried out in our laboratory have allowed the demonstration of the existence of these vesicle pools and of the cellular structure controlling the size of these pools (Vitale et al. 1995). To demonstrate that the cortical F-actin is, indeed, a barrier to secretion, and that this structure determines the size of the release-ready vesicle pool, we took advantage of our earlier observations that acute (6 min) incubation of chromaffin cells with phorbol myristate acetate (PMA) disrupts the cortical actin cytoskeleton without a concomitant change in basal catecholamine release (Vitale et al. 1992). PMA-induced changes seem to be due to PKC stimulation since 4a-PMA, an inactive phorbol ester, was ineffective. In addition, 4a-PMA did not produce any change in the distribution of PKC between cytoplasma and membranes (Vitale et al. 1992). As suspected, PMA increased the incorporation of PKC into membranes 2.5 times (Vitale et al. 1992).

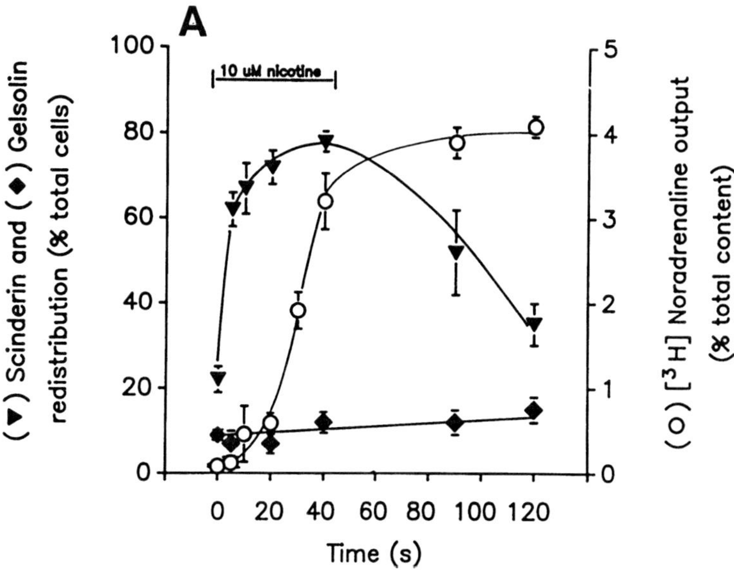

Figure 3A. Time courses of scinderin and gelsolin redistribution and [³H]-noradrenaline ([³H]NA) output in response to stimulation in cultured chromaffin cells. (A) Nicotinic stimulation: chromaffin cells cultured for 48 h were incubated for 0, 5, 10, 20, or 40 s with 10^{-5} M nicotine or for 40-s with nicotine followed by an additional 50- or 80-s period with regular Locke's solution. After these periods of incubation, cells were immediately fixed, permeabilized, and processed for immunofluorescence microscopy using either scinderin (Ñ) or gelsolin (u) antisera. 100 cells per coverslip were examined and classified as having either a "continuous cortical fluorescent pattern" (see Fig.1A) or a "discontinous cortical fluorescent pattern" (see Fig.1B). This was done without knowing whether cells were control or stimulated with nicotine. Gelsolin (another actin filament severing protein present in chromaffin cells) distribution was not affected by nicotine stimulation. Each value shown represents the mean ± SEM of the percentage of discontinuous cortical fluorescence patterns of 6-8 coverslips (600-800 cells for each value) containing cells from three different chromaffin cell cultures. [³H]NA output (¡): cultured chromaffin cells with catecholamine stores labelled with [³H]NA were incubated for 0, 5, 10, 20, 30, or 40 s with 10^{-5} M nicotine or for 40 s with 10 mM nicotine followed by an additional 50- or 80-s period with regular Locke's solution. After each of those periods media were removed and their radioactivity measured. Basal [³H]NA output was determined by incubating the cells with nicotine-free Locke's solution for the same periods of time as above. Basal values (0.7-1.0%) were subtracted from the corresponding data obtained during stimulation. Nicotine-induced [³H]NA secretion is expressed as percentage of total [³H]NA cell content. Each point represents the mean ± SEM of values obtained from three different culture dishes (Vitale et al. 1991).

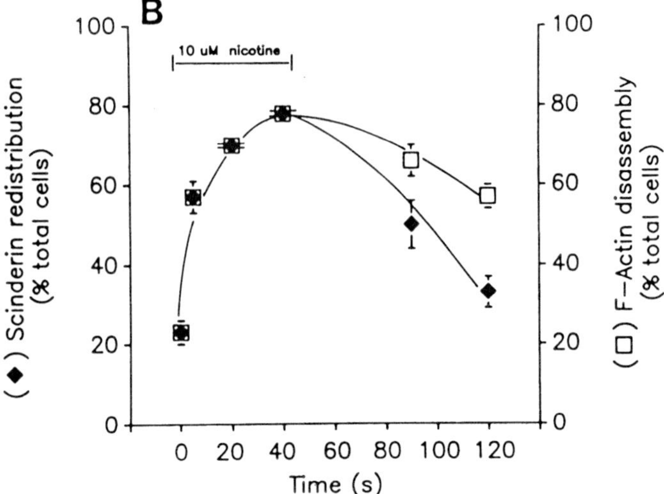

Figure 3B. Time courses of F-actin disassembly and scinderin redistribution in response to nicotine stimulation in cultured chromaffin cells. Chromaffin cells cultured for 48 h were incubated for 0, 5, 20, or 40 s with 10^{-5} M nicotine or for 40 s with nicotine followed by an additional 50 to 80 s with regular Locke's solution. After these periods of incubation cells were immediately fixed, permeabilized, and processed for fluorescence microscopy using rhodamine-phalloidin and scinderin antiserum. Upon removal of the stimulus the rate of recovery was different for scinderin and F-actin (90 and 120 s) (Vitale et al. 1991).

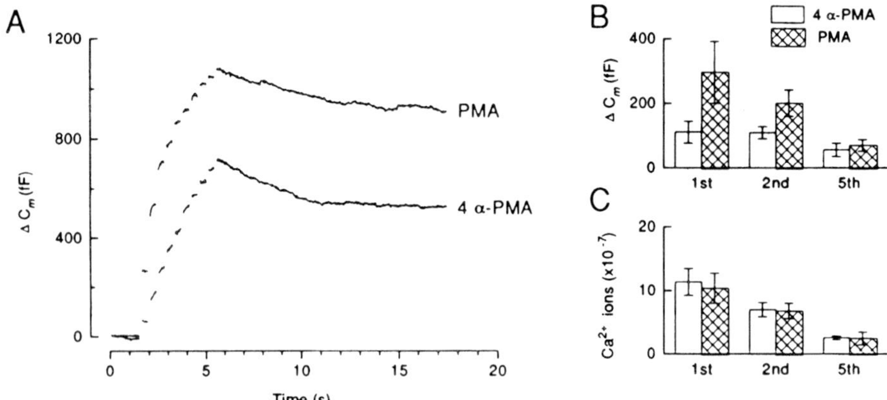

Figure 4. Determination of exocytosis by membrane capacitance.
A. Two day-old chromaffin cells were treated for 5 min with 10^{-7} M of either 4a-PMA or PMA immediately prior to establishing whole-cell recording. Secretion, measured as increases in membrane capacitance, was evoked with a train of 10 depolarizing pulses of 40-80 ms duration. Superimposed traces shown in (A) are representative of changes in membrane capacitance (C_m in Femptofarads) recorded in response to 10 pulses of 80 ms duration (gaps in a cell pretreated with 4a-PMA or PMA, as indicated). C_m recording was interrupted during application of each depolarization as indicated by gaps in the traces. PMA-treated cells consistently showed a larger membrane capacitance increase than 4a-PMA-treated cells in response to the same stimulus. B. and C. A summary of data from six paired cells. As shown (B), the average magnitude of the first and second capacitance jump is significantly longer in PMA compared with 4a-PMA pretreated cells. This potentiation is restricted to the beginning of the stimulus, by the fifth pulse, the secretory rate is nearly the same in the two populations of cells. The Ca^{2+} ion influx per pulse is summarized in (C). This was determined by integration of the corresponding Ca^{2+} currents recorded during the corresponding pulse. Ca^{2+} currents recorded in PMA and 4a-PMA treated cells were qualitatively and quantitatively similar, suggesting that the effects of PMA on the initial rate of exocytosis were not due to increases in Ca^{2+} influx. Data shown in (B) and (C) are the mean ± SEM of 6 values per experimental condition (Vitale et al. 1995).

Sphingosine, staurosporine and calphostin C (PKC inhibitors) produce a concentration-dependent inhibition of PMA-induced F-actin disassembly (Rodríguez Del Castillo et al. 1992 and Vitale et al. 1992). In resting cells, electron microscopy revealed the presence of a 200 nm wide peripheral area almost devoid of secretory vesicles and fluorescence microscopy showed that a network of actin filaments occupies this area (Vitale et al. 1995). Very few secretory vesicles are found between the F-actin network and the plasma membrane. This region, 0-50 nm is occupied by 1.24-2.4% of the total number of secretory vesicles present in chromaffin cells (Vitale et al. 1995). PMA acute treatment disrupts F-actin networks in some cortical areas and causes a 2-3 fold increase in the number of secretory vesicles within 0-50 nm of the plasma membrane (Vitale et al. 1995). PMA did not change basal catecholamine secretion but enhanced the initial rate of secretion in response to nicotine or high K^+ (Vitale et al. 1995). Using the high temporal resolution of membrane capacitance recording technique to measure exocytosis, a 3 fold increase in the membrane capacitance (i.e. a 3 fold increase in the number of vesicles fusing with the plasma membrane) during the first and second depolarization of a train, was detected in PMA pretreated cells when compared with 4a-PMA pre-treated cells (Fig.4) (Vitale et al. 1995). These occurred without increase in voltage-dependent Ca^{2+} influx (Fig.4,C). During the first 80 ms of depolarization, 4a-PMA treated cells exocytosed vesicles at the rate of 511 vesicles/sec $^{-1}$, whereas PMA-treated cells released 1240 vesicles/sec^{-1} (Vitale et al. 1995). The total number of vesicles fused with the plasma membrane derived from membrane capacitance studies correlated well with the number of vesicles occupying the 0-50 nm peripheral zone obtained in ultrastructural studies. The above discussed observations indicate that cortical F-actin disassembly allows the translocation of vesicles to the plasma membrane in preparation for exocytosis.

Role of scinderin in the control of F-actin disassembly and exocytosis

Stimulation-induced F-actin disassembly is Ca^{2+}-dependent and search for a chromaffin cell factor(s) which might be involved in the regulation of F-actin networks led to the discovery of scinderin (Sc), a protein which severs F-actin in a Ca^{2+}-dependent manner (Rodríguez Del Castillo et al 1990). Scinderin has two Ca^{2+}-binding sites (K_d 5.9×10^{-7}M, B_{max} 0.8 mol Ca^{2+}/mol protein; K_d 2.8×10^{-6}M, B_{max} 1.9 mol Ca^{2+}/mol protein). Scinderin is found in tissues with high secretory activity (chromaffin cell, anterior and posterior pituitary, brain, kidney, salivary glands, testis, platelets) and unlike gelsolin (another Ca^{2+}-dependent F-actin severing protein), it is not present in liver, plasma, heart and skeletal muscles (Rodríguez Del Castillo et al. 1990 and Tchakarov et al. 1990). Immunocytochemical studies on chromaffin cells showed an intense subplasmalemmal staining for scinderin together with a diffuse cytoplasmic distribution (Fig.1,A') (Vitale et al. 1991). Under resting conditions subplasmalemmal scinderin appears as a continuous fluorescent ring (Fig.1,A') (Vitale et al. 1991). Upon nicotinic receptor stimulation or K^+-induced depolarization, cortical F-actin and scinderin fluorescent rings are disrupted suggesting redistribution of scinderin and disassembly of F-actin (Fig.1; Fig.2; Fig.3) (Vitale et al. 1991). These dynamic changes are dependent on extracellular Ca^{2+}. We have recently cloned the scinderin gene (Marcu et al. 1994) and analysis of the nucleotide sequence revealed at least 67% and 51% homology with gelsolin and villin respectively, two other Ca^{2+}-dependent F-actin severing proteins. The N-terminal half of the molecule is the functional domain of scinderin and 2 sequences corresponding to actin-binding domains are present here together with 2 other additional phosphatidylinositol 4,5-bisphosphate

(PIP$_2$) binding domains (Fig.5,A) (Marcu et al. 1994). One of them shows the consensus sequence R(X)XXXKXRR typical of PIP$_2$ binding sites of phospholipase C, gelsolin and villin. As gelsolin, scinderin has internal repeats of shorter sequence motifs which occur six times at approximately equal intervals (Marcu et al. 1994). In summary, the sequence analysis indicates that, among the families of Ca^{2+}-dependent F-actin severing proteins, scinderin is a distinct protein (Marcu et al. 1994).

Scinderin cDNA was expressed in two systems: a) *E-coli* GM105 using glutathion-S-transferase (GST) Gene Fusion System and expression vectors pGEX4T2 and pGEX4T3 and b) the *E-coli* GI698 using TRX Thio-Fusion System and expression vector pGEX4T2 (Marcu et al. 1994). The recombinant scinderin thus obtained cross-react with native scinderin antibodies and bind phosphatidylserine, phosphatidylinositol 4,5-bisphosphate (PIP$_2$) and actin in a Ca^{2+}-dependent manner (Marcu et al. 1994 and Zhang et al. 1996). Recombinant truncated scinderin (Sc$_{274-715}$) was also prepared (Fig.5,A). This protein is recognized by scinderin antibodies but does not sever filamentous actin since the first two scinderin domains (S$_1$ and S$_2$) have been deleted (Fig.5,A) (Zhang et al. 1996).

Permeabilized cells are useful preparations to study secretory events distal to receptor and channel activation. Therefore, digitonin permeabilized cells were incubated with full-length recombinant and truncated scinderins. Ca^{2+}-induced release of catecholamine increased in a concentration-dependent manner in the presence of full-length recombinant scinderin (Fig.5,B) (Zhang et al. 1996). Similarly, serotonin release from platelets was increased by recombinant scinderin (Marcu et al. 1996). Moreover, no effects were observed when chromaffin cells were incubated with recombinant truncated scinderin (Fig.5,B). The potentiation of Ca^{2+}-evoked catecholamine release by recombinant scinderin was due to an enhanced F-actin severing activity of scinderin as demonstrated by an increase in the number of cells displaying cortical F-actin disassembly in the presence of recombinant scinderin (Zhang et al. 1996). An additional proof in favour of F-actin disassembly mediating the response of recombinant scinderin, is the fact that the increases, in both neurotransmitter release and F-actin disassembly, were inhibited by endogenous g-actin and by two peptides (Sc-ABP$_1$ and Sc-ABP$_2$) with sequences corresponding to two active actin-binding sites of scinderin (Fig.5,B) (Zhang et al. 1996). Two of the actin-binding sites of scinderin are in domains S$_1$ and S$_2$ of the molecule (Fig.5,A) (Marcu et al. 1994). These are the F-actin-severing domains of the protein and should be the domains responsible for the scinderin potentiation of Ca^{2+}-induced release of catecholamines. This concept gains support from the experiments with recombinant truncated scinderin showing that this fusion protein neither potentiates nor inhibits Ca^{2+}-evoked catecholamine release (Fig.5,B) and cortical F-actin disassembly (Zhang et al. 1996). It has been previously demonstrated and as indicated above, that PIP$_2$ binds to, and modulates the severing activity of, scinderin (Rodríguez Del Castillo et al. 1992). Consequently, the ability of recombinant scinderin to increase Ca^{2+}-evoked release of neurotransmitter and F-actin disassembly was inhibited by PIP$_2$, an effect which was reverted when a scinderin-derived PIP$_2$ binding peptide (ScPIP$_2$BP) was present in the medium (Zhang et al. 1996). ScPIP$_2$BP has a sequence present in domain S$_1$ of scinderin. One of the two PIP$_2$ binding sites of scinderin overlaps with its second actin-binding site. This will explain, at least in part, the inhibitory effect of PIP$_2$ on scinderin F-actin severing activity and the inhibition of recombinant scinderin effects on neurotransmitter release. The present results also indicate that the effects of PIP$_2$ on F-actin disassembly and Ca^{2+}-evoked exocytosis are mediated through the interaction between the intact PIP$_2$ molecule and scinderin. Therefore, the inhibitory effects of PIP$_2$ are not due to the activation of a specific PIP$_2$ transduction pathway. The fact that plasma membrane PIP$_2$ binds scinderin under resting conditions together with the inhibitory effects of PIP$_2$ on the F-actin severing activity of scinderin, will indicate that activation of the phospholipase C-PIP$_2$ pathway might release scinderin from its binding sites and remove its inhibition by PIP$_2$.

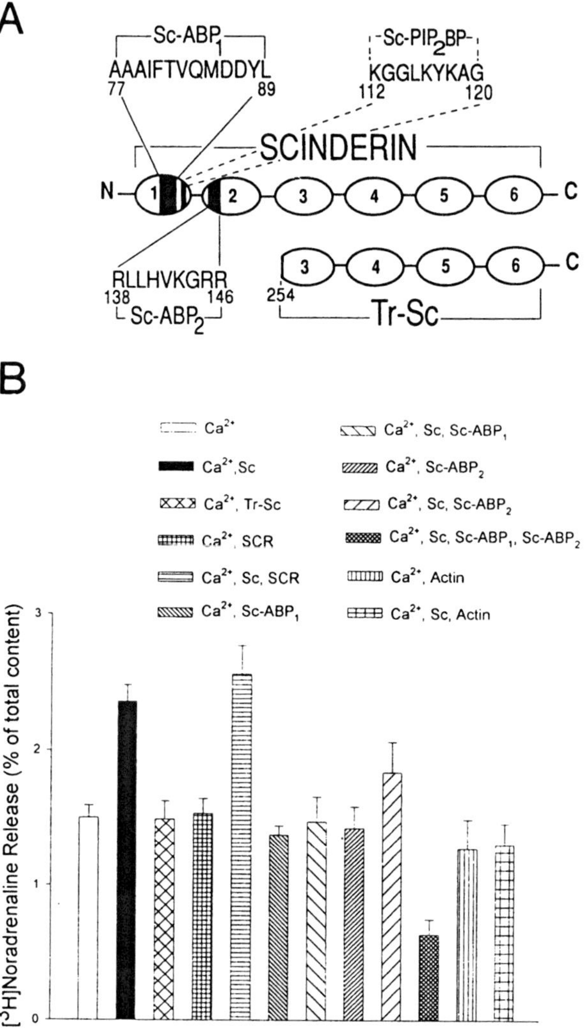

Figure 5. Effect of scinderin-derived actin-binding peptides and of exogenous actin on the potentiation of Ca^{2+}-induced [^{3}H]NA release from permeabilized chromaffin cells by recombinant scinderin. Peptides Sc-ABP$_1$, Sc-ABP$_2$ and Sc-PIP$_2$BP were prepared as described previously (Zhang et al., 1996). The sequence of these peptides and their positions within the domains (S$_1$ to S$_2$) of the scinderin molecule are shown in (A). In addition, an SCR peptide (YAALMFDI-DATQV) to be used as control was also prepared (Zhang et al., 1996). No homology for the SCR sequence was found in the sequences stored in the EMBL data library. Sc-ABP$_1$, Sc-ABP$_2$ and SCR, each at the concentration of 10 mM, were present during both the 5 min digitonin permeabilization and the 2 min stimulation with 10 mM Ca^{2+}. When indicated, 0.1 mM of either recombinant scinderin or recombinant truncated scinderin (Tr-Sc) was also present during permeabilization and stimulation (B). Tr-Sc corresponds to scinderin $_{254-715}$(A). Under the same experimental conditions, the effect of 10 mM chicken gizzard g-actin was also tested (B). The effects of the above mentioned treatments on [^{3}H]NA outputs are shown in (B). Each bar represents the mean ± SEM of at least eight chromaffin cell preparations (Zhang et al. 1996).

General inferences

It is clear that one of the sites of action of Ca^{2+} in secretion is the control of F-actin network dynamics and the interaction of secretory vesicles with the cytoskeleton. The experimental evidence discussed above indicates that the cortical F-actin network constitutes a barrier (negative control or negative clamp) to the movement of secretory vesicles to release sites and it must be locally disassembled to allow translocation of vesicles to the plasma membrane in preparation for exocytosis (Fig.6). This cycle of disassembly and assembly of the cortical actin network controls the number of vesicles present in the release-ready vesicle pool. Disassembly of cortical F-actin is brought about by activation of scinderin, a Ca^{2+}-dependent F-actin severing protein present in secretory tissues (Fig.6). There is a fine regulation of scinderin activity with PIP_2 being one of the most important regulators. Taken together, all of the results discussed above suggest that scinderin and its substrate, the cortical F-actin network are important components of the exocytotic machinery.

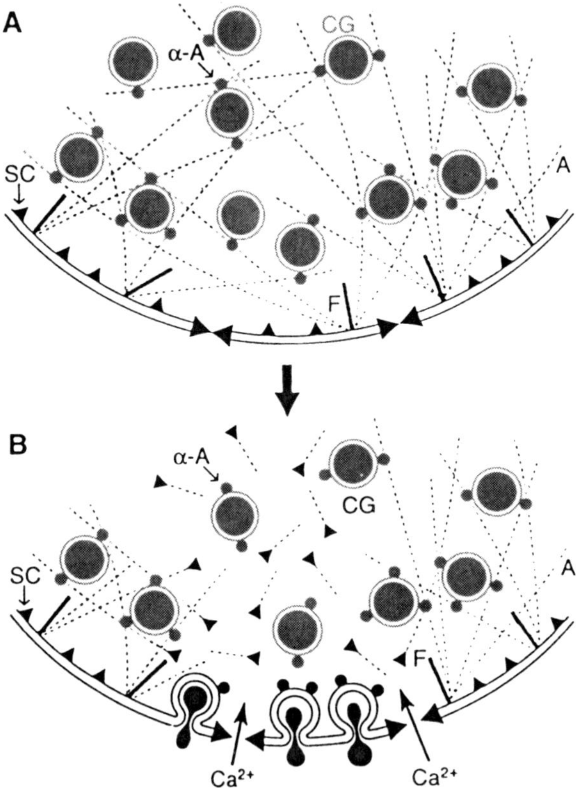

Figure 6. The possible involvement of the cortical actin filament network in secretory vesicle exocytosis from chromaffin cells. (A) In resting cells, cortical actin filaments (A) are anchored to the plasma membrane and to chromaffin granules (CG) through fodrin (F) and a-actinin (a-A). The cortical actin filament network restrains chromaffin granules from interacting with exocytotic sites on the plasma membrane. (B) Cell stimulation induces the influx of Ca^{2+}, which in turn detaches chromaffin granules bound to actin filaments and simultaneously activates scinderin (Sc), a protein that sever actin filaments. This creates subplasmalemmal areas of low viscosity in which chromaffin vesicles are highly mobile; these areas are the exocytotic sites (Trifaró and Vitale, 1993).

Acknowledgements

We are grateful to Ms. S. J. Dunn for typing the manuscript. This work was supported by grants from the Medical Research Council of Canada and the Heart and Stroke Foundation of Ontario.

Plenary discussion

Basbaum A.: What is the relationship of the protein that you have isolated (scinderin) to other synaptic/vesicle proteins, including synapsin, synaptobregin, synaptophysin, synaptotagmin, etc.?

Trifaró J.-M.: The proteins that you have just mentioned are part of the so-called "SNARE COMPLEX." This complex is a part of the fusion machinery and operates on vesicles which are locked to or are very close to the plasma membrane. The scinderin/cortical F-actin network system controls the delivery of secretory vesicles from the reserve compartment into the release-ready vesicle compartment. In other words, scinderin-induced F-actin disassembly precedes vesicle docking and fusion and, therefore, the intervention of the SNARE COMPLEX in the release reaction. Moreover, it should be pointed out, that Ca^{++} seems to have at least two sites of action in neurosecretion: a) the removal of the cortical F-actin barrier as a result of scinderin activation, and b) the removal of the inhibitory effect of synaptotagmin (a negative clamp) on the SNARE component.

Saade N.: Do you think that hypothalamic neurons that secrete hormones or neurons with classical synaptic activity (i.e. neurotransmitter release) can display both types of chemical machinery, i.e. cortical active filaments and snare proteins?

Trifaró J.-M.: The proteins which form the "SNARE COMPLEX" (fusion machinery) are expressed from yeast to man. Therefore, the fusion machinery components have been conserved throughout evolution. Consequently, the answer to your question is: Yes, hypothalamic neurons do contain the different proteins responsible for the operation of the "SNARE COMPLEX."
Regarding the operation of the F-actin microfilament network in neurons, nerve terminals also have an F-actin network which binds synaptic vesicles through synapsin I. Phosphorylation of this protein by calmodulin kinase II regulates this interaction. Moreover, work on isolated synaptosomes has demonstrated that K^{+}-induced depolarization produced, as in chromaffin cells, a Ca^{++} dependent F-actin disassembly. Therefore, dynamic cytoskeletal changes in response to stimulation also seem to operate in nerve terminals.

References

Alvarez de Toledo G, Fernández-Chacón, R and Fernández JM (1993) Release of secretory products during transient vesicle fusion. Nature 363, 554-557.

Bernstein FW and Bamburg JR (1985) Reorganization of actin in depolarized synaptosomes. J Neurosci 5, 2565-2569.

Bittner MA and Holz RW (1992) Kinetic analysis of secretion from permeabilized adrenal chromaffin cells reveals distinct components. J Biol Chem 267, 16219-16225.

Bommert K, Charlton MP, DeBello WM, Chin GJ, Betz H and Augustine GJ (1993) Inhibition of neurotransmitter release by C 2-domain peptides implicates synaptotagmin in exocytosis. Nature 363, 163-165.

Burgoyne RD, Geisow MJ and Barron J (1982) Dissection of stages in exocytosis in the adrenal chromaffin cells with use of trifluoperazine. Proc R Soc Lond (B)216, 111-115.

Burgoyne RD, Morgan A and O'Sullivan AJ (1989) The control of cytoskeeltal actin and exocytosis in intact and permeabilized adrenal chromaffin cells: role of calcium and protein kinase C Cell Signal 1, 323-334.

Cheek TR and Burgoyne RD (1986) Nicotine-evoked disassembly of cortical actin filaments in adrenal chromaffin cells. FEBS Lett 207, 110-114.

Cheek TR and Burgoyne RD (1991) Cytoskeleton in secretion and neurotransmitter release. In: The Neuronal Cytoskeleton (RD Burgoyne ed) Wiley-Liss, pp.309-329.

Douglas WW (1968) Stimulus-secretion coupling: The concept and clues from chromaffin and other cells. Br J Pharmacol 34, 451-474.

Douglas WW and Rubin RP (1961) The role of calcium in the secretory response of the adrenal medulla to acetylcholine. J Physiol 159, 40-57.

Harvey DG and MacIntoch FC (1940) Calcium and synaptic transmission in a sympathetic ganglion. J Physiol 97, 408-418.

Heinemann C, von Rüden L, Chow RH and Neher E (1993) A two-step model of secretion control in neuroendocrine cells. Pflugers Arch-Eur J Physiol 424, 105-112.

Houssay BA and Molinelli EA (1928) Excitabilité des fibres adrénalino-sécrétories du neuf grand splanchnique: fréquences, seuil et optimum des stimulus: rôle de l'ion calcium. CR Seances Soc Biol Ses Fil. 99, 172-174.

Jockush BM, Burger MM, Da Prada M, Richards JG, Chaponnier C and Gabbiani G (1977) a-actinin attaches to membranes of secretory vesicles. Nature 270, 628-629.

Lee RWH and Trifaró J-M (1981) Characterization of anti-actin antibodies and their use in immunocytochemical studies on the localization of actin in adrenal chromaffin cells in culture. Neuroscience 6, 2087-2108.

Marcu GM, Rodríguez Del Castillo A, Vitale ML and Trifaró J-M (1994) Molecular cloning and functional expression of chromaffin cell scinderin indicates that it belongs to the family of Ca^{2+}-dependent F-actin severing proteins. Mol Cell Biochem 141, 153-165.

Marcu GM, Zhang L, Nau-Staudt K and Trifaró J-M (1996) Recombinant scinderin, an F-actin severing protein, increases calcium-induced release of serotonin from permeabilized platelets, an effect blocked by two scinderin-derived actin-binding peptides and phosphatidylinositol 4,5-bisphosphate. Blood 87, 20-24.

Nakata T and Hirokawa N (1992) Organization of cortical cytoskeleton in cultured chromaffin cells and involvement in secretion as revealed by quick-freeze, deep-etching and double-label immunoelectron microscopy. J Neuroscience 12, 2186-2197.

Neher E and Zucker RS (1993) Multiple calcium-dependent processes related to secretion in bovine chromaffin cells. Neuron 10, 21-30.

Parsons TD, Coorssen JR, Horstmann H and Almers W (1995) Docked granules, the exocytotic burst, and the need for ATP hydrolysis in endocrine cells. Neuron 15, 1085-1096.

Popov SV and Poo MM (1993) Synaptotagmin: a calcium-sensitive inhibitor of exocytosis? Cell 73, 1247-1249.

Rodríguez Del Castillo A, Lemaire S, Tchakarov L, Jeyapragasan M, Doucet J-P, Vitale ML and Trifaró J-M (1990) Chromaffin cell scinderin: a novel calcium-dependent actin filament severing protein. EMBO J 9, 43-52.

Rodríguez Del Castillo A, Vitale ML and Trifaró J-M (1992) Ca^{2+} and pH determine the interaction of chromaffin cell scinderin with phosphatidylserine and phosphatidylinositol 4,5-bisphosphate and its cellular distribution during nicotinic-receptor stimulation and protein kinase C activation. J Cell Biol 119, 797-810.

Sudhof TC and Jahn R (1991) Proteins of synaptic vesicles involved in exocytosis and membrane recycling. Neuron 6, 665-677.

Tchakarov L, Vitale ML, Jeyapragasan M, Rodríguez Del Castillo A and Trifaró J-M (1990) Expression of scinderin, an actin filament-severing protein, in different tissues. FEBS Lett 268, 209-212.

Trifaró J-M (1977) Common mechanisms of hormone secretion. Annu Rev Pharmacol Toxicol 17, 27-47.

Trifaró J-M (1982) The cultured chromaffin cell: a model for the study of biology and pharmacology of paraneurons. Trends in Pharmacol Sci 3, 389-392.

Trifaró J-M (1984) The adrenal paraneuron, its biology and pharmacology. Can J Physiol Pharmacol 62, 465-466.

Trifaró J-M (1990) The 1989 Upjohn Award Lecture: cellular and molecular mechanisms in hormone and neurotransmitter secretion. Can J Physiol Pharmacol 68, 1-16.

Trifaró J-M, Bader M-F and Doucet JP (1985) Chromaffin cell cytoskeleton: its possible role in secretion. Can J Biochem Cell Biol 63, 661-679.

Trifaró J-M, Novas ML, Fournier S and Rodríguez Del Castillo A (1989) Cellular and molecular mechanisms in hormone and neurotransmitter secretion. In: Recent Advances in Pharmacology and Therapeutics (M Velasco, A Israel, E Romero and H Silva eds) Elsevier Science Publishers pp.15-20.

Trifaró J-M and Poisner AM (1982) Common properties in the mechanisms of synthesis, processing and storage of secretory products. In: The Secretory Process. (AM Poisner and J-M Trifaró eds) Vol.I The Secretory Granule Elsevier/North Holland pp.387-407

Trifaró J-M and Vitale ML (1993) Cytoskeleton dynamics during neurotransmitter release. Trends Neurosci 16, 466-472.

Vitale ML, Rodríguez Del Castillo A, Tchakarov L and Trifaró J-M (1991) Cortical filamentous actin disassembly and scinderin redistribution during chromaffin cell stimulation precede exocytosis, a phenomenon not exhibited by gelsolin. J Cell Biol 113, 1057-1067.

Vitale ML, Rodríguez Del Castillo A and Trifaró J-M (1992) Protein kinase C activation by phorbol esters induces chromaffin cell cortical filamentous actin disassembly and increases the initial rate of exocytosis in response to nicotinic receptor stimulation. Neuroscience 51, 463-474.

Vitale ML, Seward EP and Trifaró J-M (1995) Chromaffin cell cortical actin network dynamics control the size of the release-ready vesicle pool and the initial rate of exocytosis. Neuron 14, 353-363.

Zhang L, Marcu MG, Nau-Staudt K and Trifaró J-M (1996) Recombinant scinderin enhances exocytosis, an effect blocked by two scinderin-derived actin-binding peptides and PIP_2. Neuron 17, 287-296.

Peripheral and Spinal Cord Physiology

Pain Mechanisms and Management
S.N. Ayrapetyan and A.V. Apkarian (Eds.)
IOS Press, 1998

Nociceptive Pain Mechanisms and Chronification

Peter W. Reeh

*Dept. Physiology and Exp. Pathophysiology, University Erlangen-Nuremberg
Erlangen, Germany*

Chronic pain is rarely a condition of permanent ongoing pain, but rather a problem of hyperalgesia that causes ordinary loads of daily life to become painful stimuli. Hyperalgesia may build up within minutes and last for years. Apart from tuberculosis, most inflammatory diseases are associated with hyperalgesia, and this includes post-injury conditions and many malignant tumors.

The animal models of inflammation used for electrical recording from primary afferent nerve fibers differ in rather fundamental respects but, nonetheless, provide corresponding evidence that "inflamed" nociceptors abnormally exhibit ongoing activity and hypersensitivity to adequate stimulation.

The acute pain from mechanical and thermal injury can be explained by the inherent mechano- and thermo-sensitivity of nociceptors, but as soon as the pain outlasts the sheer presence of noxious forces and temperatures, the chemosensitivity comes into play. This capacity is generally accepted to be the basis for inflammatory alterations in nociception. Thus, the question arises which chemical mediator(s) cause(s) the ongoing activity and hypersensitivities of nociceptors. Which chemicals mimic the sensory effects of inflammation?

Mechanical sensitization of nociceptors

With respect to mechanical sensitization, as a cause of hyperalgesia, no simple answer can be expected, since not all classes of nociceptors and not all models of inflammation show this phenomenon on primary afferent level. It appears that the more complex--the less reductionist--an experimental model, the more different endogenous chemicals are reported to induce signs of mechanical hyperalgesia. The widely used withdrawal test to paw pressure in the rat supplies with a long, probably incomplete list of substances: bradykinin (BK), serotonin (5HT), prostaglandins, leukotriens, norepinephrin, adenosin, neurokinin A, substance P, interleukin 1b, 6, 8, tumor necrosis factor a, cyclic AMP and nerve growth factor (Davis and Perkins, 1994; Taiwo and Levine, 1992; Taiwo and Levine, 1990; Levine et al. 1986; Nakamura-Craig and Gill, 1991; Ferreira et al. 1988; Ferreira et al. 1993; Ferreira et al. 1993; Taiwo et al. 1989; Lewin et al. 1993).

All these agents are reported to rapidly reduce the withdrawal threshold, but do they all act directly on nociceptors to sensitize them against mechanical forces? Single-fiber recording studies in animals partly seem to answer in the affirmative, when chemicals were injected into the skin or into the blood stream supplying joints. So, prostaglandin E2 (PGE2) and other eicosanoids were reported to have enhancing effects on mechanosensitivity of rat cutaneous nociceptors (Pateromichelakis and Rood, 1981; Pateromichelakis and Rood, 1982; Martin et al. 1987; White et al. 1991; Wang et al. 1996). A more complete "soup" of inflammatory mediators, containing BK, 5HT, PGE and histamine (HA), was shown to lower von Frey-thresholds in monkey skin and to "awaken" part of the silent nociceptors (Davis et al. 1993; Kress et al. 1992). In joints, finally, BK was reported to enhance responsiveness to movement or indentation, and PGE2 to facilitate this BK effect (Neugebauer et al. 1989; Schaible and Schmidt, 1988; Grubb et al. 1991).

The list of substances inducing signs of mechanical hyperalgesia has become much shorter in the electrophysiological models above, but still the chemicals were injected into the complexity of living tissues with all the possibilities of secondary actions through blood- or tissue-borne mediators and cells. Indeed, many of the inflammatory mediators are chemoattractant to leukocytes, activate platelets, degranulate mast cells, induce vasodilatation and plasma extravasation. The mere edema, resulting from vascular leakage, has major impact on the biomechanical transmission properties of the tissue and can rapidly lower mechanical thresholds of particular nociceptors (Cooper et al. 1991; Cooper, 1993). A further example are activated platelets, which excite (and sensitize to heat) a large proportion of cutaneous nociceptors, in vitro, and induce pain and delayed mechanical hyperalgesia when injected into human skin (Ringkamp et al. 1994; Osiander et al. 1996; Blunk et al. 1996; Schmelz et al. 1997). Thus, the mediators may act "hyperalgesic" by inducing rather than by mimicking inflammation. This hypothesis would agree with the experimental observation that injection of large BK and PGE2 doses only resulted in behavioral hyperalgesia, if applied into the dense and highly vascularized subepidermal layer of the skin--no effect if injected into the loose subcutaneous tissue (Khasar et al. 1993).

Isolated tissues, kept viable in an organ bath, have lost most of the possibilities for secondary actions, and extracellular concentrations of chemicals can well be controlled and kept constant by superfusion (Kumazawa et al. 1987; Reeh, 1986; Cervero and Sann, 1989; Adelson et al. 1996). Under these conditions, only one agent from the above list of substances, cyclic AMP, has yet been shown to lower the von Frey threshold of the most abundant, i.e. polymodal nociceptor type (Kress et al. 1996). The effect was significant but not dramatic, and a millimolar concentration of cAMP-analog was needed. Thus, it can only be taken as indication for further work although behavioral results support the findings (Taiwo et al. 1989). A physiological increase of cAMP in the nerve terminal could result from an action of PGE2 which, however, had in vitro definitely no influence on the mechanical threshold in skin, even when combined with other mediators such as BK, 5HT and HIS (Kessler et al. 1992). These statements are based on exposure of noci-receptive fields for up to half an hour. Mediator-induced mechanical hyperalgesia in humans, however, may take much longer to develop: Ferreira performed a continuous infusion for thirty minutes of an "inflammatory soup" (BK + HIS + PGE1) into the skin, causing sustained pain and erythema, and he noticed occurrence of pressure hyperalgesia two hours later (Ferreira, 1972). Again, this may mean that inflammation was induced rather than mimicked, but even so, the time domain in question has not yet been explored in electrophysiological experiments.

Sensitization to heat and ongoing discharge

The difficulties in identifying a chemical principle mediating mechanical sensitization do not apply to nociceptor sensitization to heat. In vitro, bradykinin rapidly induced prominent heat sensitization in concentrations much lower than those needed to excite nociceptors (Kumazawa et al. 1991; Koltzenburg et al. 1992). This finding is in accord with reflex studies and with human psychophysics (Rueff and Dray, 1993; Manning et al. 1991). The interaction between heat and bradykinin sensitivity was mutual: conditioning heat stimuli enhanced bradykinin responsiveness of nociceptors and vice versa (Lang et al. 1990). This built up a large sensitizing effect which lowered the heat thresholds as far as the range of body temperatures (Koltzenburg et al. 1992). This may relate to the ongoing discharge found in all models of inflammation, and it may explain the reliable antinociceptive effect of cooling the inflamed tissue (Reeh et al. 1986; Steen and Reeh, 1993). The other classical mediators of inflammation, 5HT, HIS and PGE2 are unable to induce nociceptor sensitization to heat at pathophysiologically relevant concentrations, if at all (Mizumura et al. 1994; Mizumura et al. 1993; Rueff and Dray, 1992). They may, however, facilitate the heat-sensitizing action of bradykinin, a synergism which has not yet been investigated.

Bradykinin can also excite nociceptors directly, and 5HT and PGE2 can facilitate this action (Mizumura et al. 1987; Lang et al. 1990). However, at normal peripheral temperatures and at pathophysiologically relevant mediator concentrations, the induced nociceptor discharge fades away during minutes, due to tachyphylaxis (Handwerker and Reeh, 1991). Thus, the mediators alone cannot account for the "chronic" ongoing discharge of "inflamed" nociceptors.

It lies in the nature of nociceptors to maintain discharge activity upon sustained noxious mechanical and heat stimulation (Handwerker et al. 1987; Treede, 1995). However, only one abnormal chemical condition, low extracellular pH, is known to provide sustained excitatory drive to nociceptors and to cause pain that lasts as long as experimental tissue acidosis is maintained (Steen et al. 1992; Issberner et al. 1996). This condition is regularly found in inflamed tissues and in muscles working under ischemia. In both cases, it is the relative imbalance between increased blood flow and even more increased cellular metabolism that leads to lactic acid accumulation (Reeh and Steen, 1996; Abbot et al. 1994; Harrison et al. 1986) Pathophysiologically relevant tissue pH levels alone are sufficient to maintain nociceptor discharge; however, bradykinin and even more "inflammatory soup" can considerably enhance number and activity of nociceptors driven, and, thereby, also the pain from tissue acidosis (Steen et al. 1995; Steen et al. 1996). This sensitizing effect also shows up in a putative cellular model of nociception, the capsaicin-sensitive sensory ganglion cell in culture where bradykinin and the other mediators had no excitatory effect, in our hands, but facilitated a depolarizing inward current evoked by low pH stimulation. BK alone was sufficient in this model, but in combination with the other mediators (5HT, HIS, PGE2) it potentiated the sensitizing effect (Kress and Reeh, 1996).

By speculation, inflammatory sensitization to heat and to low pH can be put together into a daily-life scenario: Inflamed tissue may be free of pain as long as it is allowed to rest; as soon as it is forced to work, temperature and proton concentration increase and pain may result due to latent sensitization of nociceptors induced by inflammatory mediators. This could be taken as a temporary conclusion, but one problem remains to be discussed: If the excitatory effect of bradykinin underlies tachyphylaxis, would not the sensitization also be expected to decline and vanish upon repeated or prolonged exposure of the nerve endings to bradykinin? This was actually the case with the heat sensitization provoked by high PGE2 concentrations which showed prominent tachyphylaxis (Mizumura et al. 1993).

The above question has recently been scrutinized for the bradykinin-induced sensitization to heat, which turned out to be maintained at full magnitude for as long as bradykinin was present, while the excitatory effect faded away within minutes (Haake et al. 1996). The same study excluded the possibility that the sensitizing and the excitatory effect of bradykinin were mediated by different BK receptors: If present, both effects were blocked by a bradykinin antagonist (HOE140) specific for the B2 receptor subtype. However, sensitization by bradykinin was much more widespread among C-fiber nociceptors than excitation; even purely mechano-sensitive units transiently delivered proper heat responses after bradykinin treatment. Altogether about 85% of all the C-fibers tested showed BK-induced sensitization to heat, and here, among the units sensitized, but not excited, a role for the B1 receptor subtype could be fixed. In about half of these cases, sensitization could be prevented with a B1 receptor antagonist, while the other half still was sensitive to HOE140 (Haake et al. 1996). It is intriguing that, in the case of the B2 receptor subtype, one and the same transduction pathway seems to activate a tachyphylactic, excitatory process and, at the same time, a non-tachyphylactic sensitizing mechanism.

Synapsis and therapeutic consequences

The principle of sustained sensitization seems to apply to heat as well as to proton responsiveness of nociceptors (Steen et al. 1995). Thus, the above scenario may have a realistic core. In the light of this speculation, chronicity is a matter of permanent nociceptor sensitization due to permanent presence of synergistic inflammatory mediators. Remedy could be to fight the inflammation, since the sensitization does not survive, but for minutes, when the mediators are removed (Koltzenburg et al. 1992).

Interestingly, the same non-stereoidal anti-inflammatory drugs (NSAID), that are employed to fight the inflammation, seem to have a rather appreciable and specific "side effect" in reducing pH-induced nociceptor discharge and pain (Stefanidis et al. 1997; Steen et al. 1995). This effect needs local drug concentrations achievable by transcutaneous as well as oral administrations (Steen et al. 1996, and unpublished results).

To attack nociceptor sensitization more specifically, further research into its detailed mechanisms is needed. The network of mutual interactions of mediators needs to be clarified, and the intracellular transduction pathways as well as their cross-talk ought to be revealed. Previous work has focused on the excitatory actions of the inflammatory mediators, which possibly are an epiphenomenon of experimentally high doses or concentrations not even reached in pathophysiological conditions (Handwerker and Reeh, 1991). Induction of sensitization, which occurs at much lower concentrations (Mizumura et al. 1991), and of hyperalgesia may be the true sensory function of the inflammatory mediators. Thereby, metabolic and physical strains become noxious stress and a source of pain. Chronicity, in this concept, is a matter of the primary, mostly inflammatory disease rather than of the nociceptors which are victims as well as actors in the process.

Plenary discussion

Wall P.: What is the standing of bradykinin antagonists?

Reeh W.: B_2 bradykinin receptors and, to a minor extent, B_1 receptors are involved in bradykinin mediated nociceptor sensitization to heat. Behavioral evidence (Perkins et al.) suggests an increased implementation of B_1 receptors during more chronic inflammatory processes. This results in an increased anti-hyperalgesic effect of B_1 antagonists, while B_2 antagonists are more effective in acute inflammatory models.

References

Abbot NC, Beck JS, Carnochan FM, Gibbs JH, Harrison DK, James PB & Lowe JG (1994) Effect of hyperoxia at 1 and 2 ATA on hypoxia and hypercapnia in human skin during experimental inflammation. J Appl Physiol; 77: 767-773.

Adelson DW, Wei JY & Kruger L (1996) H2O2 sensitivity of afferent splanchnic C fiber units in vitro. J Neurophysiol; 76: 371-380.

Blunk J, Schmelz M, Osiander G, Ringkamp M & Reeh PW (1996) Intradermally injected human plateteles induce hyperalgesia. Pflügers Archiv – Europ J Physiol; 431: P-52

Cervero F & Sann H (1989) Mechanically evoked responses of afferent fibres innervating the guinea-pig's ureter: an in vitro study. J Physiol Lond; 412: 245-266.

Cooper B (1993) Contribution of edema to the sensitization of high-threshold mechanoreceptors of the goat palatal mucosa. J Neurophysiol; 70: 512-521.

Cooper B, Ahlquist M, Friedman RM & Labanc J (1991) Properties of high-threshold mechanoreceptors in the goat oral mucosa. II. Dynamic and static reactivity in carrageenan-inflamed mucosa. J Neurophysiol; 66: 1280-1290.

Davis KD, Meyer RA & Campbell JN (1993) Chemosensitivity and sensitization of nociceptive afferents that innervate the hairy skin of monkey. J Neurophysiol; 69: 1071-1081.

Ferreira SH (1972) Prostaglandins, aspirin-like drugs and analgesia. Nature - New Biol; 240: 200-203.

Ferreira SH, Lorenzetti BB, Bristow AF & Poole S (1988) Interleukin-1b as a potent hyperalgesic agent antagonized by tripeptide analogue. Nature; 334: 698-700.

Ferreira SH, Lorenzetti BB, Cunha FQ & Poole S (1993) Bradykinin release of TNF-alpha plays a key role in the development of inflammatory hyperalgesia. Agents Actions; 38: C7-9.

Ferreira SH, Lorenzetti BB & Poole S (1993) Bradykinin initiates cytokine-mediated inflammatory hyperalgesia. Br J Pharmacol; 110: 1227-1231.

Grubb BD, Birrell GJ, McQueen DS & Iggo A (1991) The role of PGE2 in the sensitization of mechanoreceptors in normal and inflamed ankle joints of the rat. Exp Brain Res; 84: 383-392.

Haake B, Liang Y-F & Reeh PW (1996) Bradykinin effects and receptor subtypes in rat cutaneous nociceptors, in vitro. Pflügers Archiv - Europ J Physiol; 431: O-26

Handwerker HO, Anton F & Reeh PW (1987) Discharge patterns of afferent cutaneous nerve fibers from the rat's tail during prolonged noxious mechanical stimulation. Exp Brain Res; 65: 493-504.

Handwerker HO, Kilo S & Reeh PW (1991) Unresponsive afferent nerve-fibers in the sural nerve of the rat. J Physiol Lond; 435: 229-242.

Handwerker, HO and Reeh, PW (1991) Pain and Inflammation. In: Proceedings of the Vth World Congress of Pain. (Bond MR, Charlton JE, and Woolf CJ eds.) Elsevier Science Publishers BV, Amsterdam, pp. 59-69.

Harrison DK, Spence VA, Beck JS, Lowe JG & Walker WF (1986) pH changes in the dermis during the course of the tuberculin skin test. Immunol; 59: 497-501.

Issberner U, Reeh PW & Steen KH (1996) Pain due tissue acidosis: a mechanism for inflammatory and ischemic myalgia? Neurosci Lett; 208: 191-194.

Kessler W, Kirchhoff C, Reeh PW & Handwerker HO (1992) Excitation of cutaneous afferent nerve-endings in vitro by a combination of inflammatory mediators and conditioning effect of substance-P. Exp Brain Res; 91: 467-476.

Khasar SG, Green PG & Levine JD (1993) Comparison of intradermal and subcutaneous hyperalgesic effects of inflammatory mediators in the rat. Neurosci Lett; 153: 215-218.

Koltzenburg M, Kress M & Reeh PW (1992) The nociceptor sensitization by bradykinin does not depend on sympathetic neurons. Neurosci; 46: 465-473.

Kress M, Koltzenburg M, Reeh PW & Handwerker HO (1992) Responsiveness and functional attributes of electrically localized terminals of cutaneous C-fibers in vivo and in vitro. J Neurophysiol; 68: 581-595.

Kress M. and Reeh, PW (1996) Chemical excitation and sensitization in nociceptors. In: Neurobiology of Nociceptors (Belmonte C and Cervero F eds). Oxford University Press, Oxford, pp. 258-297.

Kress M, Rödl J & Reeh PW (1996) Stable analogs of cyclic AMP but not cyclic GMP sensitze unmyelinated primary afferents in the rat skin to mechanical and heat stimuli but not to inflammatory mediators, in vitro. Neurosci; 74: 609-617.

Kumazawa T, Mizumura K, Minagawa M & Tsujii Y (1991) Sensitizing effects of bradykinin on the heat response of visceral nociceptors. J Neurophysiol; 1819-1824.

Kumazawa T, Mizumura K & Sato J (1987) Response properties of polymodal receptors studied using in vitro testis superior spermatic nerve preparation of dogs. J Neurophysiol; 57: 702-711.

Lang E, Novak A, Reeh PW & Handwerker HO (1990) Chemosensitivity of fine afferents from rat skin in vitro. J Neurophysiol; 63: 887-901.

Levine JD, Taiwo YO, Collins SD & Tam JK (1986) Noradrenaline hyperalgesiais mediated through interaction with sympathetic postganglionic neurone terminals rather than activation of primary afferent nociceptors. Nature; 323: 158-160.

Lewin GR, Ritter AM & Mendell LM (1993) Nerve Growth Factor – induced hyperalgesia in the neonatal and adult rat. J Neurosci; 13: 2136-2148.

Manning DC, Raja SN, Meyer RA & Campbell JN (1991) Pain and hyperalgesia after intradermal injection of bradykinin in humans. Clin Pharmacol & Therap; 50: 721-729.

Martin HA, Basbaum AI, Kwiat GC, Goetzl EJ & Levine JD (1987) Leukotriene and prostaglandin sensitization of cutaneous high-threshold C- and A-delta mechanonociceptors in the hairy skin of rat hindlimbs. Neurosci; 22: 651-659.

Mizumura K, Minagawa M, Koda H & Kumazawa T (1994) Histamine-Induced sensitization of the heat response of canine visceral polymodal receptors. Neurosci Lett; 168: 93-96.

Mizumura K, Minagawa M, Sato J, Tsujii Y and Kumazawa T (1991) Differences in augmenting effects of various sensitizing agents on heat and bradykinin responses of the testicular polymodal nociceptors. In: Proceedings of the VIth World Congress on Pain (Bond MR, Charlton JE and Woolf CJ eds.), Pain Research and Clin Management, Vol.4, Elsevier Science Publisher, pp. 77-82.

Mizumura K, Minagawa M, Tsujii Y & Kumazawa T (1993) Prostaglandin E2-induced sensitization of the heat response of canine visceral polymodal receptors in vitro. Neurosci Lett; 161: 117-119.

Mizumura K, Sato J & Kumazawa T (1987) Effects of prostaglandins and other putative chemical intermediaries on the activity of canine testicular polymodal receptors studied in vitro. Pflügers Archiv Europ – J Physiol; 408: 565-572.

Nakamura-Craig M & Gill BK (1991) Effect of neurokinin-A, substance-P and calcitonin gene related peptide in peripheral hyperalgesia in the rat paw. Neurosci Lett; 124: 49-51.

Neugebauer V, Schaible H-G & Schmidt RF (1989) Sensitization of articular afferents to mechanical stimuli by bradykinin. Pflügers Archiv – Europ J Physiol; 415: 330-335.

Osiander G, Schmelz M, Blunk J, Ringkamp M & Reeh PW (1996) Intradermally injected human platelets induce acute pain and flare. Pflügers Archive - Europ J Physiol; 431: P-51

Pateromichelakis S & Rood JP (1982) Prostaglandin E1-induced sensitization of A delta moderate pressure mechanoreceptors. Brain Res; 232: 89-96.

Reeh PW, Kocher L & Jung S (1986) Does neurogenic inflammation alter the sensitivity of unmyelinated nociceptors in the rat? Brain Res; 384: 42-50.

Reeh PW and Steen KH (1996) Tissue acidosis in nociception and pain. In: The polymodal Nociceptor (Kumazawa T, Kruger L and Mizumura K eds.). Elsevier Science, Amsterdam, pp. 143-151.

Ringkamp M, Schmelz M, Kress M, Allwang M, Ogilvie A & Reeh PW (1994) Activated human platelets in plasma excite nociceptors in rat skin, in vitro. Neurosci Lett; 170: 103-106.

Rueff A & Dray A (1992) 5-Hydroxytryptamine-induced sensitization and activation of peripheral fibres in the neonatal rat are mediated via different 5- hydroxytryptamine-receptors. Neurosci; 50: 899-905.

Rueff A & Dray A (1993) Sensitization of peripheral afferent-fibers in the invitro neonatal rat spinal-cord tail by bradykinin and prostaglandins. Neurosci; 54: 527-535.

Schaible H-G & Schmidt RF (1988) Time course of mechanosensitivity changes in articular afferents during a developing experimental arthritis. J Neurophysiol; 60: 2180-2195.

Schmelz M, Osiander G, Blunk J, Ringkamp M, Reeh PW, Handwerker HO (1997) Intradermal injections of human platelets cause acute pain and protracted hyperalgesia. Neurosci. Lett: in press.

Steen KH, Reeh PW & Kreysel HW (1995) Topical acetylsalicylic, salicylic acid and indomethacin suppress pain from experimental tissue acidosis in human skin. Pain; 62: 339-347.

Steen KH, Steen AE, Kreysel HW & Reeh PW (1996) Inflammatory mediators potentiate pain induced by experimental acidosis. Pain; 66: 163-170.

Steen KH & Reeh PW (1993) Sustained graded pain and hyperalgesia from harmless experimental tissue acidosis in human skin. Neurosci Lett; 154: 113-116.

Steen KH, Reeh PW, Anton F & Handwerker HO (1992) Protons selectively induce lasting excitation and sensitization to mechanical stimulation of nociceptors in the rat skin, in vitro. J Neurosci; 12: 86-95.

Steen KH, Reeh PW & Kreysel HW (1996) Dose-dependent competitive block by topical acetylsalicylic and salicylic acid of low pH-induced cutaneous pain. Pain; 64: 71-82.

Steen KH, Steen AE & Reeh PW (1995) A Domiant Role of Acid pH in Inflammatory Excitation and Sensitization of Nociceptors in Rat Skin, in vitro. J Neurosci; 15: 3982-3989.

Stefanidis D, Reeh PW, Kreysel HW & Steen KH (1997) Acetysalicylic acid and salicylic acid suppress pH-induced excitation of rat nociceptors. Prim Sens Neuron; (in press)

Taiwo YO, Bjerknes LK, Goetzl EJ & Levine JD (1989) Mediation of primary afferent peripheral hyperalgesia by the cAMP second messenger system. Neurosci; 32: 577-580.

Taiwo YO & Levine JD (1990) Effects of cyclooxygenase products of arachidonic acid metabolism on cutaneous nociceptive threshold in the rat. Brain Res; 537: 372-374.

Taiwo YO & Levine JD (1992) Serotonin is a directly acting hyperalgesic agent in the rat. Neurosci; 48: 485-490.

Thalhammer JG & LaMotte RH (1982) Spatial properties of nociceptor sensitization following heat injury of the skin. Brain Res; 231: 257-265.

Treede R-D (1995) Peripheral acute pain mechanisms. Ann Med; 27: 213-216.

Wang JF, Khasar SG, Ahlgren SC & Levine JD (1996) Sensitization of C-fibers by prostaglandin E2 in the rat is inhibited by guanosine 5'-O-(2-thiodiphophate), 2'.5'-dideoxyadenosine and Walsh inhibitor peptide. Neurosci; 71: 259-263.

White DM, Taiwo YO, Coderre TJ & Levine JD (1991) Delayed activation of nociceptors--correlation with delayed pain sensations induced by sustained stimuli. J Neurophysiol; 66: 729-734.

The Spinal Rat: A Model System for Studying the Behavioral Pharmacology of Spinal Nociceptive Reflexes

C. Advokat

Department of Psychology, Louisiana State University
Baton Rouge, LA, USA

Present views of how opiate drugs act in the central nervous system to produce analgesia originated with the groundbreaking research of Wikler and colleagues nearly 50 years ago. Their investigations showed that systemically administered morphine could suppress spinal, nociceptive, reflexes in animals that had sustained a complete spinal transection. This meant that morphine could produce analgesia by acting directly on the spinal cord. Specifically, the opiate suppressed polysynaptic responses (the flexor and crossed extensor reflexes) whereas monosynaptic pathways, i.e. the knee jerk, were unaffected by moderate analgesic doses (Wikler, 1950).

However, although systemic morphine can suppress nociceptive reflexes in spinalized animals, the doses required are greater than the doses needed to produce the same effect in intact animals. This has been shown numerous times, in studies using the thermally elicited tail-withdrawal (tail flick, TF) response of the rat or mouse (Berge and Hole, 1981, Dewey at al, 1969, Irwin et al, 1951, Wood at al, 1981). In our own replication of this classic observation, we found that the dose of subcutaneously administered morphine needed to produce a half-maximal inhibition of the TF response was 2 to 3 times greater in rats tested one day after spinalization, relative to intact rats (2.5 to 4.5 mg/kg vs 1.5 mg/kg; Advokat and Burton, 1987, Advokat and Gulati, 1991).

This decrease in the effect of systemic morphine in spinal rats led to the most prominent hypothesis of opiate analgesia (Fields and Basbaum, 1978). This model proposes that systemically administered morphine produces analgesia at the spinal level by both a direct and indirect mechanism. The direct effect is exerted either pre-and/or postsynaptically at the primary afferent synapse. The indirect effect is mediated supraspinally, through descending pathways which are known to inhibit spinal nociceptive reflexes. Exogenous opiates are proposed to activate this supraspinal system and increase the inhibitory input onto intrinsic spinal pain circuits. The decreased potency of systemic morphine in the spinal animal would be due to the fact that the contribution of this descending input is lost, leaving only the direct spinal antinociceptive effect of the opiate.

Although it provides a reasonable interpretation of the data, this hypothesis does not attempt to quantify the respective spinal and supraspinal contributions to morphine-induced analgesia. This question was subsequently addressed in an elegant series of studies by Yeung and Rudy (1980) in which they determined the relationship between the brain and spinal cord in the production of opiate analgesia. They accomplished this by systematically injecting different dose ratios of morphine simultaneously, onto the spinal cord (intrathecally, i.t.) and into the 3rd cerebral ventricle of rats, and testing the analgesic effect on the tail flick and hot plate assays. The results showed that this manipulation produced a multiplicative analgesic effect, which was maximal when equivalent doses of morphine were injected at each site (1:1 ratio). The total amount required to produce an ED_{50} was only 0.35 µg at each site, whereas the comparable values for the separate intracerebroventricular and intrathecal sites were 10.0 and 4.2 µg, respectively. It was proposed that this synergistic effect was responsible for the analgesia observed following systemic morphine administration.

We have replicated the multiplicative effect of spinal and supraspinal morphine-induced analgesia, with the modification that supraspinal injections were made into the periaqueductal gray (PAG) rather than the third ventricle (Siuciak and Advokat, 1989b). Our results are shown in Fig. 1. On the left are three dose-response functions, representing the analgesic effect of morphine on the TF reflex of intact rats. The data are plotted as the difference in latency, between the predrug baseline and the postdrug response, of the tail withdrawal reflex from a high intensity thermal stimulus. Each symbol indicates the average change in withdrawal latency of a separate group of rats. A cut-off limit of 14 sec was imposed as the maximum possible analgesic score. The results of the i.t. injections are indicated by triangles, PAG injections by squares and concurrent injections into both sites by circles. (When morphine was administered to only one site, the saline vehicle was concurrently injected into the alternate locus). It is evident that the simultaneous injections produced a much greater analgesic effect than administration at either site alone. The ED_{50} values for the PAG and spinal cord alone were 2.8 and 6.7 µg, respectively, whereas the ED_{50} for the combination was 0.196 µg, i.e. approximately 0.400 µg total.

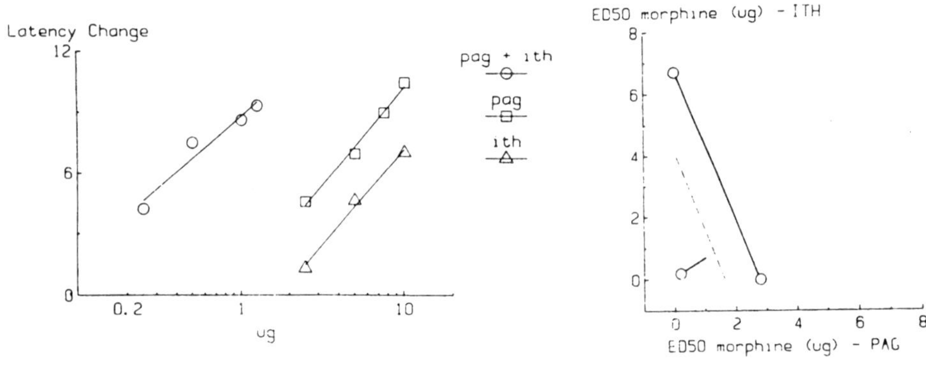

Figure 1. Synergistic effect of concurrent morphine injections into the periaqueductal gray (pag) and intrathecal space (ith) of rats. On the left side of the figure are three dose-response functions, summarizing the analgesic effect, on the tail flick, of morphine injected ith (open triangles), into the pag (open squares) or concurrently, to both sites, in a 1:1 dose ratio (open circles). On the right side is an isobolographic representation of the same data, showing the ED_{50} values for morphine administration into the pag (abscissa), the ith space (ordinate), and concurrently (lower left). The straight line indicates the theoretical ED_{50} values that would be observed if the effect at the two central sites were additive. The dashed line connects the 95% confidence limits of the ED_{50} values for the pag and ith dose-response lines. The figure shows that the 95% confidence limit of the ED_{50} value obtained after concurrent morphine injections into both sites does not cross the line connecting the 95% confidence limits of the ED_{50} values for the two separate lines. This demonstrates that the concurrent injections produced a multiplicative effect.

Although it is clear that concurrent injections potentiated the analgesic response, it cannot be determined from these data alone if they produced a synergistic or additive effect. To make that determination the data were replotted in an isobolographic format, shown on the right side of the figure. In this graph, the ED_{50} values for morphine administered to the PAG and the spinal cord are plotted on the abscissa and ordinate, respectively. The straight line connecting the spinal and supraspinal values designates the ED_{50} values that would theoretically indicate an additive interaction between the two sites. Points which lie below the line indicate a supra-additive or synergistic relationship, while points falling above the line represent an infra-additive or antagonistic interaction. The dashed line connects the 95% confidence limits of the ED_{50} values obtained from each of the two separate sites. The corresponding ED_{50} value and 95 % confidence limit for the concurrent injections clearly lies below the additive line, indicating that a multiplicative interaction was obtained.

The phenomenon of opiate analgesic synergy provides behavioral evidence that both spinal and supraspinal actions are involved in mediating analgesia following systemic morphine administration, but it does not indicate the nature of that interaction. However, subsequent results from our laboratory led us to consider one possible hypothesis. In these experiments, we compared spinal opiate antinociception in intact and spinal rats, produced by intrathecal, rather than peripheral administration (Siuciak and Advokat, 1989a). We reasoned that the effect of intrathecal morphine might not be altered by spinal transection. That is, in both intact and spinal rats, the local effect of morphine on the spinal cord would not be accompanied by a corresponding influence of the drug at supraspinal sites. Therefore, the effect of intrathecal morphine in spinal animals should not differ from that seen in intact rats.

However, the results did not support this prediction. These data are presented in Fig. 2, which shows dose-response functions for i.t. morphine on the TF test, of intact rats (open circles) and acute spinal rats, tested one day after spinal transection (filled circles). Analysis of the regression lines indicated an ED_{50} of 5.9 (g (95% confidence limits, 3.8-9.1 (g) and 0.125 (g (95% confidence limits 0.109-0.145 (g), respectively. These data show that the effect of intrathecal morphine is significantly enhanced one day after spinal transection. Furthermore, these results, from acutely spinalized rats, were remarkably similar to the values obtained when morphine was concurrently administered to the PAG (or cerebral ventricle) and the spinal cord of intact rats. The implication was that spinal transection and intracerebral morphine injections could act in the same manner, to reduce a descending inhibitory influence that is normally exerted on spinal opiate activity.

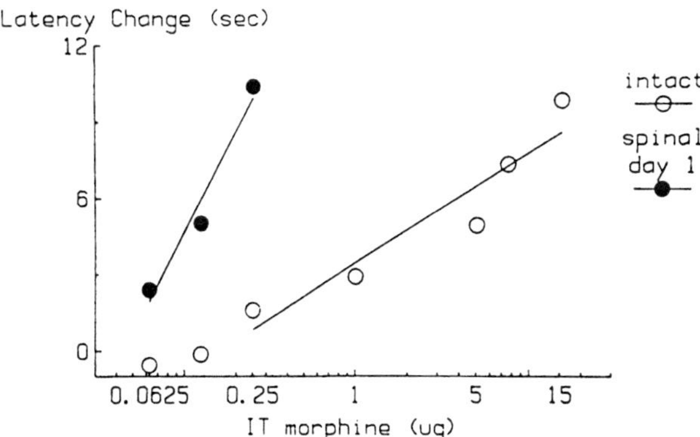

Figure 2. Dose-response functions, on the tail flick test, to intrathecal morphine in intact rats (open circles) and rats that were spinally transected one day previously (filled circles).

A schematic representation of this hypothesis is depicted in Fig. 3 (Advokat, 1988). This diagram represents a simplified version of the generally accepted view of spinal nociceptive processing. Nociceptive input, produced by painful stimulation, enters the dorsal horn of the spinal cord, and is transmitted via the primary afferent synapse (Advokat and Gulati, 1991) to the brain (Advokat, 1988) and, via interneurons, to nociceptive reflex pathways (Advokat et al, 1996). Descending supraspinal pathways (Advokat and Burton, 1987) exert tonic inhibitory control over spinal nociceptive input. The potency of morphine at each site is indicated by the size of the number representing that site. In Part A of the figure, the direct effect of morphine on the spinal cord (indicated by the filled neuron symbols) is tonically suppressed by inhibitory descending pathways. Intrathecal morphine administration is more effective in spinal rats (Part B) because descending pathways are interrupted. When morphine is simultaneously administered into the brain and onto the spinal cord (Part C), the opiate acts in the brain to reduce the magnitude of the descending inhibition exerted on its action at the spinal level. As a result, the analgesic effect of spinal morphine is enhanced. This hypothesis can account for the increased potency of i.t. morphine in acute spinal rats, the phenomenon of opiate synergy in intact rats and, by inference, the analgesic effect of systemic morphine administration.

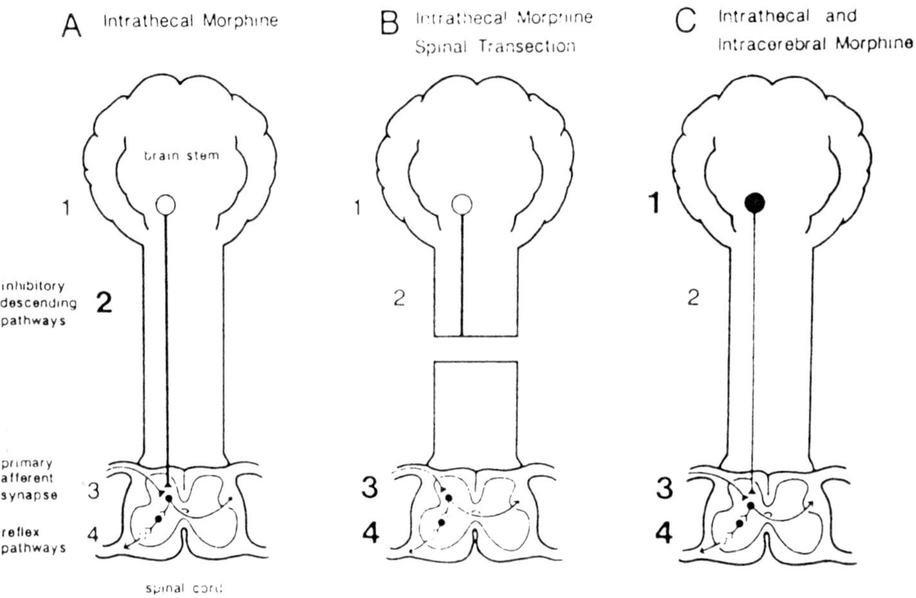

Figure 3. The proposed hypothesis, illustrating the role of descending inhibition in morphine-induced analgesia. A: The analgesic effect of intrathecal (spinal) morphine is normally suppressed by descending inhibitory input. B: Descending inhibitory control is removed by spinal transection. As a result, the antinociceptive effect of intrathecal morphine is enhanced. C: Descending inhibitory control is removed by concurrent intracerebral morphine administration. As a result, the analgesic effect of intrathecal morphine is enhanced. The decrease in descending inhibition could account for the potent analgesic effect of concurrent spinal and supraspinal morphine injections, as well as the analgesic effect of systemic morphine administration.

However, one prediction from this model is that the effect of systemic morphine in spinal rats should be the same as that in intact rats, because in each case spinal opiate effects are expressed in the absence of descending inhibition. Why then is the antinociceptive response to systemic morphine reduced after spinal transection, while the same response to intrathecal morphine is potentiated? One possibility is that the pharmacokinetics of systemic morphine is disturbed by the trauma of spinalization. As a result, the amount of drug that reaches the spinal cord after subcutaneous injection is less than the amount that reaches the cord in intact animals. Consequently, the behavioral response is reduced.

We then conducted experiments designed to examine this possibility (Advokat and Gulati, 1991). Separate groups of intact and spinal rats (transected one day earlier) were injected subcutaneously with different doses of morphine and assessed on the TF. Immediately after the test, the rats were killed and the brains, spinal cords, and trunk blood samples were collected and subsequently assayed for morphine. The results showed that the concentration of morphine in the brains and spinal cords of acute spinal rats was significantly lower than that of intact rats, whereas morphine levels in the blood did not differ. The data were consistent with the suggestion that the decreased antinociceptive effect of subcutaneous morphine in acute spinal rats was due to a decrease in opiate concentration in the central nervous system. The outcome of this study was consistent with our model, which proposed that in the acute spinal rat the antinociceptive effect of intrathecal morphine is enhanced because descending inhibition of spinal opiate activity is removed, and the effect of systemic morphine is reduced because the movement of morphine from the blood into the CNS is impaired.

Additional support for our interpretation was obtained independently, in an elegant study by Sinclair et. al. (1988). In their experiment, the TF reflex was elicited in intact rats after either systemic or intrathecal morphine injections. However, in each of these two conditions, the latency was measured both before and after the spinal cord was reversibly cooled, to 2°C. It was found that the reversible cold block of the spinal cord decreased the antinociceptive effect of systemic morphine on the TF. However, the antinociceptive effect of intrathecal morphine was increased. This is the same response pattern seen in our acute, spinally transected rats. These results support the conclusion that the decreased effect of systemic morphine in the acute spinal rat is not simply due to the trauma of spinalization, but is related to a disturbance in the distribution of the drug to the CNS.

Up to this point, our experiments had only evaluated the effect of morphine in the acute spinal rat. However, the results of those studies led to additional questions regarding the duration of the pharmacological changes. Was the enhanced antinociceptive effect of morphine on spinal reflexes permanent? If not, how long would it last? These questions were addressed by assessing the effect of a single dose of morphine on the TF, in separate groups of rats, at different time points after they were spinally transected. The results of those experiments are shown in Fig. 4. On the top part of the figure are the dose-response functions for subcutaneous morphine injections in rats tested either 1, 3, 10, 20 or 30 days after spinalization (Advokat and Burton, 1987). As indicated in the graph, during the first three weeks after spinalization, the potency of morphine gradually declined. At that time, the response appeared to stabilize, in that the dose-response functions at 20 and 30 days did not differ from each other. Because these results suggested that the decline in morphine-induced antinociception reached asymptote within 3 to 4 weeks, subsequent experiments with intrathecal morphine were conducted at those intervals (Siuciak and Advokat, 1989a). As shown on the bottom half of Fig. 4, the antinociceptive effect of spinal morphine also declined within approximately 3-4 weeks.

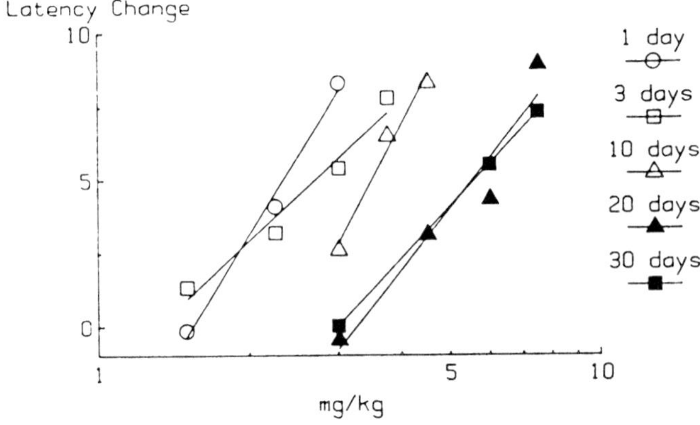

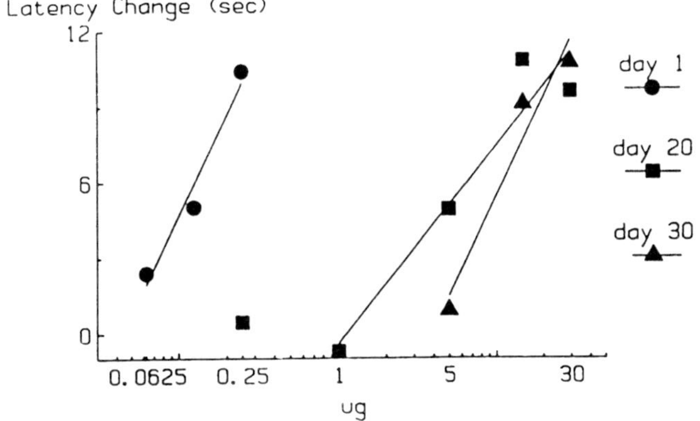

Figure 4. Antinociceptive effect of morphine, on the tail flick reflex, of rats tested at different times after spinal transection. The top part of the figure shows the results of subcutaneous administration, to separate groups of rats, at 1, 3, 10, 20 or 30 days after spinalization. The bottom part shows the results of intrathecal injection, in separate groups of rats tested 1, 20 or 30 days after spinalization.

The fact that the antinociceptive effect of morphine declined after spinal as well as systemic administration indicates that the decrease in potency was not due to a continued disturbance of opiate pharmacokinetics. Intrathecal injection bypasses the processes of absorption and distribution and directly exposes the spinal cord to the drug. Nor are the animals physically deteriorating. On the contrary, the rats are able to eat and drink as soon as they regain consciousness. With appropriate postoperative care (see Bertman and Advokat, 1995) they recover rapidly during the first two weeks after spinalization and by the third week they no longer require supportive maintenance. On gross examination during necropsy, the spinal cord tissue appears quite healthy, both above and below the lesion. By all evidence, our chronic spinal rats are very healthy subjects and the decrease in morphine-induced antinociception on the TF reflex cannot be attributed to a deterioration in their physical condition.

This conclusion is also supported by studies showing that, in fact, morphine has very potent effects in the chronic spinal subject, even though its ability to block the TF is greatly reduced. This was demonstrated by Wiesenfeld-Hallin and colleagues, who compared the effect of the opiate on the hindlimb flexor reflex of acute and chronic spinal rats (Hao et al, 1990). Their procedure consists of applying supramaximal electric shocks (0.5 ms, 10 mA) to the sural nerve innervation area of the left foot (1/min). The resulting EMG is recorded with stainless steel needles inserted into the ipsilateral biceps femoris/semitendinosus muscles and is integrated over 2 sec. Using this technique, they reported that the depressive effect of intravenous morphine on the electrophysiological index of the flexor reflex was unchanged during the first 1-3 days after spinalizaton, but, that after about 4-6 days there was an increase in sensitivity which was still evident for at least "30 to 60 days." The ED_{50} for morphine-induced depression of the flexor reflex was about 1.0 mg/kg at 1-3 days, and 0.17 mg/kg at 7-10 days posttransection.

This outcome is similar to the results of Willer and co-workers, who studied the nociceptive flexor reflex and the corresponding pain reaction, elicited by sural nerve stimulation, in human subjects (Willer, 1985). They found that, in normal individuals, intravenous doses of 0.2 and 0.3 mg/kg of morphine produced a 45% and 70% depression of nociceptive reflexes, respectively, whereas the same doses produced a 70% and 90% depression in paraplegic patients. "These data would suggest that the spinal cord neurones responsible for the nociceptive transmission are more sensitive to the effects of morphine when they are free from some supraspinal influences" (Willer, 1985).

In summary, it has been known for nearly 50 years that the antinociceptive effect of morphine on the TF decreases in the chronic spinal animal (Irwin et al, 1951), whereas recent studies show that the depressive effect of morphine on the nociceptive flexor reflex increases in this same preparation (Hao et al, 1990). What is responsible for this apparent contradiction? We believe that some of our recent results may provide an answer. In our research with the chronic spinal preparation, we observed that such rats gradually became spastic during the post-transection recovery period. This condition also develops in paraplegic patients. It therefore occurred to us that the increased potency of morphine against the flexor reflex in these situations represented an electrophysiological correlate of an antispastic, rather than an antinociceptive, response. There are, in fact, reports in the clinical literature describing the antispastic action of morphine (Erickson et al, 1985, Herman et al, 1988) and another opiate, fentanyl (Chabal et al, 1991). Accordingly, we investigated the possibility that in the same chronic spinal rats, morphine would exert an antispastic effect at doses that were no longer antinociceptively effective (Advokat et al, 1996).

In these studies, reflex spasticity was elicited with an innocuous stimulus, a metal probe pressed against the abdomen at four specific sites. The spastic reaction was evaluated at each site using a scale ranging from 0 to 4 (0 = no spastic response at any of the four sites and 4 = a maximum, tonic, clonic reaction elicited at all four sites). Hindlimb spasticity was assessed at the same time points as TF latency, i.e. prior to, and 30, 60 or 90 min after drug administration. All spasticity scores were transformed to indicate the percent spasticity, such that a score of 0/4 = 0%, 1/4 = 25%, etc. To determine whether drug treatment altered this value, the post-drug scores were normalized to the pre-drug baseline. This provided a measure of the % decrease in spasticity for each rat at each time point.

The results of this study are summarized in Fig. 5. The top part of the figure shows the effect of an i.t. injection of morphine (5 µg) or saline in intact or chronic spinal (21-28 days) rats on the TF reflex. As indicated, although this dose produced a significant analgesic effect in intact rats, it had no antinociceptive effect in chronic spinal rats, and the response of those animals to the opiate was no different than that produced by saline. The bottom half of the figure summarizes the effect of morphine on the spastic response of those same chronic spinal rats. Unlike the TF, which was not affected by this treatment, spasticity was significantly depressed by morphine, relative to the effect of saline. These data show that, in the same chronic spinal animals, the antinociceptive potency of morphine is lost after administration of a dose that exerts a significant antispastic effect. Such results may reconcile previous contradictory reports regarding the effects of opiates in chronic spinal animals.

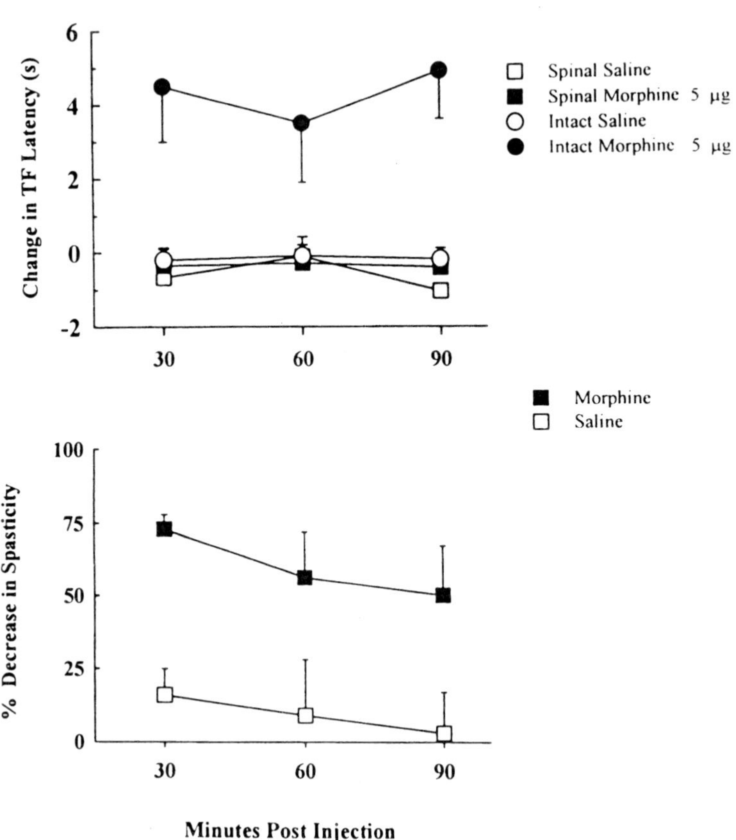

Figure 5. Comparison of the antinociceptive and antispastic effect of intrathecal morphine in chronic (21-28 days) spinal rats. The top part of the figure shows the antinociceptive response, on the tail flick test, of separate groups of intact (circles) or spinal (squares) rats to an intrathecal injection of 5 µg of morphine (filled symbols), or saline (open symbols). Unlike intact rats, there is no antinociceptive reaction of chronic spinal rats to this dose. The bottom part of the figure shows that in the same chronic spinal animals, morphine produces a significant antispastic response.

Furthermore, these results indicate that the decrease in antinociception is not due to a general loss of pharmacological activity. Rather, the data suggest that the loss of antinociceptive sensitivity may represent an alteration in opiate function that is selective to nociceptive processing. If so, this phenomenon may be relevant to a similar loss of analgesic efficacy that occurs after trauma to the human nervous system. It is generally accepted that such neuropathic injury in humans, produced by damage or disease of the peripheral or central nervous system, may induce clinical pain syndromes that are refractory to opiate analgesics (Arner and Myerson, 1988, Dickenson, 1994, Hamman, 1993). In this regard, the chronic spinal preparation may be a useful model with which to study such changes in opiate analgesic efficacy. Ultimately, the results of such investigations may help us to understand the cause of such a devastating loss of therapeutic benefit from opiate analgesics.

Up to this point, our experiments had only examined the effect of acute and chronic spinalization on morphine-induced depression of spinal reflexes. But we soon began to consider the possibility that morphine might not be unique in this respect, and that the effect of other drugs on the spinal cord might also be modulated by descending supraspinal input. We chose to begin our investigation of this question by assessing the drug baclofen in our spinal rats (Bertman and Advokat, 1995). Baclofen was chosen for several reasons. First, it is an agonist at the $GABA_B$ receptor subtype, and GABA (gamma-aminobutyric acid-the primary inhibitory neurotransmitter in the central nervous system), is found in high concentration in the spinal cord. Second, baclofen has been used clinically for nearly 25 years as a muscle relaxant and antispastic agent, particularly against spasticity caused by spinal damage. Third, although baclofen has been studied in non-human, animal experiments, most of these examined the antinociceptive effect of the drug, rather than its antispastic properties (probably because there are few whole animal models of spasticity available) (Bertman and Advokat, 1995, Malcangio and Bowery, 1995). With our paradigm, we were able to investigate the antinociceptive effect of systemic and intrathecal (-) baclofen (the more active isomer) in intact, acute and chronic spinal rats, and its antispastic effect in the same groups of chronic spinal animals.

Our results are shown in Figs. 6 and 7. Fig. 6 summarizes the effect of subcutaneous, s.c., (Part A) and i.t. (Part B) (-)baclofen on the TF reflex, in separate groups of intact (open circles), acute (filled circles) and chronic spinal (filled squares) rats. The data are plotted as the Area Under the Curve, obtained by calculating the total area (i.e. the integral) under the time-effect curve for each group.

Statistical analyses indicated that, compared to intact rats, the antinociceptive effect of s.c. (-)baclofen was reduced one day after spinalization, but that no further decline occurred during the next three weeks. In contrast, antinociception produced by low doses of i.t. (-)baclofen was increased one day after spinal transection, relative to intact rats. However, three weeks later this effect was essentially lost. At the same time, as shown in Fig. 7, in spite of this differential decrease in antinociception after i.t., relative to s.c. administration, both routes were effective against spasticity.

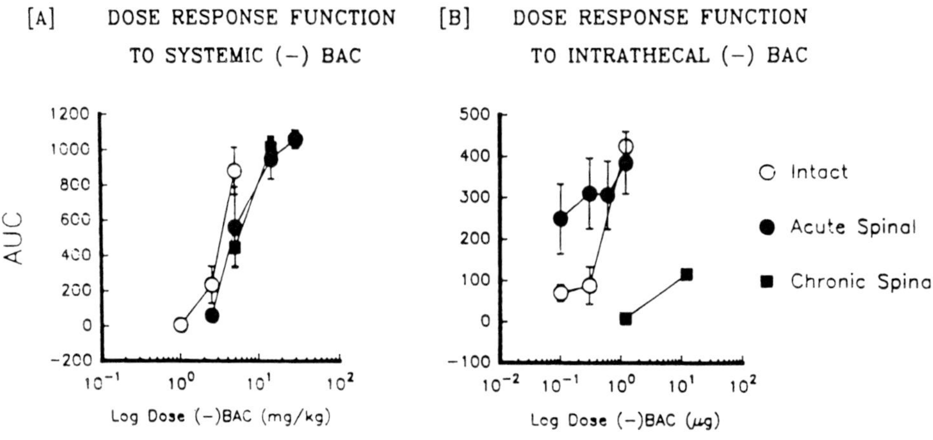

Figure 6. Antinociceptive dose-response functions, on the tail flick reflex, for (-)baclofen in intact, acute and chronic spinal rats, after subcutaneous (Part A) or intrathecal (Part B) injection. Each point summarizes the mean ± SEM of the area under the time-effect curve (AUC) of separate groups of rats at the indicated doses.

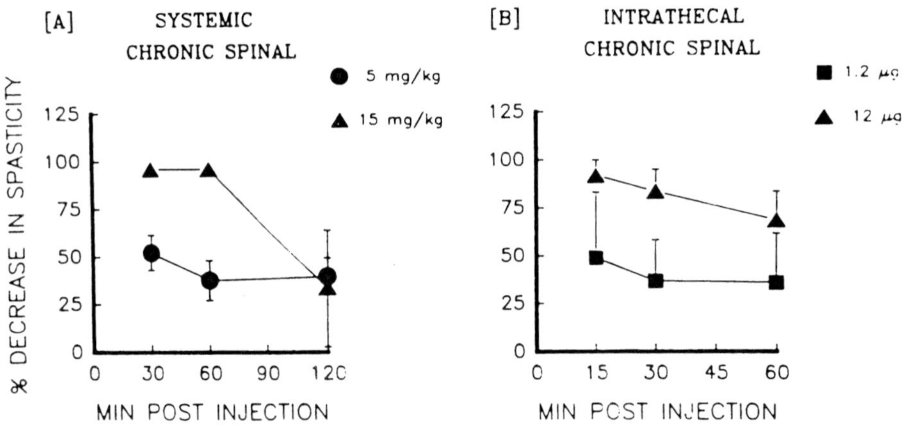

Figure 7. Antispastic effect of (-)baclofen in separate groups in chronic spinal rats after subcutaneous (Part A) or intrathecal (Part B) injection. The data are presented as the mean (SEM of the % decrease in spasticity (pre - post drug spasticity / pre-drug spasticity x 100) at the indicated time points and doses.

These data present an unusual pattern of results. Like morphine, there was a decrease in antinociception after s.c. injection and an increase after i.t. injection, in acute spinal rats. This outcome could be due to the same respective mechanisms proposed for the opiate: an impairment in the movement of (-)baclofen from the blood into the CNS, and the removal of a descending supraspinal inhibitory influence exerted on the spinal action of (-)baclofen. However, the results obtained from the chronic spinal groups differed from those seen with morphine. That is, after s.c. injection there was no loss of potency in chronic versus acute spinal rats, whereas after i.t. injection there was a dramatic loss of efficacy; yet, in both cases the antispastic action was retained.

One possible (although incomplete) explanation for these results is that the antinociceptive effect of s.c. (-)baclofen may be mediated by a local action of the drug in the periphery. In this regard, it has been shown that $GABA_B$ receptors are located on prejunctional terminals of nociceptive afferent fibers (e.g. in the skin). Agonists acting at these sites have been proposed to exert an anti-inflammatory effect by inhibiting the release of excitatory neurotransmitters, particularly substance P (Barnes et al, 1990). Experiments designed to test this hypothesis are currently in progress.

The acute and chronic spinal animal has played a significant role in the development of our present concepts of opiate pharmacology. Recent investigations with other neuropharmacological agents indicate that this classic paradigm continues to be a valuable preparation for pharmacological analyses of spinal reflex function.

Acknowledgements

This research was supported by PHS grant DA-02845 from the National Institute on Drug Abuse

References

Advokat C (1988) The role of descending inhibition in morphine-induced analgesia. Trends in Pharmacol Sci 9:330-334.

Advokat C and Burton P (1987) Antinociceptive effect of systemic and intrathecal morphine in spinally transected rats. Eur J Pharmacol 139:335-343.

Advokat C and Gulati A (1991) Spinal transection reduces both spinal antinociception and CNS concentration of systemically administered morphine in rats. Brain Res 555:251-258.

Advokat C, Mosser H and Hutchinson K (1996) Morphine and dextrorphan lose antinociceptive potency but exhibit an antispastic action in chronic spinal rats. Pain, submitted

Arnér S and Myerson BA (1988) Lack of analgesic effect of opioids on neuropathic and idiopathic forms of pain. Pain 33:11-23.

Barnes PJ, Belvisi MG and Rogers DF (1990) Modulation of neurogenic inflammation:novel approaches to inflammatory disease. Trends in Pharmacol Sci 11:185-189.

Berge O-G and Hole K (1981) Tolerance to the antinociceptive effect of morphine in the spinal rat. Neuropharmacol 20:653-657.

Bertman LJ and Advokat C (1995) Comparison of the antinociceptive and antispastic action of (-)baclofen after systemic and intrathecal administration in intact, acute and chronic spinal rats. Brain Res 684:8-18.

Chabal C, Jacobson L and Schwid HA (1991) An objective comparison of intrathecal lidocaine versus fentanyl for the treatment of lower extremity spasticity. Anesthesiol 74:643-646.

Dewey WL, Snyder JW, Harris LS and Howes JF (1969) The effect of narcotics and narcotic antagonists on the tail-flick response in spinal mice. J Pharm Pharmacol 21:548-550.

Dickenson AH (1994) Neurophysiology of opioid poorly responsive pain. Cancer Surveys, vol.21:Palliative Medicine:Problem Areas in Pain and Symptom Management, Imperial Cancer Research Fund pp. 5-16.

Erickson DL, Blacklock JB, Michaelson M, Sperling KB and Lo JN (1985) Control of spasticity by implantable continuous flow morphine pump. Neurosurg 16:215-217.

Fields HL and Basbaum AI (1978) Brainstem control of spinal pain-transmission neurons. Ann Rev Physiol 40:217-248.

Hamman W (1993) Neuropathic pain: A condition which is not always well appreciated. Brit J Anaesthesiol 71:779-781.

Hao J, Wiesenfeld-Hallin Z and Xu X (1990) Depression of the flexor reflex by systemic morphine increases in chronically spinalized rats. Eur J Pharmacol 191:407-416.

Herman RM, Wainberg MC, delGiudice PF and Willscher MK (1988) The effect of a low dose of intrathecal morphine on impaired micturition reflexes in human subjects with spinal cord lesions. Anesthesiol 69:313-318.

Irwin S, Houde R, Bennett D R, Hendershot LC and Seevers MH (1951) The effects of morphine, methadone and meperidine on some reflex responses of spinal animals to nociceptive stimulation. J Pharmacol Exp Therapeutics 101:132-143.

Malcangio M and Bowery NG (1995) Possible therapeutic application of $GABA_B$ receptor agonists and antagonists. Clin Neuropharmacol 18:285-305.

Sinclair JG, Main CD and Lo GF (1988) Spinal vs. supraspinal actions of morphine on the rat tail-flick reflex. Pain 33:357-362.

Siuciak JA and Advokat C (1989) Antinociceptive effect of intrathecal morphine in tolerant and nontolerant spinal rats. Pharmacology, Biochem Behavior 34:445-452.

Siuciak JA and Advokat C (1989) The synergistic effect of concurrent spinal and supraspinal opiate agonisms is reduced by both nociceptive and morphine pretreatment. Pharmacology, Biochem Behavior 34:265-273.

Wikler A (1950) Sites and mechanisms of action of morphine and related drugs in the central nervous system. Pharmacol Rev 2:435-506.

Wood PL, Rackham A and Richard J (1981) Spinal analgesia:comparison of the mu agonist morphine and the kappa agonist ethylketazocine. Life Sci 28:2119-2125.

Willer J-C (1985) Studies on pain. Effects of morphine on a spinal nociceptive flexion reflex and related pain sensation in man. Brain Res 331:105-114.

Yeung JC and Rudy TA (1980) Multiplicative interaction between narcotic agonisms expressed at spinal and supraspinal sites of antinociceptive action as revealed by concurrent intrathecal and intracerebroventricular injections of morphine. J Pharmacol Exp Therapeutics 215:633-642.

Pain Mechanisms and Management
S.N. Ayrapetyan and A.V. Apkarian (Eds.)
IOS Press, 1998

Spinal Facilitation and the Post Tissue Injury Pain State

Tony L. Yaksh
*Department of Anesthesiology, University of California, San Diego
La Jolla, CA, USA*

The response to an unconditioned stimulus which injures, or potentially injures, tissue is defined by the afferent pathways which are activated, and the characteristics of the integrative processes lead to organized escape behaviors. One of the important advances that has arisen in the past three decades has been first an appreciation that the input-output function of these systems is subject to considerable modulation, and second the characterization of the pharmacology of these processes, particularly as they apply to the spinal level of organization. This identification of the transmitters and receptors has provided insights into not only the organization, but has led to advances that promise to profoundly alter the tools available for the regulation of nociceptive processing. In the following sections, I will consider several components of this modulation. At the outset, it is appreciated in the normal organism that stimuli which are adequate to produce a pain state serve to induce activity in populations of small primary afferents (Aδ/C). For heuristic purposes, we can functionally define at least two postsynaptic components to the dorsal horn response generated by persistent afferent activity.

Acute activation of a C fiber volley will evoke the release of transmitters from C fiber terminals such as glutamate, and certain peptides such as sP and CGRP (See Yaksh and Malmberg, 1994). This in turn leads to the depolarization of several classes of dorsal horn neurons. The frequency of the response of the dorsal horn neuron to the acute stimulus is believed to be proportional to the release of transmitter, which is proportional to the frequency of activity in the primary afferent, which itself is proportional to stimulus intensity. Thus, with brief high intensity stimuli, the response of the second order neuron is strongly linked to the intensity of the stimulus (see Figure 1).

Psychophysical studies carried out in humans undergoing percutaneous cordotomy emphasized that the reported intensity of the stimulus correlated with the frequency of the discharge in the ascending pathways (Mayer, et al, 1975). In short, we may presume that, within limits, factors increasing the output function of spinal projection systems will enhance the pain response, while those reducing the output will reduce the pain response.

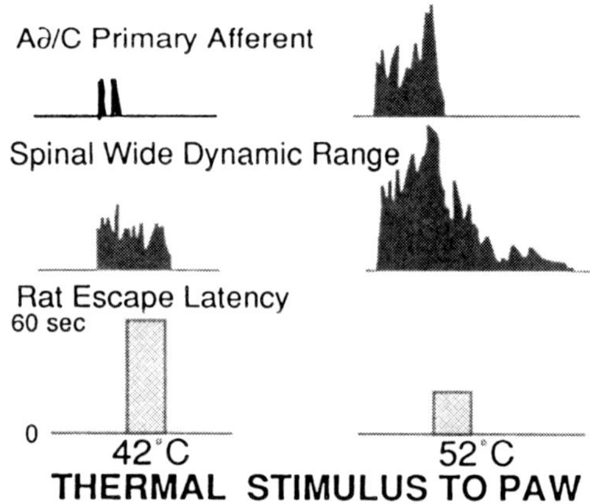

Figure 1. Cartoon indicating response of small primary afferents (top), spinal wide dynamic range neuron (middle) and escape latency (bottom) of a rat in response to application of a thermal stimulus of 42°C (left) and 52°C (right) to the paw.

In contrast to the fixed relationship between input (afferent traffic) and output (frequency of activity in ascending pathways), early studies by Mendell and Wall (1965), suggested that repetitive stimulation of C fibers would evoke an increasingly exaggerated response to a given stimulus in dorsal horn neurons. Termed "windup," this state of activity was perceived to reflect upon an increase in the responsiveness of the spinal cord to subsequent afferent input. Other work has shown that such afferent input may not only lead to an exaggerated response but also to increases in receptive field size and composition (Owens et al, 1992) (See Figure 2).

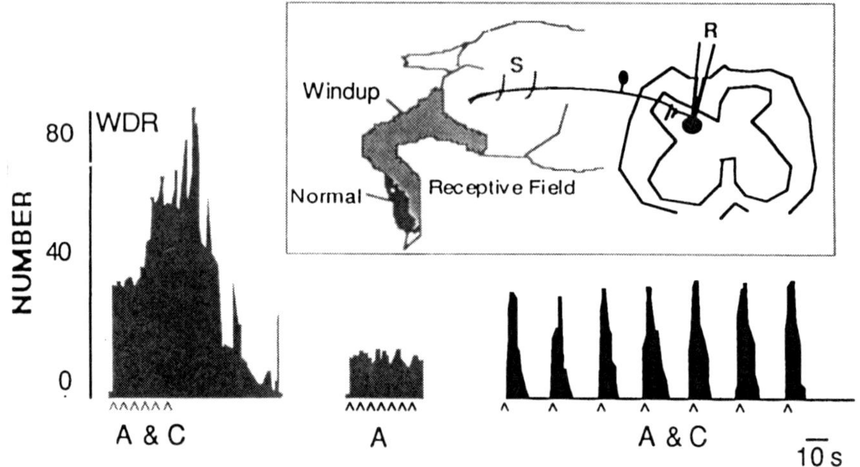

Figure 2. Schematic showing a single unit recording from a wide dynamic range neuron in response to an electric stimulus delivered at 0.1Hz (right). A very reliable, stimulus-linked response is evoked at this frequency. In contrast, when the stimulation rate is increased to 0.5 Hz, there is a progressive increase in the magnitude of the response generated by the stimulation (left). This facilitation results from the C-fiber input, not an A-fiber input (middle), and is called "wind-up". (Adapted from Dickenson and Sullivan, 1987a).

Functional correlates of central facilitation

It should be strongly emphasized that in the face of tissue injury, the typical profile of afferent input is not that of an acute stimulus, rather it is characterized by a high frequency ongoing bursting discharge. Under these circumstances, we would presume that in the post injury condition that the persistent afferent input would lead to a state of central (spinal) facilitation that would serve to increase the input-output function and produce a condition what would correspond to a behavioral state of hyperalgesia.

There are behavioral parallels to both the acute and facilitated afferent processing suggested by electrophysiology. The injection of an irritant in the paw of a rat will evoke an acute burst of C fiber activity for about 10 min followed by an extended period of low levels of afferent traffic (Heapy et al, 1985). In the unanesthetized animal, this treatment results in an initial transient appearance of pain behavior corresponding to the initial C fiber activity, but this early behavior is followed shortly by a second phase of behavior, the magnitude of which exceeds that predicted by the modest C-fiber activity present at that time (Wheeler, Aceto and Cowan, 1991) (Figure 3). The dissociation between afferent traffic and behavior is considered to reflect an exaggerated state of afferent processing.

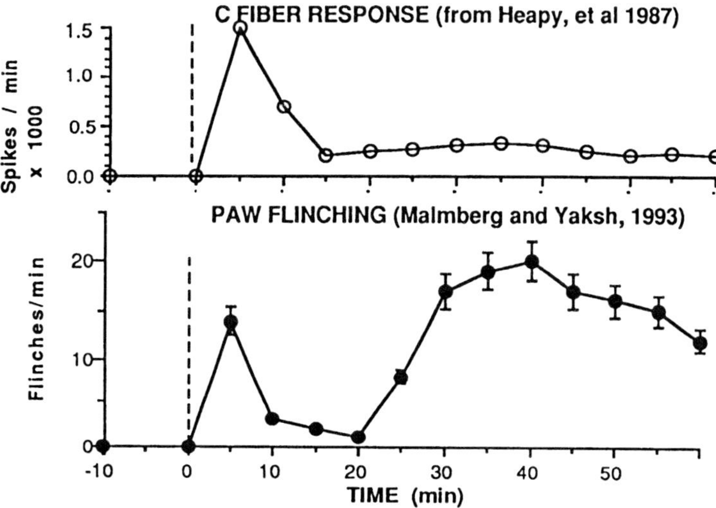

Figure 3. C-fiber activity (top) measured in the saphenous nerve of the anesthetized rat and number of flinches in the unanesthetized rat measured before and after the ipsilateral subcutaneous injection of formalin (5% / 50 μl) into the hindpaw at the time indicated by the vertical dashed line. Note the low level of input during the second phase, where behavior suggestive of pain is particularly high.

The relevance of this C fiber-evoked facilitation to humans has been emphasized by psychophysical studies. In observers, the activation of C fibers by the intradermal injection of capsaicin will lead to an initial pain state followed for an extended period of time by a large region of profoundly enhanced mechanical and thermal sensitivity. This phenomena is referred to as secondary hyperalgesia (LaMotte et al, 1991; Torebjork et al, 1992). Thus, in humans, following local injury where C fibers are similarly activated, there is every reason to believe that similar processes apply and that important components of the post-injury pain state are the events consequent to the afferent barrage and not, strictly speaking, the input present in the post-injury phase.

The absolute dependency of the hyperalgesia on the conditioning afferent input makes it reasonable that a blockade of afferent traffic, during the conditioning phase (i.e. phase 1 of the formalin test) should diminish the secondary response. Indeed, in recent studies, lidocaine given only during the phase 1 of the formalin test prevents the manifestation of the second phase, while the delivery of the same dose of lidocaine only during the second phase was without effect upon the second phase (Abram and Yaksh, unpublished observations). In humans, the blockade of the intradermal site of injection of capsaicin similarly prevents the development of the experimentally induced secondary hyperesthesia noted above (Torebjork et al, 1992).

Spinal pharmacology of post tissue injury evoked hyperalgesia

Current studies have emphasized the complexity of the spinal systems that regulate facilitated processing induced by the post injury pain state. A schematic of this - organization, to be discussed below, is presented in Figure 4.

A number of classes of agents are known to influence the processing of this dorsal horn system. These are summarized below:

1. Opiates: Intrathecal opiate agonists diminish the second phase of the formalin response, presumably by their ability to block release of transmitter from C fibers (Yaksh, 1993). These behavioral results correspond with single unit studies in spinal cord (Dickenson and Sullivan, 1987a-, Woolf and Wall, 1986). Importantly delivery of the opiate after the first phase, but prior to the second phase has been shown to have a diminished potency (Dickenson and Sullivan, 1987b).

2. NMDA antagonists: Ketamine, 2-amino5-phonovalorate or MK801, can block "wind-up" by virtue of their ability to block the NMDA receptor (Haley et al, 1990), and such agents will prevent the second phase of the formalin test, if they are administered before the formalin injection (Yamamoto and Yaksh, 1992). This reflects upon the fact that agonist occupation of the NMDA site leads to biochemical changes within the neuron which must persist after the occupancy of the NMDA receptor has passed.

3. NK1 antagonists: The spinal delivery of agents which block the NK1 site for substance P can diminish wind-up and significantly reduce the second phase (Yamamoto and Yaksh, 1991; De Koninck and Henry, 1991). Importantly, as with the NMDA antagonists, the post treatment with the NK1 antagonists reduced their efficacy at blocking the second phase.

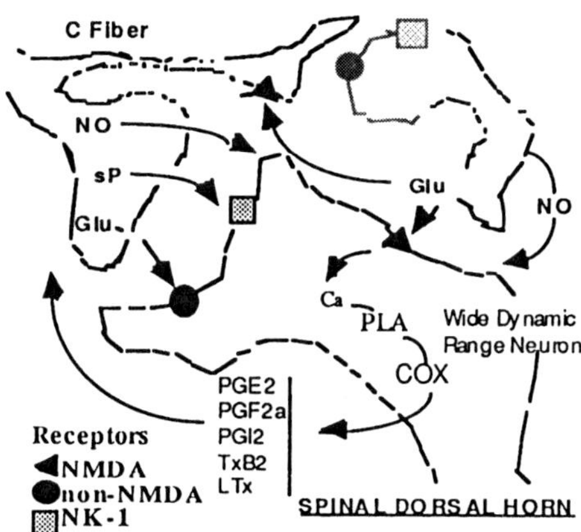

Figure 4. Schematic organization of the neurotransmitter responses discussed in the text. C-fiber input results in the release of peptides including sP and excitatory amino acids such as glutamate. sP and glutamate act post-synaptically on second order neurons to evoke their direct discharge via NK-1 and non-NMDA sites. In addition, this release interacts with interneurons in the upper lamina of the substantia gelatinosa, to evoke the release of additional agents, including glutamate from interneurons, which interact with NMDA receptors. The activation in the dorsal horn results in the increase in intracellular Ca, leading to activation of phospholipase A2 (PLA), formation of arachidonic acid (AA) and the several prostanoids which move extracellularly. These prostanoids have been shown to be both directly excitatory and to increase the Ca current in the primary afferents, leading to further transmitter release. In addition, this activation leads to the formation of nitric oxide (NO) by NO synthase, present in both primary afferent C-fibers and in second order dorsal horn neurons. NO is known also to facilitate transmitter release.

4. NSAIDS: Cyclooxygenase inhibitors have been shown to act spinally to diminish the hyperalgesic component (Malmberg and Yaksh, 1992a,b). This reaction reflects upon the important role of prostaglandins released from the spinal cord, where they can act to facilitate the release of C fiber transmitters, such as sP (see Malmberg and Yaksh, 1992a). Consistent with the observation that NMDA antagonists can block a hyperalgesic state, spinal NMDA agonists can evoke a hyperalgesic state and this hyperalgesia can also be blocked by spinal cyclooxygenase inhibitors. Such observations suggest that spinal NMDA receptor occupancy can evoke the release of prostanoids that in turn can augment spinal nociceptive processing (see Malmberg and Yaksh, 1992b).

5. Nitric oxide (NO): This agent is released following activation of NO synthase and has been shown to play a role in the LTP phenomena induced by activation of the glutamate receptor in the hippocampus. Similarly, in the spinal cord, NO synthase inhibitors have been shown to prevent hyperalgesia (Meller et al 1992; Malmberg and Yaksh, 1993).

Volatile anesthesia and afferent evoked hyperalgesia

The above observations provide insight into the potential means by which certain drug treatments might diminish the contribution of secondary hyperalgesia to the post-injury pain state. But, we must pause and consider that the concept of preemptive analgesia is always in the context of surgical patients that are typically anesthetized.

This leads to the supposition that volatile agents may induce a state clearly adequate to produce a loss of reported sensation and to block certain reflexes, but this may not be adequate to prevent the development of post-injury hyperalgesia. In recent studies, we have in fact demonstrated that high concentrations of isoflurane (2.3%) or isoflurane + N20 only during the phase 1 of the formalin response failed to prominently diminish phase 2 (the hyperalgesic component) of the formalin response (see Figure 2). In contrast, the addition of morphine and the delivery of naloxone between phases 1 and 2 resulted in a significant reduction in the phase 2 response (see Figure5).

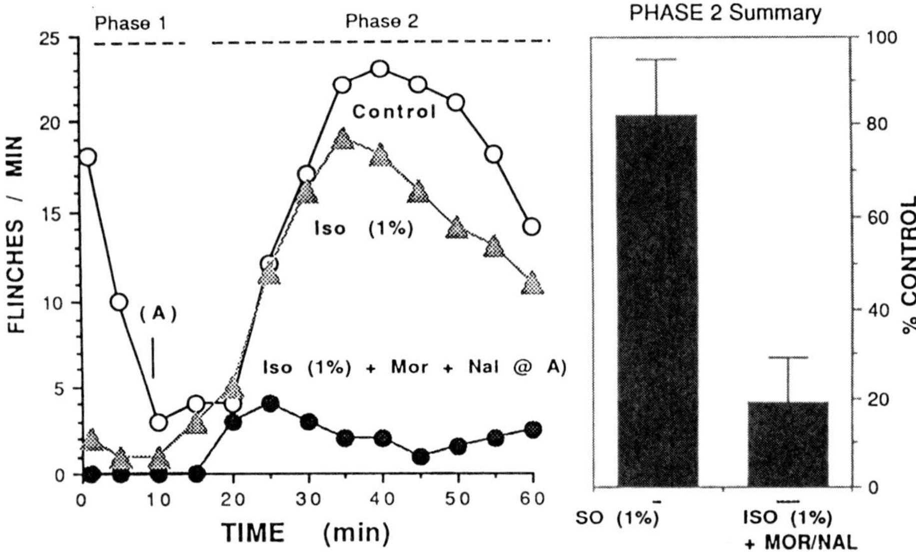

Figure 5. Left : Time course of the flinching induced by intraplantar formalin injection at time 0 in animals 1) under a very brief anesthetic (Control); 2) in animals anesthetized with isoflurane (Iso 1%) before (15 min) and after (+6 min) formalin and 3) in animals anesthetized with isoflurane (1%) (as in group 2) and in addition, receiving an intrathecal injection of morphine (30 µg) 15 min prior to the formalin injection. To block the effect of morphine, naloxone was administered at 6 min after formalin (time A).
Right: Histogram presents the effects as percent of control (i.e. no anesthetic or opioid). As indicated, isoflurane given alone only during the phase 1 of the formalin test alone resulted in a modest suppression of the phase 2 response, but morphine, active only during the phase 1 (i.e. prior to naloxone) served to abolish the second phase response (adapted from Abram and Yaksh, 1993).

These results are consistent with the fact that wind up and other such changes in dorsal horn function, including transmitter release can be readily demonstrated in halothane anesthetized animals (see Dickenson and Sullivan, 1987a,b), and that there is no reason to suspect that volatile anesthetics will alter either the binding of these transmitters to their respective receptors or alter the post-synaptic biochemical changes which occur secondary to those receptors activation--for example the increase in intracellular Ca mediated by the NMDA site. The failure of volatile anesthetics in the animal model to alter significantly the hyperalgesic component thus likely reflects upon the fact that volatile agents, at surgically usable concentrations, do not block the spinal processes set into play by the acute activation of C fibers secondary to the local injury.

Concluding comments

After tissue injury, small afferents display a persistent barrage. In human and animal models, this ongoing input has been shown to lead to a facilitated state of processing at the spinal level. The important observation is that absolute blockade of small afferent input with either local anesthetics or opioids (but not certain volatile anesthetics) will prevent the evolution of this facilitated state. Additionally, it has been shown that the facilitated state has a unique pharmacology, with agents that are unable to block the initial activation, showing the ability to block the facilitated state. Such drugs likely have important consequences for managing post trauma pain states, though they are not classically considered to be analgesics (rather they are anti-hyperalgesics). One clear example of this is the widely appreciated efficacy of cyclooxygenase inhibitors in the post surgical and cancer pain state (McCormack and Brune, 1991). As noted above, considerable data suggests that the post injury pain state possesses a strong component of facilitated processing that is mediated in part by the spinal release of Prostaglandins. These results are in accord with a clinical literature that, while controversial suggests that the continued management of small afferent-evoked activity can significantly alter the evolution of the post operative pain state (see for example, McQuay et al, 1988).

References

Abram SE, Yaksh TL (1993) Morphine, but not inhalation anesthesia, blocks post-injury facilitation: the role of preemptive suppression of afferent transmission. Anesthesiology 78:713-21.

De Koninck Y, Henry JL (1991) Substance P-mediated slow excitatory postsynaptic potential elicited in dorsal horn neurons in vivo by noxious stimulation. Proceedings of the National Academy of Sciences USA 88: 11344-11348.

Dickenson AH, Sullivan AF (1987a) Evidence for a role of the NMDA receptor in the frequency dependency potentiation of deep rat dorsal horn nociceptive neurones following C fibre stimulation. Neuropharmacol 26: 1235-1238.

Dickenson AH, Sullivan AF, (1987b) Subcutaneous formalin-induced activity of dorsal horn neurones in rat: differential response to an intrathecal opiate administered pre or post formalin. Pain 30:349-360.

Haley JE, Sullivan AF, Dickenson AH (1990) Evidence for spinal N-meth I D-aspartate receptor involvement in prolonged chemical nociception in the rat. Brain Res 518:218-26.

Heapy CG, Jamieson A, Russell NJW (1985) Afferent C fiber and A-delta fiber activity in models of inflammation. Br J Pharmacol 90: 164P.

LaMotte R, Shain C, Simone D, Tsai EF (1991) Neurogenic hyperalgesia: psychophysical studies of underlying mechanisms. J Neurophysiol 66:190-21 1.

Malmberg AB, Yaksh TL (1992a) Hyperalgesia mediated by spinal glutamate and sP receptor blocked by spinal cyclooxygenase inhibition. Science 257: 1276-1279.

Malmberg AB, Yaksh TL (1992b) Antinociceptive actions of spinal non-steroidal antiinflammatory agents on the formalin test in the rat. Journal of Pharmacology and Experimental Therapeutics 263: 136-146.

Malmberg AB, Yaksh TL (1993) Spinal nitric oxide synthesis inhibition blocks NMDA induced thermal hyperalgesia and produces antinociception in the formalin test in rats. Pain 54: 291-300.

Mayer DJ, Price DD, Becker DP (1975) Neurophysiological characterization of the anterolateral spinal cord neurons contributing to pain perception in man. Pain 1:51-8. McCormack K, Brune K (1991) Dissociation between the antinociceptive and antiinflammatory effects of the nonsteroidal anti-inflammatory drugs. A survey Of their analgesic efficacy. Drugs 41:553-547.

McQuay HJ, Carroll D, Moore RA, (1988) Postoperative orthopedic pain--the effect of opiate premedication and local anesthetic blocks. Pain 33:291-295.

Meller ST, Dykstra C, Gebhart GF (1992) Production of endogenous nitric oxide and activation of soluble guanylate cyclase are required for N-methyl-D-aspartate-produced facilitation of the nociceptive tail-flick reflex. Dissociation between the antinociceptive and antiinflammatory effects of the nonsteroidal anti-inflammatory drugs. A survey of their analgesic efficacy. Drugs, 41:533-47.

Mendell LM, Wall PD (1965) Response of single dorsal cord cells to peripheral cutaneous unmyelinated fibres. Nature 206: 97-99.

Owens C, Zhang D, Willis W (1992) Changes in the response states of primate spinothalamic tract cells caused by mechanical damage of the skin or activation of descending controls. J Neurophysiol 67:1509-27.

Torebjork H, Lundberg L, LaMotte R (1992) Central changes in processing of mechanoreceptive input in capsaicin-induced secondary hyperalgesia in humans. J Physiol 448:765 780.

Wheeler-Aceto H, Cowan A (1991) Standardization of the rat paw formalin test for the evaluation of analgesics. Psychophannacol 104: 35-44.

Woolf CJ, Wall PD (1986) Morphine-sensitive and morphine-insensitive actions of C-fibre input on the rat spinal cord. Neurosci Lett 221-225.

Yaksh TL (1993) The spinal actions of opioids. Hdbk of Expert Pharmacology 104:53-89 Yaksh TL, Malmberg AB (1994) Central pharmacology of nociceptive transmission. In: Textbook of Pain. (Melzack R and Wall P eds.): 3E, Churchill Livingstone, UK, pp. 165-200.

Yamamoto T, Yaksh TL, (1991) Stereospecific effects of a nonpeptidic NK1 selective antagonist, CP,96-345: antinociception in the absence of motor dysfunction. Life Sci 49: 1955-1963.

Yamamoto T, Yaksh TL (1992) Comparison of the antinociceptive effects of pre- and post treatment with intrathecal morphine and MK801, an NMDA antagonist, on the formalin test in the rat. Anesthesilog 77: 757-763.

Changes in Nociceptive Processing in the Setting of Persistent Injury: Insights from an Analysis of the Interaction of Substance P with its Receptor in the Rat Spinal Cord

Allan I. Basbaum
Departments of Anatomy and Physiology
and
W.M. Keck Center for Integrative Neuroscience
University of California San Francisco
San Francisco, CA, USA

Traditional diagrams of the pathways through which injury stimuli are processed in the nervous system illustrate a relatively hard-wired system. Primary afferent nociceptors activate subpopulations of neurons in the dorsal horn of the spinal cord; these in turn project to several supraspinal sites and through a totally enigmatic mechanism, pain can arise. Recent studies, however, indicate that the nervous system of the animal, and thus presumably the patient, that has experienced injury and pain, is very different from that of the normal animal. Of particular interest is the evidence that a process of central sensitization occurs through which a state of hyperexcitability develops in the spinal cord (Woolf, 1983; Woolf and Thompson, 1991). In the present paper I will address recent evidence that comparable changes occur at the level of the interaction between the primary afferent neurotransmitter, substance P (SP) and its target, the neurokinin-1, or substance P, receptor.

A host of previous studies has implicated SP in the transmission of nociceptive messages Levine et al., 1993). Of importance to the present discussion are the immunhistochemical studies that have clearly established that SP, which derives predominantly from small diameter dorsal root ganglion (DRG) cells, is concentrated in the superficial laminae of the dorsal horn, laminae I and II (Hokfelt et al., 1975). On the other hand, when the pattern of staining of the substance P receptor (SPR) is studied, a very different pattern is revealed (Brown et al., 1995; Liu et al., 1994). Specifically, using antisera directed against the C terminal of the substance P receptor, we found that although there is dense receptor staining in a subpopulation of neurons in lamina I, there is almost no labelling in lamina II, the substantia gelatinosa. The only staining in lamina II is in dorsally directed dendrites of large SPR positive neurons in lamina III. There are many SPR positive neurons in lamina V and VI and around the central canal. Thus, there is a mismatch in the pattern of staining between SP and its receptor. EM studies underscored the mismatch. Neurons that synthesize the SPR express it over almost their entire somatic and dendritic surfaces. Quantitative analysis revealed that at most 15 % of the surface SPR is apposed by SP-containing synapses.

Since it is possible that the only functional receptor is that which apposes the SP-containing synaptic input, we turned to functional studies of the interaction between SP and its receptor. Our analysis was based on studies in other receptor systems, which demonstrated that when ligand binds receptor, there is an internalization of the receptor, with either rapid recycling of the receptor to the membrane, or degradation in lysosomes. Our first studies were performed in the striatum, which contains a relatively homogenous population of SPR containing neurons (Mantyh et al., 1995). Using confocal microscopy, we found that when substance P was injected into the striatum, there was a rapid movement of the receptor from the membrane to the cytoplasm. The internalization peaked at five minutes after SP injection; within 60 minutes, the receptor was relocated to the surface of the neurons. Importantly, receptor internalization was found over the entire surface of the cell soma and dendrites, was dose-dependent, and could be blocked by selective substance P receptor antagonists. This result established that the "nonsynaptic" receptor is functional over the entire surface of the neuron.

Having established the functionality of the receptor, we turned our attention to the spinal cord and evaluated the effects of noxious stimulation (Mantyh et al., 1995). Our initial studies used anesthetized rats. As noted above, in the normal rat, and in the absence of stimulation, the receptor is distributed largely on the surface of cell bodies and dendrites. Within five minutes of noxious stimulation, for example, capsaicin injection into the hindpaw, noxious pinch of the hindpaw or temperatures greater than 45°C, we found significant receptor internalization in cell bodies and dendrites of the superficial dorsal horn. Of particular interest was the observation that there while there was significant internalization in the dorsally-directed dendrites of the large SPR-immunoreactive neurons in lamina III, the internalization was *only* found in that part of the dendrite located in lamina I and the outer part of the substantia gelatinosa. Despite the presence of large numbers of SPR-immunoreactive neurons located in lamina V and X, we never found internalization in these neurons in the normal animal. As in the striatum, we also studied the changes in receptor distribution over time. We found that the receptor returned to the surface of the neurons within 60 minutes of stimulation.

More recently, we determined that the most effective "natural" stimulus for internalization is noxious mechanical pinch of the hindpaw. Even very short stimuli produced internalization in the majority of SPR-immunoreactive neurons in lamina I. On the other hand, to evoke significant internalization by noxious heat, we had to use temperatures of at least 48°C. What is considered a traditional noxious thermal threshold (namely 45°C) was without effect. Since we performed these experiments under anesthesia, it is possible that the efficacy of thermal stimulation was reduced, however, our results are consistent with earlier studies that reported that there is a relatively selective release of SP in response to noxious mechanical, but not noxious thermal stimulation (Duggan et al., 1988; Kuraishi et al., 1985; Morton et al., 1989). It may be the case that noxious thermal stimulation only evokes significant release of SP when the temperatures are sufficiently high, or maintained for a sufficient duration to induce inflammation.

The fact that the locus of receptor internalization was limited to the superficial dorsal horn indicates that the receptor changes are only found in the immediate vicinity of the major termination of SP containing primary afferents, namely laminae I and outer II. Importantly, since the receptor internalized over the entire surface of lamina I neurons, we conclude that there is diffusion of SP from its site of release. However, the distance over which the diffusion takes place in the normal rat is rather limited.

We next turned our attention to the changes that occur in the setting of persistent injury. We used two different models, persistent inflammation produced by hindpaw injection of complete Freund's adjuvant and a nerve injury model produced by section of the sciatic nerve (Abbadie et al., 1996). In both models, we found that there was a significant increase in the density of SP receptor in the superficial dorsal horn; it was our impression that there was also an increase in lamina III-VI; however, this was not quantitated. This result is consistent with an earlier study that found increased SPR message in the dorsal horn under persistent inflammation conditions (McCarson and Krause, 1994). The fact that we found increases in both inflammation and nerve injury conditions was, however, surprising because these two models are respectively associated with an increase and a decrease in the levels of SP in the DRG and the dorsal horn (Jessell et al., 1979; Lembeck et al., 1981; Noguchi et al., 1988).

Importantly, we also found that the distribution of the receptor was found in regions of the dorsal horn outside of the topographic distribution of the afferents from the paw. For example, in the L4 and L5 segments, we found increased SPR in the lateral part of the dorsal horn, as well as in the medial half, which is the target of afferents from the hindpaw. We also found increases at segments rostral and caudal to L4 and L5. Although it is possible that the increase in these non-topographic regions is in dendrites of neurons with cells in the topographically appropriate region, it is our impression that increases also occurred in cell bodies in these regions. Of interest is, however, that despite the increase in SPR density, we found no evidence of increased cytoplasmic receptor. We first established this at the light microscopic analysis and confirmed it by electron microscopy.

Based on these observations, it was clearly of interest to determine whether the functional consequences of the increased internalization were manifest when stimuli are administered in the persistent injury state. As noted above, there is considerable evidence that the injury state is associated with significant changes in the processing of nociceptive information. Of particular interest to the present series of studies is the demonstration of central sensitization produced by intense peripheral stimulation or persistent injury (Woolf, 1983). The major features of central sensitization are manifest in the firing of dorsal horn neurons, including decreased threshold, increased receptive field size, and enhanced spontaneous activity. These physiological features correlate with the behavioral manifestation of the injury, namely hyperalgesia and allodynia, i.e. increased pain responses with noxious stimulation and pain induction by non-noxious stimuli, respectively. Although most studies have implicated glutamate acting at the NMDA receptor in the induction of central sensitization (Dickenson and Sullivan, 1987; Woolf and Thompson, 1991), there is also evidence for a contribution of SP. With a view to visualizing the changes that occur in the setting of inflammation, we thus next evaluated the effects of hindpaw stimulation on SP receptor internalization in the setting of inflammation (Abbaddie et al, in preparation).

Our first studies compared the effects of mechanical stimulation in the rat with unilateral inflammation of the hindpaw. We tested the rats at 3 days after induction of inflammation, which is the point where we found maximal expression of the receptor (Abbadie, et al., 1996). The major result from these studies is that in contrast to the normal rat, where SPR internalization was restricted to the superficial dorsal horn, noxious mechanical stimulation of the inflamed paw produced significant receptor internalization in neurons of laminae III-VI. Most importantly, under persistent inflammatory conditions, we could also evoke internalization with prolonged brushing of the hindpaw, a stimulus that is totally without effect in the normal rat. The latter result could have arisen from the activation of C fibers whose mechanical threshold had decreased as a result of a peripheral cyclooxygenase-dependent process. It is also possible that the receptor changes were induced by activation of large diameter fibers, which can excite dorsal horn neurons that have undergone central sensitization. Recent evidence that cell bodies of large diameter neurons begin to synthesize SP after nerve injury (Noguchi et al., 1994) or inflammation (Neumann et al., 1996) may be relevant.

The effective shift in the dose response curve for mechanical stimulation to induce receptor internalization and the greatly increased rostro-caudal distribution of SPR-immunoreactive neurons that showed internalization in rats with chronic inflammation was not observed when we used thermal stimulation. That is, the temperature dependence of the internalization was not altered in the rats with chronic inflammation; only at the highest temperature did we record any internalization in regions of the cord ventral to the superficially dorsal horn.

What could account for the appearance of internalization in neurons distant from the predominant location of SP containing primary afferents, namely laminae I and outer II? Two possibilities can be considered: The simplest explanation is that there is an activation of intrinsic neurons of the dorsal horn that express SP. There is little information on the distribution of these neurons, and almost no information on their axonal targets, however, their possible contribution cannot be ruled out. An alternative explanation is that under conditions of inflammation, there is much more extensive diffusion of SP in response to stimulation. As noted above, since ligand binding is essential for receptor internalization, the fact that receptors internalize over the entire surface of the neurons, indicates that there must be diffusion of SP, and that this diffusion has consequences. It is not a big jump, therefore, to suggest that peptide diffusion with functional consequences is exacerbated in the animals with persistent inflammation. There is, of course, considerable evidence that SP can diffuse considerable distances through tissue. For example, noxious stimulation evokes the release of SP into the spinal cord CSF (Yaksh et al., 1980); this must have arisen from diffusion of the peptide from the primary afferent terminals, dorsally into the CSF. Studies with labelled peptide injected in spinal CSF also demonstrated significant diffusion into the spinal tissue (Cridland et al., 1987). Using antibody coated microelectrodes, Duggan and colleagues found that there is diffusion of tachykinins in the dorsal horn (Duggan et al., 1992; Hope et al., 1990) and that this is increased in persistent injury conditions (Schaible et al., 1990). Interestingly, there is much greater diffusion of NKA, the tachykinin that co-occurs with SP in primary afferent terminals, apparently because NKA is not a substrate for the neutral endopeptidase that degrades SP (Duggan, et al., 1992). Finally, the fact that intrathecal injection of SP can evoke pain behavior provides additional evidence that SP can diffuse relatively quickly within the spinal cord tissue (Hylden and Wilcox, 1981).

Taken together, these results indicate that there are significant changes in the interaction of SP with its receptor in normal rats and in rats with persistent inflammation. Our results suggest that upregulation of SP receptor as well as diffusion of SP from the superficial laminae of the dorsal horn greatly increase the population of neurons that are influenced by peptide release from the primary afferent. The question of the long-term consequences of the internalization remains. Clearly, receptor desensitization is not the purpose of internalization; desensitization occurs before the receptor has been internalized (Garland et al., 1994; Grady et al., 1996). One possibility is that internalization and recycling regulate the time course of resensitization; this will depend also on the extent to which the receptor is completely stripped from the membrane. On a longer time scale, we suggest that the consequences of SP interaction with its receptor contribute to central sensitization, which will significantly influence the response properties of dorsal horn nociresponsive neurons. The duration over which this occurs will also depend on the molecular consequences of the SP-SP receptor interaction.

Our next series of studies examined the effects of analgesic doses of morphine on the pattern and magnitude of receptor internalization in normal rats and in rats with persistent inflammation. There is considerable evidence that morphine exerts its analgesic action in part via blockade of the release of SP from primary afferents (Jessell and Iversen, 1977). The presence of opioid receptors on primary afferents provides a substrate for this action (Ji et al., 1995; Lamotte et al., 1976). Our first studies used systemic injection. Morphine was administered twenty minutes prior to application of the noxious stimulus. Five minutes after the noxious stimulus, the rats were perfused and the tissue processed for SPR immunoreactivity. Thus, the noxious stimulus was presented at a time when morphine action is at its peak. Although these studies were performed under general anesthesia, we used a dose that our previous studies demonstrated to be analgesic (10 mg/kg). To our surprise, we found almost no effect of systemic morphine on the percentage of cells that showed internalization of the SP receptor in response to noxious pinch (Abbadie et al, in preparation). This was true for normal rats and rats with hindpaw inflammation. At most we found a 10% inhibition of receptor internalization. This result suggests that the analgesia produced by systemic morphine (at least at the dose used) does not involve significant inhibition of release of SP from primary afferents. Interestingly, our results are in agreement with a release study that also found no change in SP release after systemic injection of morphine (Morton et al., 1990).

Since the concentration of morphine given systemically may not effectively block primary afferent receptors, we also attempted to block release by intrathecal injection of opioids. Neither morphine, nor more selective ligands were effective. Although these results were unexpected, they provided interesting confirmation of a conclusion that we drew concerning the persistence of information processing in the spinal cord in the setting of morphine analgesia. Specifically, our earlier studies demonstrated that noxious stimulus-evoked Fos expression is not completely blocked in rats made analgesic by systemic or supraspinal injection of opioids (Gogas et al., 1996; Gogas et al., 1991; Jasmin et al., 1994; Presley et al., 1990). It is conceivable, in fact, that downstream consequences of SP interaction with its receptor and internalization are related to the induction of molecular changes exemplified by the induction of the c-fos proto-oncogene. It follows that despite complete analgesia, there may be persistent and profound cell biological consequences of a noxious stimulus. These changes may underlie a persistent central sensitization that can influence subsequent responses to noxious stimulation.

In summary, by following the interaction of SP with its receptor, and by using internalization of the receptor to monitor the responsiveness of neurons of the dorsal horn, our results emphasize that there are important and possibly long lasting differences between the transmission of nociceptive messages in the normal rat and in the rat that experiences persistent injury. Preventing these changes may be an effective approach to preventing long term negative consequences of injury.

Acknowledgements

This work was supported by grants from the National Institutes of Health: DE08973, NS21445 and NS14627.

Plenary discussion

Basmadjian G.: You mentioned that morphine systemically does not block substance P, but intrathecally it does. Is the mechanism of this blockage known? Are there other drugs known to block substance P when given systemically?

Basbaum A.: I believe that intrathecal morphine must be working by presynaptic block of substance P release from primary afferents. Systemic morphine since it doesn't block substance P receptor internalization must be working via postsynaptic mechanisms.
The answer to the second part of your question is: "Not yet."

Wall P.: Is the communication from dorsal to ventral via intra- or extra-cellular mechanisms?

Basbaum A.: We believe that it is extracellular but cannot rule out a contribution of substance P-containing interneurons.

Saade N.: Have you looked into a possible rostro-caudal migration of substance P receptor expression?

Basbaum A.: There is definitely a rostro-caudal approach, beyond the primary afferent projection.

Saade N.: Could this migration of substance P receptor from marginal to deep laminae be related to autonomic manifestations related to inflammatory pain?

Basbaum A.: We have no data on this point.

Besson J.-M.: I am not contesting your data on the lack of effect of systemic morphine on substance P internalization, it is in agreement with other approaches. What do you think in general of the role of substance P in controlling nociception processes at the spinal cord level?

Basbaum A.: I do not believe that it is the primary contributor to nociceptive transmission; glutamate is almost certainly the key player. Substance P, however, exacerbates and prolongs the effects produced by glutamate.

Reeh W.: What is the evidence for hyperalgesic behavior of rats injected with formalin, apart from their paws being inflamed?

Basbaum A.: We have found mechanical allodynia. Others find hypo or hyperalgesia in thermal tests.

Amassian V.: Are the two phases of nociceptive responses you describe determined by the initial flurry of impulses when you inject the formalin? It would be hard in the mouse, but easy in the cat, to do a nerve block soon after the injection to see if you get the first phase without the second.

Basbaum A.: Although some studies argue that activity during the first phase drives the second phase; our data using remifentanil (a short acting opiate) during the first phase suggest that the second phase is independent.

Berkley K.: How long after injury is "internalization" evident?

Basbaum A.: The substance P receptor recycles to the membrane within one hour.

Berkley K.: Would you expect to see this internalization in a spinalized rat?

Basbaum A.: I would expect it to persist and possibly increase, if spinalization reduces presynaptic inhibitory controls.

Panossian A.: Do your results mean that components which inhibit PKC activity will relieve the pain induced by chronic inflammation?

Basbaum A.: Our results suggest that selective PKC (antagonists might be particularly useful for neuropathic pain.

Ayrapetyan S.: What allows you to conclude that your observation in receptor dynamics is specific for substance P?

Basbaum A.: In the striatum we showed:
1. a dose-dependent effect of substance P;
2. blockade by selective substance P receptor (NK-1) antagonists;
3. that NKA does not provoke SP receptor internalization.
Finally, the noxious stimulus-evoked changes are mimicked by intrathecal injection of SP, which also produces a dose-dependent internalization.

Morpurgo C.: Which is the dose of morphine you consider appropriate for intrathecal administration as compared with the intravenous one?

Basbaum A.: We use 10mg/kg systematically and 10mg (i.e. about 30mg/kg) intrathecally.

References

Abbadie C, Brown J L, Mantyh P W and Basbaum A I (1996) Spinal cord substance P receptor immunoreactivity increases in both inflammatory and nerve injury models of persistent pain. Neuroscience 70:201-209.

Brown J L, Liu H, Maggio J E, Vigna S R, Mantyh P W and Basbaum A I (1995) Morphological characterization of substance P receptor-immunoreactive neurons in the rat spinal cord and trigeminal nucleus caudalis. J Comp Neurol 356:327-344.

Cridland R A, Yashpal K, Romita V V, Gauthier S and Henry J L (1987) Distribution of label after intrathecal administration of 125I-substance P in the rat. Peptides 8:213-221.

Dickenson A H and Sullivan A F (1987) Evidence for a role of the NMDA receptor in the frequency dependent potentiation of deep rat dorsal horn nociceptive neurons following C fiber stimulation. Neuropharmacol. 26:1235-1238.

Duggan A W, Hendry I A, Morton C R, Hutchison W D and Zhao Z Q (1988) Cutaneous stimuli releasing immunoreactive substance P in the dorsal horn of the cat. Brain Res 451:261-273.

Duggan A W, Schaible H G, Hope P J and Lang C W (1992) Effect of peptidase inhibition on the pattern of intraspinally released immunoreactive substance P detected with antibody microprobes. Brain Res 579:261-269.

Garland A M, Grady E F, Payan D G, Vigna S R and Bunnett N W (1994) Agonist-induced internalization of the substance P (NK1) receptor expressed in epithelial cells. Biochem J 303:177-186.

Gogas K R, Cho H J, Botchkina G I, Levine J D and Basbaum A I (1996) Inhibition of noxious stimulus-evoked pain behaviors and neuronal Fos-like immunoreactivity in the spinal cord of the rat by supraspinal morphine. Pain 65:9-15.

Gogas K R, Presley R W, Levine J D and Basbaum A I (1991) The antinociceptive action of supraspinal opioids results from an increase in descending inhibitory control: Correlation of nociceptive behavior and c-fos expression. Neuroscience 42:617-628.

Grady E F, Gamp P D, Jones E, Baluk P, McDonald D M, Payan D G and Bunnett N W (1996) Endocytosis and recycling of neurokinin 1 receptors in enteric neurons. Neuroscience 75:1239-1254.

Hokfelt T, Kellerth J -O, Nilsson G and Pernow B (1975) Substance P: Localization in the central nervous system and in some primary sensory neurons. Science 190:889-890.

Hope P J, Jarrott B, Schaible H G, Clarke R W and Duggan A W (1990) Release and spread of immunoreactive neurokinin A in the cat spinal cord in a model of acute arthritis. Brain Res 533:292-299.

Hylden J L and Wilcox G L (1981) Intrathecal substance P elicits a caudally-directed biting and scratching behavior in mice. Brain Res 217:212-215.

Jasmin L, Wang H, Tarczy-Hornoch K, Levine J D and Basbaum A I (1994) Differential effects of morphine on noxious stimulus-evoked Fos-like immunoreactivity in subpopulations of spinoparabrachial neurons. J Neurosci 14:7252-7260.

Jessell T, Tsunoo A, Kanazawa I and Otsuka M (1979) Substance P: depletion in the dorsal horn of rat spinal cord after section of the peripheral processes of primary sensory neurons. Brain Res 168:247-259.

Jessell T M and Iversen L L (1977) Opiate analgesics inhibit substance P release from rat trigeminal nucleus. Nature (Lond.) 268:549-551.

Ji R R, Zhang Q, Law P Y, Low H H, Elde R and Hökfelt T (1995) Expression of mu-, delta-, and kappa-opioid receptor-like immunoreactivities in rat dorsal root ganglia after carrageenan-induced inflammation. J Neurosci 15:8156-8166.

Kuraishi Y, Hirota N, Sato Y, Hino Y, Satoh M and Akagi H (1985) Evidence that substance P and somatostatin transmit separate information related to pain in the spinal dorsal horn. Brain Res 325:294-298.

Lamotte C, Pert CB and Snyder S H (1976) Opiate receptor binding in primate spinal cord: distribution and changes after dorsal root section. Brain Res 112:407-412.

Lembeck F, Donnerer J and Colpaert F C (1981) Increase of substance P in primary afferent nerves during chronic pain. Neuropeptides 1:175-180.

Levine J D, Fields H L and Basbaum A I (1993) Peptides and the primary afferent nociceptor. J Neurosci 13:2273-2286.

Liu H, Brown J L, Jasmin L, Maggio J E, Vigna S R, Mantyh P W and Basbaum A I (1994) Synaptic relationship between substance P and the substance P receptor: Light and electron microscopic characterization of the mismatch between neuropeptides and their receptors. Proc Natl Acad Sci (USA) 91:1009-1013.

Mantyh P W, Allen C J, Ghilardi J R, Rogers S D, Mantyh C R, Liu H, Basbaum A I, Vigna S R and Maggio J E (1995) Rapid endocytosis of a G protein-coupled receptor: Substance P-evoked internalization of its receptor in the rat striatum in vivo. Proc Natl Acad Sci (USA) 92:2622-2626.

Mantyh P W, DeMaster E, Malhotra A, Ghilardi J R, Rogers S D, Mantyh C R, Liu H, Basbaum A I, Vigna S R, Maggio J E and Simone D A (1995) Receptor endocytosis and dendrite reshaping in spinal neurons after somatosensory stimulation. Science 268:1629-1632.

McCarson K E and Krause J E (1994) NK-1 and NK-3 type tachykinin receptor mRNA expression in the rat spinal cord dorsal horn is increased during adjuvant or formalin-induced nociception. J Neurosci 14:712-720.

Morton C R, Hutchison W D, Duggan A W and Hendry I A (1990) Morphine and substance P release in the spinal cord. Exp Brain Res 82:89-96.

Morton C R, Hutchison W D, Hendry I A and Duggan A W (1989) Somatostatin: Evidence for a role in thermal nociception. Brain Res 488:89-96.

Neumann S, Doubell T P, Leslie T and Woolf C J (1996) Inflammatory pain hypersensitivity mediated by phenotypic switch in myelinated primary sensory neurons. Nature (Lond). 384:360-364.

Noguchi K, Dubner R, De L M, Senba E and Ruda M A (1994) Axotomy induces preprotachykinin gene expression in a subpopulation of dorsal root ganglion neurons. J Neurosci Res 37:596-603.

Noguchi K, Morita Y, Kiyama H, Ono K and Tohyama M (1988) A noxious stimulus induces the preprotachykinin-A gene expression in the rat dorsal root ganglion: a quantitative study using in situ hybridization histochemistry. Mol Brain Res 4:31-35.

Presley R W, Menétrey D, Levine J D and Basbaum A I (1990) Systemic morphine suppresses noxious stimulus-evoked Fos protein-like immunoreactivity in the rat spinal cord. J Neurosci 10:323-335.

Schaible H G, Jarrott B, Hope B J and Duggan A W (1990) Release of immunoreactive substance P in the spinal cord during development of acute arthritis in the knee joint of the cat: A study with antibody microprobes. Brain Res 529:214-223.

Woolf C J (1983) Evidence for a central component of post-injury pain hypersensitivity. Nature (Lond). 308:686-688.

Woolf C J and Thompson S (1991) The induction and maintenance of central sensitization is dependent on N-methyl-D-aspartic acid receptor activation; Implications for the treatment of post-injury pain hypersensitivity states. Pain 44:293-299.

Yaksh T L, Jessell T M, Gamse R, Mudge A W and Leeman A E (1980) Intrathecal morphine inhibits substance P release from mammalian spinal cord in vivo. Nature (Lond.) 286:155-157.

Pain Mechanisms and Management
S.N. Ayrapetyan and A.V. Apkarian (Eds.)
IOS Press, 1998

Morphine and Noxiously Evoked Spinal Fos Expression Induced by Carrageenin Inflammation

Prisca Honoré and Jean-Marie Besson
Physiopharmacologie du Système Nerveux
INSERM U 161
and
Laboratoire de Physiopharmacologie de la Douleur (EPHE)
Paris, France

The discovery of the proto-oncogene *c-fos* at the beginning of the 80's had a lot of important consequences in various research fields such as oncology but also neurobiology (Dragunow and Robertson 1987, Hunt et al. 1987, Morgan et al. 1987, Sagar et al. 1988). The induction of proto-oncogenes is rapid, transient and protein synthesis independent (see references in Hughes and Dragunow 1995, Morgan 1991). In the field of pain research, Hunt et al. (1987) has been the first to show that cutaneous stimulations could induce *c-fos* protein (Fos) expression in neurons of the dorsal horn of the spinal cord in the rat. After this original study, numerous other studies have clearly demonstrated that spinal Fos expression is essentially induced by various types of nociceptive processes (see references in Abbadie et al. 1994b, Zieglgänsberger and Tölle 1993). In addition, at the level of the spinal cord, the basal Fos expression is negligible and animal handling or injection of saline does not induce spinal Fos expression. Thus, since in the absence of peripheral stimulation in freely moving rats there is virtually no background activity, the immunohistochemical study of the level of spinal Fos protein following various types of noxious stimuli is ideal. Furthermore c-fos is one of the first IEGs to be induced, the half life of which is relatively short, and the resultant rapid speed of onset/offset of *c-fos* induction following stimulation means that the level of Fos follows closely the intensity/duration of the noxious stimulation.

Morphine is a well established potent analgesic which is efficient when considering all classical nociceptive tests. Therefore it is considered to be a drug of reference when studying various types of nociceptive responses. The depressive effects of morphine upon the transmission of nociceptive messages at the level of the dorsal horn of the spinal cord is well established and documented (see references in Basbaum and Besson 1991, Dickenson 1994, Duggan and North 1984) and it has been clearly established that the effect of morphine is selective for noxiously evoked responses of dorsal horn (Duggan et al. 1977, Le Bars et al. 1975).

After the first study of Presley et al. (1990), numerous pharmacological studies have shown that the intravenous (i.v.), intracerebroventricular (i.c.v.) or subcutaneous (s.c.) injection of morphine decreases the number of Fos-like immuoreactive (Fos-LI) neurons observed in the dorsal horn of the rat spinal cord after various types of nociceptive stimulations such as noxious heat, noxious cold, intraplantar injection of formalin, mechanical stimulation the polyarthritic rat, intraperitoneal injection of acetic acid, nociceptive colorectal distention and chemical stimulation of the meninges (see Table 1 for references). In general, the majority of these studies have demonstrated dose-related effects of morphine which are blocked by naloxone.

Table 1. Effects of morphine on noxiously evoked spinal Fos expression.

Studies	route	doses	Effects (reduction)	stimulation
Abbadie et al. 1994c	s.c.	10mg/kg	53%	3min., -20°C
Hammond et al. 1992	s.c.	10mg/kg	100%	acetic acid i.p. 3.5% 0,5ml
Presley et al. 1990	s.c.	10mg/kg	79%	formalin 5% 150μl
Jasmin et al. 1994	s.c.	10+5mg/kg	60%	formalin 5% 100μl
Nozaki et al. 1992	s.c.	15μmol/kg	63%	meninges stimulation
Abbadie et Besson 1993a	i.v.	3mg/kg	96%	mechanical (arthritic rat)
Abbadie et al. 1994a	i.v.	7.5mg/kg	75%	15sec., 52°C
Honore et al. 1995	i.v.	3mg/kg	60%	carrageenin 6% 150μl
Tölle et al. 1990, 1994a,b	i.v.	10mg/kg	71%	noxious heat stimulation
Traub et al. 1995	i.v.	5mg/kg	58%	colorectal distension
Gogas et al. 1996	i.c.v.	14.5nmol	75%	formalin 5% 100μl

As shown in Table 1, the results of these studies on the effects of morphine are not homogeneous, with morphine being more or less potent depending on the study. This large variability in the effects of morphine may be related to the type of noxious stimulation employed in addition to the varying intensity and duration of noxious stimuli, relative to the time course of the effects of systemic morphine. Taken together, these results are difficult to compare, but the effects of morphine seem more pronounced when an inflammatory stimulation is applied.

In the laboratory, we have started an extensive study on the effects of morphine on noxiously evoked spinal Fos expression, evaluating the time course of these effects, their specificity, but also the effects of the peripheral administration of morphine, the development of tolerance to these peripheral anti-nociceptive effects and the numerous interactions between the effects of morphine and other compounds influencing the transmission of nociceptive informations at the spinal level. In order to realize all these studies, we have used as nociceptive stimulation, the intraplantar injection of λ-carrageenin (Winter et al. 1962) in the rear paw of freely moving rats, which produces an acute restricted inflammation associated with thermal and mechanical hyperalgesia and allodynia (Hargreaves et al. 1988, Iadarola et al. 1988, Joris et al. 1990, Kayser and Guilbaud 1987) and spinal Fos expression (Draisci and Iadarola 1989, Honoré et al. 1995, Noguchi et al. 1991, 1992).

As you can see in Figure 1A, three hours after intraplantar carrageenin injection (6mg/150 µl), Fos-LI neurons are present in the dorsal horn of the spinal segments L2-L6, ipsilateral to the site of injection, with a maximal number of Fos-LI neurons observed in lumbar segments L4-L5, equally distributed between the superficial laminae (I and II) and deep laminae (V and VI) of the spinal dorsal horn. These results are in agreement with the spinal projections of the primary afferent innervating the rear paw of the rat (LaMotte et al. 1991, Molander et al. 1984, Molander and Grant 1986).

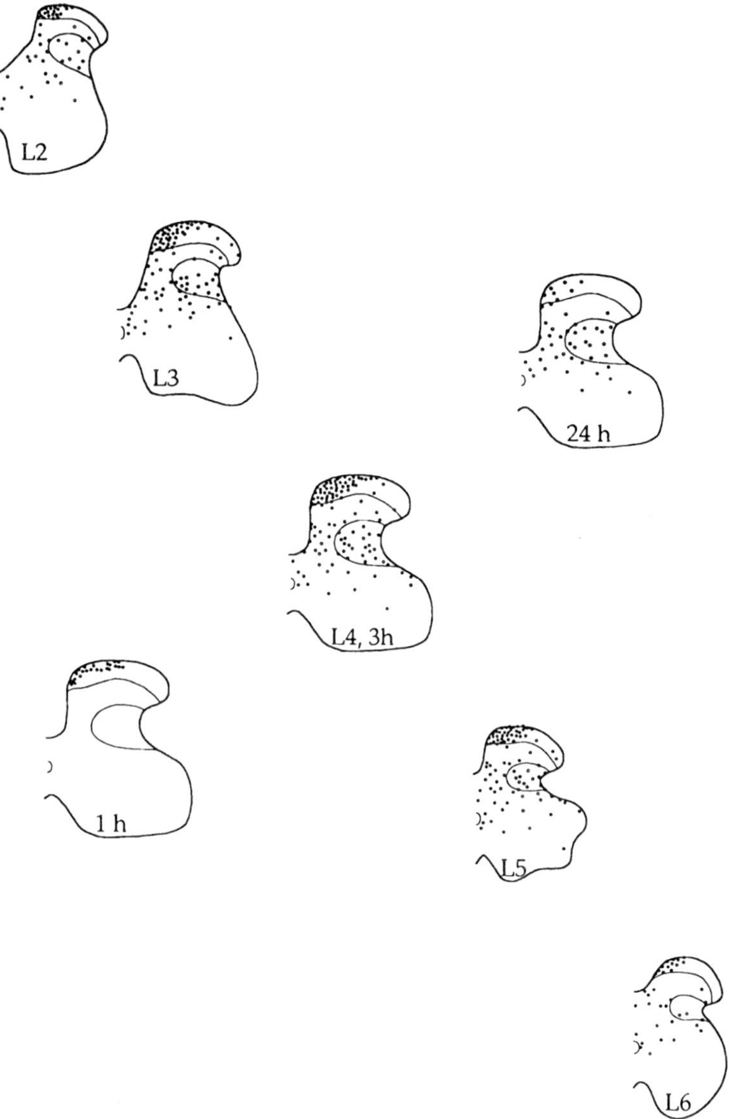

Figure 1. Intraplantar carrageenin induced spinal Fos expression. Each schema includes all Fos-LI neurons in one 40 (m section; each dot represents one Fos-LI neuron. This figure is showing the distribution of Fos-LI neurons 3 hours after intraplantar carrageenin in spinal lumbar segment L2-L6 and the spinal Fos expression at the level of the lumbar segment L4 1 hour, 3 hours and 24 hours after intraplantar carrageenin injection.

The number of Fos-LI neurons and their laminar distribution vary depending on the time point observed after intraplantar carrageenin (Figure 1B). Very few Fos-like immunoreactive (Fos-LI) neurons were observed 0.5 h after carrageenin. However, spinal Fos expression increased initially (at 1 hr), in the superficial laminae (I-II) of the spinal dorsal horn, and incrementally increased both in the superficial and deep (V-VI) laminae at later time points after carrageenin to reach a maximum at 3 to 4 hours. When looking at 24 hours, the total number of Fos-LI neurons has decreased and the remaining neurons are preferentially located in the deep laminae of the spinal dorsal horn. This time course of spinal Fos expression is parallel to the increase of mRNA of *c-fos* (Draisci and Iadarola 1989) and the development of peripheral inflammation observed after intraplantar carrageenin injection.

Time course of the effects of morphine

As already mentioned, there are some discrepancies concerning the degree of effect of morphine on spinal Fos expression which may be related to the type, the intensity and the duration of noxious stimulation used, the route of morphine administration, the use or absence of anesthesia, and the delay between stimulation and perfusion. With regards to this latter point, we have recently evaluated the effects of morphine on spinal Fos expression induced at various time points after carrageenin injection (Honoré et al. 1996c). In this study, pre-administered morphine (3mg/kg i.v.) strongly reduced carrageenin evoked spinal Fos expression in the superficial laminae at 1.5 hrs after carrageenin (58±3% reduction of control), but was significantly less efficacious at 2.5 hrs after carrageenin injection (34±6% reduction of control; Figure 2). Thus, the peak effect of pre-administered morphine on carrageenin evoked spinal Fos expression was observed 1.5 hrs and 2 hrs after intraplantar carrageenin, with a weaker effect observed at 2.5 hrs after carrageenin. Furthermore, since spinal Fos expression increased in a parallel fashion between 2 hrs and 2.5 hrs in both the control and morphine groups, these results strongly suggest that the differences seen between the two groups are merely a reflection of the earlier suppression of spinal Fos expression and that morphine is no more active. These results clearly illustrate the importance of multiple considerations both in terms of the onset and duration of drug action relative to the time of spinal Fos expression when determining the optimum time point of the action of morphine, or of other analgesic compounds.

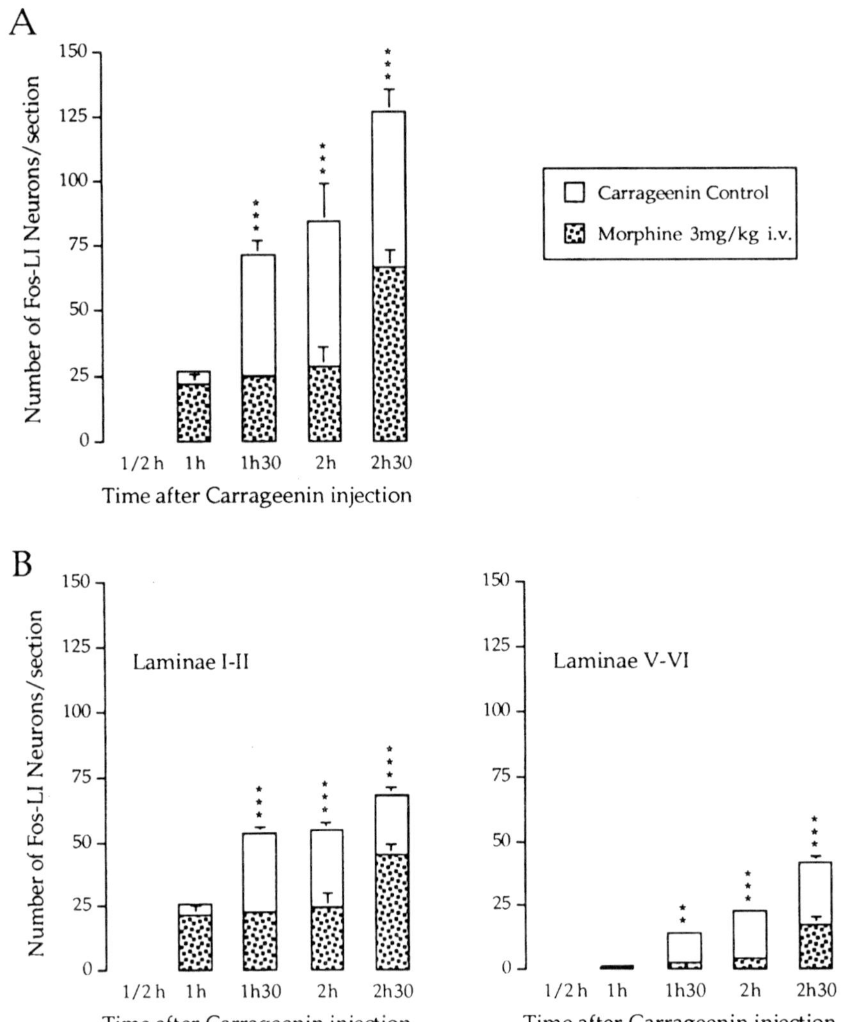

Figure 2. Time course of the effects of morphine (3mg/kg i.v.) on carrageenin induced spinal Fos expression. Results are expressed as number of Fos-LI neurons/section (mean ± s.e.m.) (A) for the total number and (B) for the superficial or deep laminae in the spinal segments L4-L5. Anova and PLSD, **p<0.01; ***p<0.001 as compared to control).

Specificitiy of the effects of morphine

As already mentioned, the effects of morphine are usually blocked by a coadministration of naloxone, which is a low specificity opioid receptor antagonist. We have demonstrated, in another experiment, that pre-administered morphine (3mg/kg i.v.) decreased spinal Fos expression induced 2 hrs after intraplantar carrageenin (55±5% reduction, p<0.0001), these effects being completely blocked by pre-administered β-Funaltrexamine (10mg/kg i.v., 24 hrs prior to stimulation) a selective long-lasting μ-opioid receptor antagonist (Portoghese et at. 1980). In conclusion, these results clearly demonstrate that the effects of morphine on noxiously-evoked spinal Fos expression are essentially mediated via μ-opioid receptors (Honoré et al. 1996b). This major role of μ-opioid receptor activation in the effects of morphine has been confirmed showing that both antagonists of the delta or kappa opioid receptors such as naltrindole or norbinaltorphimine do not significantly modify the effects of morphine on carrageenin induced spinal Fos expression.

The ability of systemic morphine to reduce noxiously evoked spinal Fos expression is in keeping with the well established depressive effect of morphine at the spinal level (see references in Dickenson 1994a). Although the direct action of morphine at the dorsal horn level is well documented there is additional controversial electrophysiological evidence concerning the ability of morphine to increase (for review see Basbaum and Fields 1978), or not (Bouhassira et al. 1988), the activity of the descending inhibitory controls. In keeping with the former concept it has been shown that i.c.v. administered morphine or DAMGO dose-dependently reduced formalin evoked spinal Fos expression, at the lumbar level, in a naloxone reversible manner (Gogas et al. 1991, 1996). These findings were interpreted as suggesting that the analgesic action of supraspinally administered opiates results from an increase in descending inhibitory controls that regulate the firing of certain populations of spinal neurons.

Peripheral effects of morphine

Traditional thought has associated anti-nociceptive effects of opiates with activation of opioid receptors located in the central nervous (for recent review see Dickenson 1994a). However, there is accumulating experimental and clinical evidence that, in particular under inflammatory conditions, exogenous opioids can also produce anti-nociceptive effects by interacting with peripheral opioid receptors (for review see Stein 1993, 1995). We have addressed this issue by considering the effect of intraplantar injection of morphine on spinal Fos expression evoked by intraplantar injection of carrageenin as compared to noxious heat stimulation (Honoré et al. 1996a). Intraplantar morphine (10-50 μg/ 50 μl) dose-dependently reduced carrageenin (Table 2), but not noxious heat (52°C during 15 seconds) evoked spinal Fos expression. We have clearly demonstrated that these effects were opioid receptor mediated and strictly peripheral since there is an effect after local administration but not after systemic administration of an equal dose of morphine. In addition, the effects of intraplantar morphine are dose-dependent and blocked by intraplantar methiodide naloxone, which does not cross the blood brain barrier.

Table 2. Effects of i.pl. morphine on carrageenin induced spinal Fos expression. Results are expressed as percentages of control values ± s.e.m. observed 1.5hr and 3hrs after the intraplantar carrageenin injection for the total number of Fos-LI per section (Total) and in the various laminae of the dorsal horn. Significance is expressed as compared to the control group (*p<0.05; **p<0.01; ***p<0.001).

		1h30		3h		
Drugs	Dose (μg)	Total	Laminae I-II	Total	Laminae I-II	Laminae V-VI
Morphine	10 (i.pl.)	81±8%	77±9% *	84±2% ***	75±3% ***	87±3% *
	25 (i.pl.)	74±6%	63±5% **	82±2% ***	78±2% ***	84±5% *
	50 (i.pl.)	55±4% **	53±2% ***	63±3% ***	58±1% ***	67±4% ***
Morphine + Meth Nx	50 (i.pl.) 20 (i.pl.)	121±22%	109±12%	110±3% *	108±4%	110±5%
Meth Nx	20 (i.pl.)	124±4%	116±3%	90±3% *	93±3%	87±4% *
Morphine	50 (i.v.)	88±9%	88±9%	———	———	———

Such results confirmed that peripheral effects of morphine preferentially occur during inflammatory states and strongly outline the interest of using peripheral opioids in clinical inflammatory pain states.

Tolerance to the effects of morphine

The development of tolerance associated with repeated injection of morphine is well documented. Numerous studies have shown that tolerance develops to both systemically (see references in Cox 1991, Detweiler et al. 1995, Gold et al. 1994, Kissin et al. 1991, Paronis and Holzman 1992) and spinally administered μ-opioid agonists (Advokat et al. 1987, Kalso et al. 1993, Nishino et al. 1990, Stevens and Yaksh 1989, 1992, Yaksh et al. 1977). However, in the literature, there is controversy about the appearance of tolerance to the anti-nociceptive effects of intraplantar μ-opioid agonists (Aley et al. 1995 for DAMGO; see however Ferreira et al. 1984 for morphine).

In addition, there is evidence that the phenomenon of opioid tolerance can be detected by the Fos technique. It has previously been shown that the level of noxious heat evoked spinal Fos expression in rats rendered tolerant to morphine is not different from the level evoked in naive rats (see however Rohde et al. 1993), nevertheless the ability of systemic morphine to reduce Fos expression in tolerant rats was reduced by 50% as compared to naive rats (Abbadie et al. 1994a).

In a recent study, the effects of intravenous (3 mg/kg i.v.) and intraplantar (50 μg/μl.) morphine were investigated on spinal Fos expression induced 2 hrs after intraplantar carrageenin (6 mg/150 μl), and on carrageenin (2 mg/150 μl) induced mechanical allodynia, at day 4, in both naive and chronic morphine treated rats (80 mg/kg/day s.c. on days 1, 2 and 3; Honoré et al. 1997). In naive rats, i.v. and i.pl. morphine significantly decreased spinal Fos expression and mechanical allodynia which only developed in carrageenin injected paw. Both treatments were ineffective in chronic morphine treated rats.

These studies based on spinal Fos expression as an indirect marker of spinal nociceptive processes and on behavioral experiments clearly revealed that chronic treatment with systemic morphine induced tolerance to both its systemic and peripheral effects.

Opioid receptor mediated effects do not occur in isolation, but there is considerable interaction with other spinal transmitters. We have used the Fos technique to investigate the eventual interactions of the opioidergic systems with the various other transmitter systems implicated in nociceptive processing at the level of the dorsal horn. In the following section we will present evidence in favor of such interactions which are in agreement with, and extend, previous electrophysiological and behavioral observations.

Morphine and cholecystokinin B receptor antagonists

The antinociceptive effects of morphine at the level of the spinal cord have been shown to be subject to an ongoing modulation by cholecystokinin (CCK), with CCK attenuating the effects of μ-opioid agonists at the spinal level (Barbaz et al. 1989, Faris et al. 1984, Magnuson et al. 1990, Wiesenfeld-Hallin and Duranti 1987) and selective CCK_B receptor antagonists enhancing morphine analgesia (Dourish et al. 1990, Wiesenfeld-Hallin et al. 1990, Xu et al. 1994, Zhou et al. 1993).

We have investigated whether an interaction between the effect of morphine and L-365,260, a CCK_B receptor antagonist, can the noxiously evoked spinal Fos expression

(Chapman et al. 1995). In this study the effects of two concentrations of systemically administered morphine with, and without, prior administration of a standard concentration of L-365,260 on carrageenin evoked spinal Fos expression were assessed.

The administration of an inactive dose of L-365,260 (0.2mg/kg s.c.) reveals the antinociceptive effects of a previously inactive dose of morphine (0.3 mg/kg i.v., Figure 3) but does not increase the strong antinociceptive effects of a high dose of morphine (3 mg/kg i.v.).

These results demonstrating the ability of a normally ineffective dose of morphine to reduce the spinal expression of Fos when co-administered with L-365,260, are in agreement with the well documented potentiation between morphine and CCK_B receptor antagonists as shown by behavioral and electrophysiological studies (see references above). However the effect of a higher concentration of morphine was not enhanced by L-365,260, suggesting that either the effects of the higher dose of morphine are less open to CCK modulation or that a different dose of L-365,260 is required to modulate the effect of this dose of morphine. It is important to note that none of the various drug administrations influenced the peripheral carrageenin evoked edema suggesting spinal and / or supra-spinal sites of action.

In conclusion these results provide evidence that CCK_B receptor antagonism enhances the ability of a low dose of morphine to reduce the longer term intracellular events, the induction and expression of Fos, associated with prolonged pain processing.

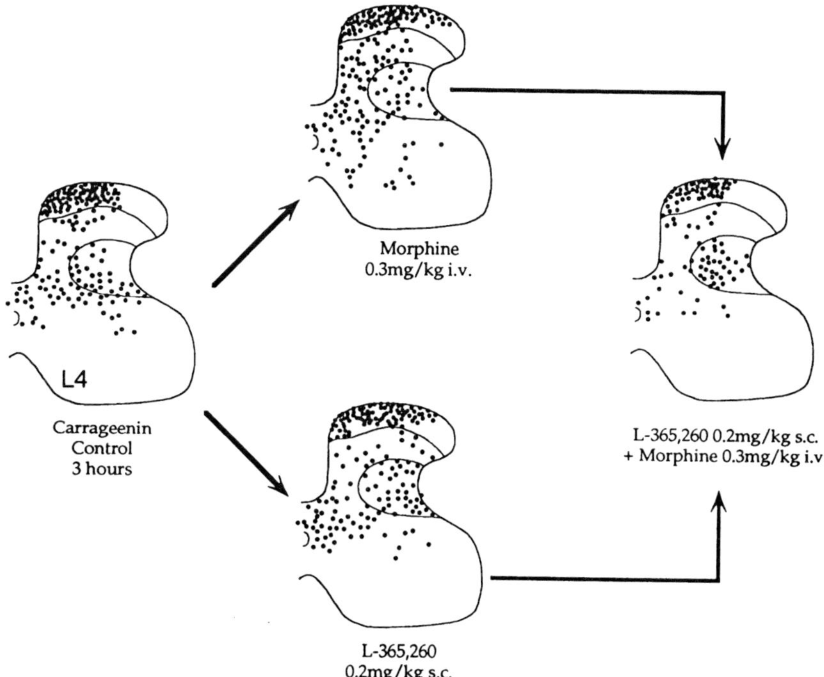

Figure 3. A comparison of the effect of morphine, versus L-365,260, a CCK_B receptor antagonist, versus morphine plus L-365,260 on carrageenin evoked spinal Fos expression. Individual example section of the spinal cord (L4-L5 segment) are presented. Each drawing includes all Fos-LI neurons in one 40 (m section; each dot represents one Fos-LI neuron.

Morphine and α2-adrenoceptor agonists

Previous studies have clearly demonstrated the modulation of nociceptive transmission, at the spinal level, by descending noradrenergic systems (see referenes in Yaksh 1985), which is predominantly mediated by α2-adrenoceptors (see references in Proudfit 1988). The spinal administration of α2-adrenoceptor agonists, mimicking the descending antinociceptive systems produces anti-nociception both in terms of behavioral (Fischer et al. 1991, Kalso et al. 1991, Puke and Wiesenfeld-Hallin 1993) and neuronal (Fleetwood-Walker et al. 1985, Pertovaara et al. 1991, Sullivan et al. 1987, 1992) responses. An early study implicated both α1- and α2 -adrenoceptor subtypes in the attenuating effect of norepinephrine on spinal Fos-LI neurons following noxious heat stimulation (Jones 1992). Subsequently we have demonstrated that systemic administration of medetomidine, a selective α2-adrenoceptor agonist, dose-dependently reduces carrageenin evoked spinal Fos expression, effects associated with a parallel reduction of the peripheral edema (Honoré et al.1996d). These effects were blocked by the selective (α2-adrenoceptor antagonist atipamezole) (see also Pertovaara et al. 1993).

In addition to the independent anti-nociceptive effect of α2-adrenoceptor agonists, it is well documented that co-administration of an α2-adrenoceptor agonist with opioids, predominantly morphine, results in dramatically enhanced anti-nociceptive effects as compared to the individual effect of either drug (Loomis et al. 1987, Monasky et al. 1990, Ossipov et al. 1990, Pertovaara et al. 1993, Sullivan et al. 1987, 1992, and see references in Yaksh 1985). We have recently investigated the effect of co-administration of the selective α-adrenoceptor agonist medetomidine and morphine on carrageenin evoked spinal Fos expression and inflammation (Honoré et al. 1996d).

In this study, we have shown that the co-administration of an inactive dose of morphine (1.5 mg/kg i.v.) and a weakly effective dose of medetomidine (12.5 µg/kg i.v.) significantly and strongly decreased the total number of Fos-LI neurons (51±8%, reduction as compared to control carrageenin Fos-LI expression, Table 3). The effects of this co-administration were significantly greater than that of medetomidine alone (p<0.001) and morphine alone (p<0.0001). Both atipamezole (75 µg/kg i.v.) and the combined injection of atipamezole and naloxone (1 mg/kg i.v.) significantly blocked the effects of co-administered medetomidine and morphine on the total number of Fos-LI neurons (p<0.05 and p<0.05 as compared to co-administered medetomidine and morphine group, respectively).

Interestingly, the enhanced effect of morphine and medetomidine on spinal Fos expression was not paralleled by an enhancement of the effects of medetomidine, by morphine, on the peripheral edema, thus suggesting that the effects of this co-administration represent a central site of interaction.

In conclusion, we found that co-administration of low doses of morphine plus medetomidine greatly reduced the level of carrageenin evoked spinal Fos expression, thus illustrating that the well established potentiation between opiates and α2-adrenoceptor systems (see references in Dickenson1994a) influences one of the down-stream consequences of nociceptive transmission, the spinal expression of Fos.

Table 3. A comparison of the effect of morphine, versus Medetomidine, an α2-adrenoceptor agonist, versus morphine plus Medetomidine on carrageenin evoked spinal Fos expression. Results are expressed as percentages of control values $\pm$ s.e.m. observed 3 hrs after the intraplantar carrageenin injection for the total number of Fos-LI per section (Total) and in the various laminae of the dorsal horn. Significance is expressed as compared to the control group (*), the morphine treated group (+) and the medetomidine treated group (°). (***p<0.001).

Drugs	Dose (iv)	3h		
		Total	Laminae I-II	Laminae V-VI
Medetomidine	12.5µg/kg	87±4%	100±3%	73±7%
Morphine	1.5mg/kg	100±9%	100±4%	100±13%
Medetomidine + Morphine	12.5µg/kg 1.5mg/kg	49±8% *** +++ ooo	60±5% *** +++ ooo	38±11% *** +++ o

Morphine and NMDA receptor antagonists

It has been shown that NMDA receptor mediated events such as wind-up and the second phase of the formalin are poorly responsive to opioids, however high concentrations of morphine can ultimately reduce NMDA receptor mediated events although this may be associated with an increased side-effect liability (Chapman et al. 1994, and see references therein). However, co-therapy with sub-threshold doses of morphine and of an antagonist of the glycine site of the NMDA receptor has been shown to considerably reduce electrically evoked windup (Chapman and Dickenson 1992). In our study, we have used a relatively new antagonist at the glycine site of the NMDA receptor, (+)-HA966, which has been extensively investigated (Millan and Seguin 1994), shown to cross the blood brain barrier, and produce analgesic effects in the absence of side effects.

In this series of experiments we have studied the effect of coadministration of morphine and (+)-HA966 on carrageenin evoked spinal Fos expression at 1.5 hrs and 3 hrs after carrageenin injection (Honoré et al. 1996e).

Prior co-administration of systemic morphine (0.3 mg/kg) and subcutaneous (+)-HA966 (2.5 mg/kg) significantly reduced spinal Fos expression induced 1.5hr (Figure 4), but not 3 hrs, after carrageenin. However, coadministration of a larger dose of morphine (3 mg/kg) with (+)-HA966 (2.5 mg/kg) reduced spinal Fos expression at 3 hrs after carrageenin, in a partial naloxone reversible manner. The effect of morphine and (+)-HA966 on spinal Fos expression were significantly different from the effect of morphine alone and the lack of effect of (+)-HA966 alone.

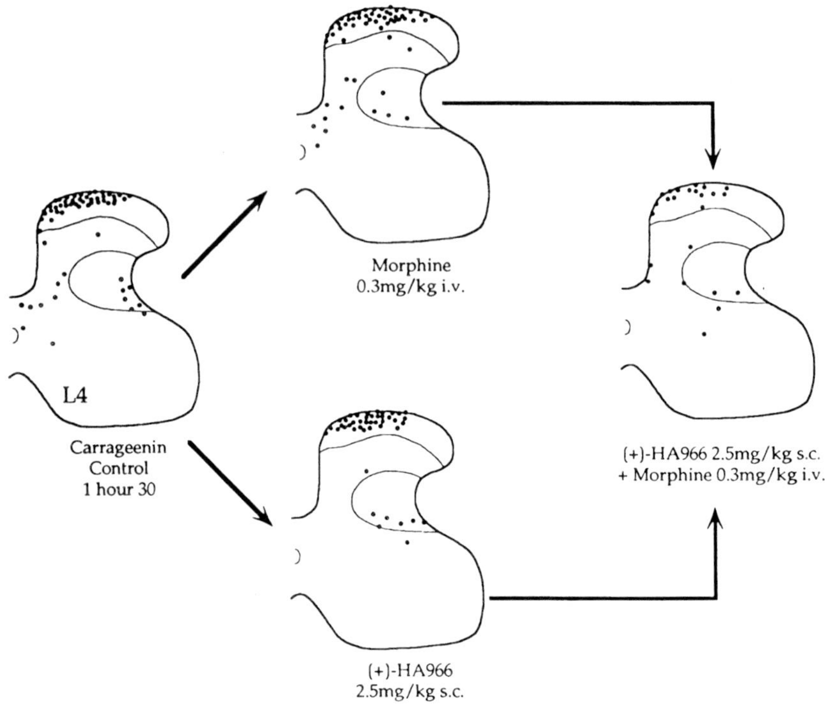

Figure 4. A comparison of the effect of morphine, versus (+)-HA966, an NMDA receptor antagonist, versus morphine plus (+)-HA966 on carrageenin evoked spinal Fos expression

These results suggest that the interaction between these two drugs are not based on a modification of the pharmacokinetic parameters of the action of morphine (i.e. increasing the duration of action), but support the presence of pharmacodynamic interactions. The peripheral edema was not influenced by the co-administration of morphine and (+)-HA966, suggesting that the location of the potentiation is at the spinal cord level or/and higher brain centers.

Our results suggesting, at least, supra-additive reductory effects of coadministered morphine and (+)-HA966 on carrageenin-induced spinal Fos expression are in good agreement with previous studies showing a potentiation between the effects of intrathecal morphine and an NMDA antagonist on windup (Chapman and Dickenson 1992) and on the thermal hyperalgesia in a model of neuropathic pain (Yamamoto and Yaksh 1992).

Conclusion

Our studies have demonstrated that the Fos technique provides some alternative information related to spinal nociceptive processing to that obtained by either behavioral or electrophysiological methods. This technique can be considered as a high resolution photographic image of the level of neuronal activity of different populations of neurons at a given time point. With such a technique, it is possible to observe drug effects on different neuronal populations simultaneously (superficial versus deep laminae neurons), and therefore this technique is complementary to electrophysiological methods applied at the spinal level.

This technique was especially suitable to study the interactions between the effects of morphine and other compounds acting on various systems implicated in the transmission or modulation of nociceptive informations at the spinal level. We have shown that there is an enhanced anti-nociceptive effect of morphine co-administered with either α2-receptor agonists, CCK_B receptor antagonists or NMDA antagonists and that these interactions have important therapeutic implications for the reduction, or prevention of the long term manifestations associated with sustained nociceptive processing, with a reduced side effect liability.

Acknowledgements

We would like to thank C. Abbadie, G. Catheline, J. Buritova, V. Chapman and S. Le Guen who greatly participated in these studies. These studies were supported by l'Institut National de la Santé et de la Recherche Médicale (INSERM), le Ministere de la Recherche et de l'Enseignement Supérieur and an unrestricted grant from Bristol-Myers Squibb.

Plenary discussion

Reeh W.: I may have missed something, but did you provide evidence for a direct neuronal action of NSAIDs separate from their anti-inflammatory effect?

Besson J.-M.: We didn't provide direct evidence for a neuronal action of NSAIDs, but we reported a very positive correlation between the anti-inflammatory effect of these compounds and their ability to reduce, dose dependently, the number of FOS-like immunoreactive neurons. The next step will be to compare the effects of stereoisomers of Ibuprofin.

Berkley K.: As basic scientists, could we not help in the development of new drugs by adding to our experiments the study of the conditions in which drugs were given? For example:
a) time of the day;
b) presence of other rats;
c) conditions of stress (etc.).

Besson J.-M.: The answer is "Yes," but unfortunately, only few groups are interested in these aspects of the problem.

Basbaum A.: Although you clearly demonstrated a correlation between FOS expression and paw diameter, and a decrease of both with NSAIDs, it would still be valuable to study the effects of intrathecal injections of NSAIDs. This is particularly true because COX_2 is probably concentrated in spinal cord astrocytes.

Besson J.-M.: I agree with you, in the experiments using NSAIDs COX_2 inhibitors we never rejected a possible central effect, i.e. the spinal cord but also other probable central sites of action.

Amassian V.: You showed a nice slide exhibiting in chronic inflammation not only more FOS expression dorsally, but also in intermediate regions of the gray. Are these intermediate level neurons related to reflex effects of chronic inflammation, either inhibitory to antigravity alpha motoneurons, or excitatory to flexors?

Besson J.-M.: The FOS-like immunoreactive neurons located in the deep dorsal horn or in the intermediate region of the spinal cord are particularly numerous during chronic inflammation (i.e. chronic arthritis induced by the administration of Freund's adjuvent). We didn't use double or triple labeling to characterize these neurons, but according to the literature some of them are probably wide dynamic range neurons some of them being at the origin of ascending tracts while others are probably interneurons. In our experimental conditions motoneurons didn't express FOS.

Lima D.: Contrary to mechanical stimulation, in which repeated stimulation produces very easily hypersensitization of spinal cord neurons, repeated thermal stimuli lead very often to desensitization. You have seen a large increase in FOS expression when thermal stimulation was sustained for 2 min. when compared to short duration stimulation. Would you like to comment on it ?

Besson J.-M.: In these experiments we used a single noxious heat stimulation (generally 15 seconds); the large increase in the number of FOS-like immunoreactivity we observed for a stimulation of 2 minutes probably reflects temporal and spatial convergence of dorsal horn neurons.

References

Abbadie C, Besson JM (1993a) Effects of morphine and naloxone on basal and evoked Fos-like immunoreactivity in lumbar spinal cord neurones of arthritic rats. Pain 52: 29-39.

Abbadie C, Honoré P, Fournié-Zaluski MC, Roques BP, Besson JM (1994a) Effects of opioids and non opioids on *c-fos*-like immunoreactivity induced in rat lumbar spinal cord neurones by noxious heat stimulation. Eur J Pharmacol 258:215-227.

Abbadie C, Honoré P, Besson JM (1994b) Postsynaptic changes during sustained primary afferent fiber stimulation as revealed by *c-fos* immunohistochemistry in the rat spinal cord. In L. Urban, A. Dray, S. Jeftinija, P. Reeh and C.J. Woolf (Eds.), The cellular mechanisms of sensory processing, Laszlo Urban, Berlin 449-471.

Abbadie C, Honoré P, Besson JM (1994c) Intense cold noxious stimulation of the rat hindpaw induces *c-fos* expression in lumbar spinal cord neurones. Neuroscience 59: 457-468.

Advokat C, Burton P, Tyler CB (1987) Investigation of tolerance to chronic intrathecal morphine infusion in the rat. Physiol Behav 39: 161-168.

Aley KO, Green PG, Levine JD (1995) Opioid and adenosine peripheral antinociception are subject to tolerance and withdrawal. J Neurosci 15: 8031-8038.

Barbaz BS, Hall NR, Liebman JM (1989) Antagonism of morphine analgesia by CCK-8-S does not extend to all assays nor all opiate analgesics. Peptides 9: 1295-1300.

Basbaum AI, Besson JM (1991) Towards a new pharmacotherapy of pain. In: Basbaum AI, Besson JM (eds). Dahlem Workshop Reports, Life Sciences Research Report 49, John Wiley & Sons, Chichester.

Basbaum AI and Fields HL (1978) Endogenous pain control mechanisms: Review and hypothesis. Annals of Neurology 4: 451-462.

Bouhassira D, Villanueva L, Le Bars D (1988) Intracerebroventricular morphine decreases descending inhibitions acting on lumbar dorsal horn neuronal activities related to pain in the rat. J Pharmacol Exp Ther 247: 332-342.

Chapman V, Dickenson AH (1992) The combination of NMDA antagonism and morphine produces profound anti-nociception in the rat dorsal horn. Brain Res: 573: 321-323.

Chapman V, Haley JE, Dickenson AH (1994) Electrophysiologic analysis of preemptive effects of spinal opioids on N-methyl-D-aspartate receptor-mediated events. Anaesthesiology 81: 1429-1435.

Chapman V, Honoré P, Buritova J, Besson JM (1995) Cholecystokinin B receptor antagonism enhances the ability of a low dose of morphine to reduce *c-fos* expression in the spinal cord of the rat. Neuroscience 67: 731-739.

Cox BM (1991) Molecular and cellular mechanisms of opioid tolerance. In: A.I. Basbaum and J.-M. Besson (Eds.), Towards a new pharmacotherapy of pain. John Wiley and Sons, Chichester, pp 137-156.

Detweiler DJ, Rhode DS, Basbaum AI (1995) The development of opioid tolerance in the formalin test in the rat. Pain 63: 251-254.

Dickenson AH (1994) Where and how do opioids act? In: Gebhart GF, Hammorid DL, Jensen TS (eds) Progress in Pain Research Management, IASP Press, Seattle p 525.

Dickenson AH (1994) NMDA receptor antagonists as analgesics. In: Fields HL, Liebeskind JC (eds) Progress in Pain Research Management, IASP Press, Seattle p 173.

Dourish CT, Hawley D, Iversen SD (1988) Enhancement of morphine and prevention of morphine tolerance in the rat by the cholecystokinin antagonist L-364, 718. Eur J Pharmacol 147: 469-472.

Dourish CT, O'Neill MF, Coughlan J, Kitchener SJ, Hawley D, Iversen SD (1990) The selective CCK-B receptor antagonist L-365,260 enhances morphine analgesia and prevents morphine tolerance in the rat. Eur J Pharmacol 176: 35-44.

Dragunow M, Robertson HA (1987) Kindling stimulation induces *c-fos* protein(s) in granule cells of the rat dentate gyrus. Nature 329: 441-442.

Draisci G, Iadarola MJ (1989) Temporal analysis of increases in *c-fos*, preprodynorphin and preproenkephalin mRNAs in rat spinal cord. Molecular Brain Research 6: 31-37.

Duggan AW, Hall JG, Headley PM (1977) Suppression of transmission of nociceptive impulses by morphine: selective effects of morphine administered in the region of the substantia gelatinosa. Brit J Pharmacol 61: 65-76.

Duggan AW, North RA (1984) Electrophysiology of opioids. Pharmacol Rev 35: 219.

Faris PL, McLaughlin CL, Baile CA, Olney JW (1984) Morphine analgesia potentiated but tolerance not affected by active immunisation against cholecystokinin. Science 226: 1215-1217.

Ferreira SH, Lorenzetti BB, Rae GA (1984) Is methylnalorphinium the prototype of an ideal peripheral analgesic? Eur J Pharmacol 99: 23-29.

Fisher B, Zomow MH, Yaksh TL, Peterson BM (1991) Antinociceptive properties of intrathecal dexmedetomidine in rats. Eur J Pharmacol 192: 221-225.

Fleetwood-Walker SM, Mitchell R, Hope PJ, Molony V, Iggo A (1985) An a2 receptor mediates the selective inhibition by noradrenaline of nociceptive responses of identified dorsal horn neurones. Brain Res 334: 243-254.

Gogas KR, Presley RW, Levine JD, Basbaum AI (1991) The antinociceptive action of supraspinal opioids results from an increase in descending inhibitory control: correlation of nociceptive behaviour and *c-fos* expression. Neuroscience 42: 617-628.

Gogas KR, Cho HJ, Botchkina GI, Levine JD, Basbaum AI (1996) Inhibition of noxious stimulusevoked pain behaviors and neuronal fos-like immunoreactivity in the spinal cord of the rat by supraspinal morphine. Pain 65: 9-15.

Gold LH, Stinus L, Inturrisi CE, Koob GF (1994) Prologed tolerance, dependence and abstinence following subcutaneous morphine pellet implantation in the rat. Eur J Pharmacol 253: 45-51.

Hammond DL, Presley RW, Gogas KR, Basbaum AI (1992) Morphine or U-50,488 suppresses Fos protein-like immunoreactivity in the spinal cord and nucleus tractus solitarii evoked by a noxious visceral stimulus in the rat. J Comp Neurol 315: 244-253.

Hargreaves K, Dubner R, Brown F, Flores C, Joris J (1988) A new and sensitive method for measuring thermal nociception in cutaneous hyperalgesia. Pain 32: 77-88.

Honoré P, Buritova J, Besson JM (1995) Carrageenin-evoked *c-fos* expression in rat lumbar spinal cord: the effects of indomethacin. Eur J Pharmacol 272: 249-259.

Honoré P, Buritova J, Besson JM (1996a) Intraplantar morphine depresses spinal *c-fos* expression induced by carrageenin inflammation but not by noxious heat. Brit J Pharmacol 118: 671-680.

Honoré P, Buritova J, Besson JM (1996b) The effects of morphine on carrageenin-induced spinal *c-fos* expression are completely blocked by β-Funaltrexamine, a selective μ-opioid receptor antagonist. Brain Res 732: 242-246.

Honoré P, Catheline G, Le Guen S and Besson JM (1997) Chronic treatment with systemic morphine induced tolerance to the systemic and peripheral antinociceptive effects of morphine on both carrageenin induced mechanical hyperalgesia and spinal *c-fos* expression in awake rats. Pain 71: 99-108

Honoré P, Chapman V, Buritova J, Besson JM (1996c) When is the maximal effect of preadministered systemic morphine on carrageenin evoked spinal *c-fos* expression in the rat. Brain Research 705: 91-96.

Honoré P, Chapman V, Buritova J, Besson JM (1996d) To what extent do spinal interactions between α2-adrenoceptor and μ-opioid agonists influence noxiously evoked *c-fos* expression in the rat? A pharmacological study. J.P.E.T. 278: 393-403.

Honoré P, Chapman V, Buritova J, Besson JM (1996e) Concomitant administration of morphine and an N-Methyl-D-Aspartate receptor antagonist profoundly reduced inflammatory evoked spinal *c-fos* expression. Anesthesiology 85: 150-160.

Hughes P, Dragunow M (1995) Induction of immediate-early genes and the control of neurotransmitter-regulated expression within the nervous system. Pharmacol Reviews: 47(1): 133-178.

Hunt SP, Pini A, Evan G (1987) Induction of *c-fos*-like protein in spinal cord neurones following sensory stimulation. Nature 328: 632-634.

ladarol MJ, Brady LS, Draisci G, Dubner R (1988) Enhancement of dynorphin gene expression in spinal cord following experimental inflammation: stimulus specificity, behavioral parameters and opioid receptor binding. Pain 35: 313-326.

Jasmin L, Wang H, Tarcy-Hornoch K, Levine JD, Basbaum I (1994) Differential effects of morphine on noxious stimulus-evoked Fos-like immunoreactivity in subpopulations of spinoparabrachial neurones. J Neurosci 14: 7252-7260.

Jones SL (1992) Noradrenergic modulation of noxious heat-evoked fos-like immunoreactivity in the dorsal horn of the rat sacral spinal cord. J Comp Neurol 325: 435-445.

Joris J, Costello A, Dubner R, Hargreaves K (1990) Opiates supress carrageenan-induced edema and hyperthermia at doses that inhibit hyperalgesia. Pain 43: 95-103.

Kalso EA, Poyhia R and Rosenberg PH (1991) Spinal anti-nociception by dexmedetomidine, a highly selective (2-adrenergic agonist. Pharmacol Toxicol 168: 140-143.

Kalso EA, Sullivan AF, McQuay HJ, Dickenson A, Roques BP (1993) Cross-tolerance between μ-opioid and α2 adrenergic receptors, but not between μ- and δ-opioid receptors in the spinal cord of the rat. J Pharmacol Exp Ther 265: 551-558.

Kayser V, Guilbaud G (1987) Local and remote modifications of nociceptive sensitivity during carrageenin-induced inflammation in the rat. Pain 28: 99-107.

Kissin I, Brown PT, Robinson C, Bradley EL (1991) Acute tolerance in morphine analgesia: continuous infusion and single injection in rats. Anesthesiology 74: 166-171.

LaMotte C, Kapadia SE, Shapiro CM (1991) Central projections of the sciatic, saphenous, median, and ulnar nerves of the rat demonstrated by transganglionic transport of choleragenoid-HRP (B-HRP) and wheat germagglutinin-HRP (WGA-HRP). J Comp Neurol 311: 546-562.

LeBars D, Menetrey D, Conseiller C, Besson JM (1975) Depressive effects of morphine upon lamina V cells activities in the dorsal horn of the spinal cat. Brain Res 98: 261-277.

Loomis CW, Jhamandas K, Milne B, Cervenko F (1987) Monoamine and opioid interactions in spinal analgesia and tolerance. Pharmacol Biochem Behav 26: 445-451.

Magnuson DSK, Sullivan AF, Simonnet G, Roques BP, Dickenson AH (1990) Differential interactions of cholecystokinin and FLFQPQRF-NH2 with μ- and δ-opioid anti-nociception in the rat spinal cord. Neuropeptides 16: 213-218.

Millan MJ, Seguin L (1994) Chemically-diverse ligands at the glycine B site coupled to N-methyl-D-aspartate (NMDA) receptors selectively block the late phase of the formalin-induced pain in mice. Neurosci Letts 178: 139-143.

Molander C, Grant G (1986) Laminar distribution and somatotopic organization of primary afferent fibers from hindlimb nerves in the dorsal horn. A study by transganglionic transport of horseradish peroxidase in the rat. Neuroscience 19 (1): 297-312.

Molander C, Xu Q, Grant G (1984) The cytoarchitectonic organization of the spinal cord in the rat: I: The lower thoracic and lumbosacral cord. J Comp Neurol 230:133-141.

Monasky MS, Zinsmeister AR, Stevens CW, Yaksh TL (1990) Interaction of intrathecal morphine and ST91 on anti-nociception in the rat: dose-response analysis, antagonism and clearance. J Pharmacol Exp Ther 234: 383-392.

Morgan JI (1991) Discussions in Neuroscience, Proto-oncogene expression in the nervous system Vol. Vll, No 4, Elsevier, Amsterdam Holland.

Morgan JI, Cohen DR, Hempstead JL, Curran T (1987) Mapping patterns of *c-fos* expression in the central nervous system after seizure. Science 237: 192-197.

Nishino K, Su YF, Wong CS, Watkins WD, Chang KJ (1990) Dissociation of mu opioid tolerance from receptor down-regulation in rat spinal cord. J Pharmacol Exp Ther 253: 67-72.

Noguchi K, Dubner R, Ruda MA (1992) Preproenkephalin mRNA in spinal dorsal horn neurones is induced by peripheral inflammation and is co-localised with Fos and Fos-related proteins. Neuroscience 46: 561-570.

Noguchi K, Kowalski K, Traub R, Solodkin A, Iadarola MJ, Ruda MA (1991) Dynorphin expression and Fos-like immunoreactivity following inflammation induced hyperalgesia are colocalised in spinal cord neurones. Mol Brain Res 10: 227-233.

Nozaki K, Moskovitz MA, Boccalini P (1992) CP-93129, sumatriptan, dihydroergotamine block *c-fos* expression within rat trigeminal nucleus caudalis caused by chemical stimulation of the meninges. Br J Pharmacol 106: 409-415.

Ossipov MH, Harris S, Lloyd P, Messineo E, Lin BS, Bagley J (1990) Antinociceptive interaction between opioids and medetomidine: systemic additivity and spinal synergy. Anesthesiology 73: 1227-1235.

Paronis CA, Holtzman SG (1992) Development of tolerance to the analgesic activity of mu agonists after continuous infusion of morphine, meperidine or fentanyl in rats. J Pharmacol Exp Ther 262: 1-9.

Pertovaara A, Kaupila T, Jyväsjärvi E, Kalso E (1991) Involvement of supraspinl and spinal segmental α2-adrenergic mechanisms in the medetomidine-induced antinocieption. Neuroscience 44: 705-714.

Pertovaara A, Bravo R, Herdegen T (1993) Induction and suppression of immediate-early-genes in the rat brain by a selective α2-adrenoceptor agonist and antagonist following noxious peripheral stimulation. Neuroscience 44: 705-714.

Presley RW, Menétrey D, Levine JD, Basbaum AI (1990) Systemic morphine suppresses noxious stimulus-evoked Fos protein-like immunoreactivity in the rat spinal cord. J Neurosci 10: 323-335.

Proudfit HK (1988) Pharmacologic evidence for the modulation of nociception by noradrenergic neurones. In: H.L. Fields and J.M. Besson (eds) Progress in Brain Research. Elsevier Science Publishers BV, Amsterdam Holland p 357.

Puke MJC, Wiesenfeld-Hallin Z. (1993) The differential effects of morphine and the α2-adrenoceptor agonists clonidine and dexmedetomidine on the prevention ad treatment of experimental neuropathic pain. Anesth Analg 77: 104-109.

Rohde DS, Detweiler DJ, Basbaum AI (1993) Spinal cord fos-like immunoreactivity (FLI) during precipitated abstinence: comparison with patterns evoked by noxious stimulation. Neuroscience Abstract 19: 1247.

Sagar SM, Sharp FR, Curran T (1988) Expression of *c-fos* protein in brain: metabolic mapping at the cellular level. Science 240: 1328-1331.

Sakurada T, Katsumata K, Yogo H, Tan-NO K, Sakurada S, Ohba M, Kisera K (1995) The neurokinin-1 receptor antagonist, sendide, exhibits anti-nociceptive activity in the formalin test. Pain 60: 175-180.

Stanfa L, Dickenson AH (1993) Cholecystokinin as a factor in the enhanced potency of spinal morphine following carrageenin inflammation. Br J Pharmacol 108: 967-973.

Stein C (1993) Peripheral mechanisms of opioid analgesia. Anest Analg 76: 182-191.

Stein C (1995) Peripheral opioid analgesia: mechanisms and therapeutic applications. In: Besson JM, Guilbaud G, Ollat H (eds) Peripheral neurons in nociception. John Libbey Eurotext, Paris, p 157.

Stevens CW, Yaksh TL (1989) Time course characteristics of tolerance development to continuously infused antinociceptive agents in rat spinal cord. J Pharmacol Exp Ther 251: 216-223.

Stevens CW, Yaksh TL (1992) Studies of morphine and D-ala^2-D-leu^5-enkephalin (DADLE) cross tolerance after continuous intrathecal infusion in the rat. Anesthesiology 76: 596-603.

Sullivan AF, Dashwood MR, Dickenson AH (1987) α2-adrenoceptor modulation of nociception in rat spinal cord: location, effects and interactions with morphine. Eur J Pharmacol 138: 169-177.

Sullivan AF, Kalso EA, McQuay HJ and Dickenson AH (1992) The antinociceptive actions of dexmedetomidine on dorsal horn neuronal responses in the anaesthetised rat. Eur J Pharmacol 215: 127-133.

Tölle TR, Castro-Lopes JM, Coimbra A, Zieglgänsberger W (1990) Opiates modify induction of *c-fos* proto-oncogene in the spinal cord of the rat following noxious stimulation. Neuroscience Letters, 4651.

Tölle T,R, Castro-Lopes JM, Evan, G, Zieglgänsberger W (1991) *C-fos* induction in the spinal cord following noxious stimulation prevention by opiates but not by NMDA antagonists. In: Bond, Charlton, Woolf (eds) Proceedings of the IVth World Congress on Pain. Elsevier, Amsterdam p 299.

Tölle TR, Herdegen T, Schadrack J, Bravo R, Zimmermann M, Zieglgänsberger W (1994a) Application of morphine prior to noxious stimulation differentially modulates expression of Fos, Jun and Krox-24 proteins in rat spinal cord neurones. Neuroscience 58: 305-321.

Tölle TR, Schadrack J, Castro-Lopes JM, Evan G, Roques BP, Zieglgänsberger W (1994b) Effects of Kelatorphan and morphine before and after noxious stimulation on immediate-early gene expression in rat spinal cord neurones. Pain 56: 103-112.

Traub RJ, Stitt S, Gebhart GF (1995) Attenuation of *c-fos* expression in the rat lumbosacral spinal cord by morphine or tramadol following noxious colorectal distention. Brain Res 701: 175-182.

Wiesenfeld-Hallin Z, Duranti R (1987) Intrathecal cholecystokinin interacts with morphine but not substance P in modulating the nociceptive flexion reflex in the rat. Peptides 8: 153-158.

Wiesenfeld-Hallin Z, Xu X-J, Hughes J, Horwell DC, Hökfelt T (1990) PD134308, a selective antagonist of cholecystokinin type B receptor, enhances the analgesic effect of morphine and synergistically interacts with intrathecal galanin to depress spinal nociceptive reflexes. Pro Natl Acad Sci USA 87: 7105-7109.

Winter CA, Risley EA, Nuss GW (1962) Carrageenan-induced edema in hind paw of the rat as an assay for antiinflammatory drugs. Proc Soc Exp Biol Med 111: 544-547.

Xu X-J, Hökfelt T, Hughes J, Wiesenfeld-Hallin Z (1994) The CCK-B antagonist C1988 enhances the effect of the reflex-depressive effect of morphine in axotomized rats. NeuroReport 5: 718-720.

Yaksh TL (1985) Pharmacology of spinal adrenergic systems which modulate spinal nociceptive processing. Pharmacology Biochemistrv and Behavior 22: 845-858.

Yamamoto T, Yaksh TL (1992) Comparison of the antinociceptive effects of pre- and post-treatment with morphine and MK-801, an NMDA antagonist, on the formalin test in the rat. Anesthesiology 77: 757-763.

Zhou Y, Sun Y-H, Zhang Z-W, Han J-S (1993) Increased release of immunoreactive cholecystokinin octapeptide by morphine and potentiation of μ-opioid analgesia by CCK_B receptor antagonist L365,260 in the rat spinal cord. Eur J Pharmacol 234: 147-154.

Zieglgänsberger W, Tölle TR (1993) The pharmacology of pain signalling. Current Opinion in Neurobiology 3: 611-618.

Pain Mechanisms and Management
S.N. Ayrapetyan and A.V. Apkarian (Eds.)
IOS Press, 1998

The Role of Signal Transduction Pathways in Sensitization of Primate Spinothalamic Tract Neurons

Wm. D. Willis, Jr.
Department of Anatomy & Neurosciences and Marine Biomedical Institute
University of Texas Medical Branch
Galveston, TX, USA

Introduction

Brief noxious stimuli usually produce pain of brief duration. This is our everyday experience when encountering sharp surfaces or accidentally bumping into immovable objects. However, even in such cases, our bodies often remember the abuses inflicted by an unaccommodating world. For instance, after stumbling into a table in a darkened room in search of the bathroom or a nighttime snack, the pain is long outlasted by the tenderness surrounding a bruise. Until healing has progressed, a feeling of pain is provoked by relatively gentle manipulation of the bruised tissue. This tenderness does not reside only in the memory of the event, but also in a reluctant shin which provides a constant reminder that you should avoid risking further stumbles. Similar experiences may follow other painful events: burns, surgery, a visit to the dentist, athletic injuries, and the onslaught of many illnesses such as arthritis, peripheral nerve damage, cancer and many more.

The following is a discussion of how pain states may linger following injury. First, definitions are given for pain, hyperalgesia, and allodynia. A distinction is then made between primary hyperalgesia and secondary hyperalgesia, and allodynia. Next, there is a discussion of the use of capsaicin injections to produce hyperalgesia and allodynia in human subjects and central sensitization in experimental animals. This approach provides an opportunity to examine the role of particular neurotransmitters and of signal transduction cascades in mediating central sensitization and presumably hyperalgesia and allodynia.

Definitions

The International Association for the Study of Pain defines pain (Merskey & Bogduk, 1994) as "an unpleasant sensory and emotional experience associated with actual or potential tissue damage, or described in terms of such damage." "Hyperalgesia" is "an increased response to a stimulus which is normally painful." "Allodynia" is "pain due to a stimulus which does not normally provoke pain." Bumping one's shin may result in the triad of pain, hyperalgesia, and allodynia. After the initial pain has receded, strong compression of the skin over the bruise results in far more pain than would be produced by the same stimulus under normal conditions. This is hyperalgesia. Furthermore, even gentle caressing of the skin may cause pain (or "tenderness"). This is allodynia. The hyperalgesia and allodynia can long outlast the pain.

An important distinction was drawn by Lewis (1942) and then more clearly by Hardy, Wolff and Goodell (1967) between primary and secondary hyperalgesia (see also Willis, 1992). Primary hyperalgesia is hyperalgesia distributed in the region of damage, whereas secondary hyperalgesia is that distributed in the surrounding undamaged area. Presumably, the term "secondary" allodynia can be used to describe the region of allodynia having a distribution similar to that of "secondary hyperalgesia."

In recent years, experimental evidence has accumulated that promises an explanation of these lingering states of hyperalgesia and allodynia.

Primary Hyperalgesia

Although once controversial, it is now recognized that there are specialized primary afferent neurons, the nociceptors, that serve to detect noxious stimuli (reviewed in Willis, 1985; Willis & Coggeshall, 1991). Nociceptors are found in peripheral nerves supplying skin, muscle, joints, and viscera. Direct activation of nociceptive afferent fibers in human subjects through a microneurographic electrode elicits pain (Ochoa & Torebjörk, 1989), and blocking conduction in these nerve fibers with local anesthetic results in analgesia (Torebjörk & Hallin, 1974).

Many nociceptors are very difficult to excite under normal circumstances. However, when the tissue they innervate undergoes inflammation, these "sleeping" nociceptors awaken and become exquisitcly responsive even to gentle mechanical stimuli (Schaible & Schmidt, 1985). Although first described in the knee joint, comparable "sleeping" nociceptors have now been described in cutaneous and visceral nerves (Davis et al., 1993; Häbler et al., 1990; Handwerker et al., 1991). The change in these nociceptors from a relatively unresponsive to a highly responsive state is determined by the activation of second messenger systems with inflammatory mediators, such as bradykinin, prostaglandins, serotonin and histamine (Birrell et al., 1993; Davis et al., 1993; Dray et al., 1988; Schepelmann et al. 1992). It has been proposed that protein kinase C is involved in the sensitization of primary afferent nociceptors, since phorbol ester has a stimulatory action and the protein kinase inhibitor, staurosporine, prevents this (Dray et al., 1988; Schepelmann et al., 1993).

It is believed that the sensitization of nociceptors, whether "sleeping" or initially responsive, is the neural basis for primary hyperalgesia (Meyer & Campbell, 1981; LaMotte et al., 1983; see Willis, 1985; 1992; Willis & Coggeshall, 1991).

Secondary Hyperalgesia and Allodynia

Hyperalgesia and allodynia of the skin spread from a region of damage into the surrounding undamaged skin. Lewis (1942) thought that this spread resulted from the release of substances from peripheral nerve fibers by axon reflexes. However, Hardy et al. (1967) argued that these processes had to be attributed to changes that take place within the dorsal horn of the spinal cord. Recent experiments support the contention of Hardy et al. (1967).

The capsaicin model of hyperalgesia and allodynia

A reproducible way to elicit pain, hyperalgesia and allodynia is to inject a small amount of capsaicin into the skin (Simone et al., 1989; LaMotte et al., 1991; 1992;

Torebjörk et al., 1992; see review by Buck & Burks, 1986). The pain is immediate and intense, but it diminishes to a low level in a few minutes and disappears in 10-30 minutes (LaMotte et al., 1991). The pain is succeeded by primary and secondary hyperalgesia and allodynia. At the injection site, there is a small region of analgesia where the capsaicin has desensitized nociceptors. Surrounding this is an area of primary hyperalgesia and allodynia where there is enhanced pain from normally painful mechanical or heat stimuli, as well as pain from normally nonpainful stimuli. It has been difficult to demonstrate that nociceptors supplying this area of primary hyperalgesia and allodynia are sensitized by the capsaicin, but such a change seems likely, since topical application of capsaicin does produce sensitization of nociceptors (Baumann et al., 1991; LaMotte et al., 1992). There is no evidence for sensitization of mechanoreceptors (Baumann et al., 1991), and so allodynia in the area of primary hyperalgesia may result from central sensitization (see below and LaMotte et al., 1992). If so, this would presumably represent secondary allodynia in the area of primary hyperalgesia.

Secondary hyperalgesia and allodynia following capsaicin injection spread across the skin in concentric fashion from the area of primary hyperalgesia. The maximum spread occurs after about 15-20 minutes (Hardy et al., 1967; LaMotte et al., 1991). After this, the areas of secondary hyperalgesia and allodynia recede. However, the time course of resolution of secondary hyperalgesia differs from that of allodynia. The secondary hyperalgesia may persist for as long as a day, whereas the allodynia disappears after 1-6 hours (LaMotte et al., 1991). No heat hyperalgesia is observed in the area of secondary mechanical hyperalgesia following an injection of capsaicin (Simone et al., 1991).

Under the cross-species assumption that pain states in humans will be reflected by changes in the activity of identified spinothalamic tract (STT) neurons in monkeys, recordings were made by Simone et al. (1991) from STT cells before and after intradermal injection of capsaicin within the receptive field. Prior to the injection of capsaicin, the STT cells were classified as wide dynamic range (WDR) neurons if they responded to weak mechanical stimuli, as well as to noxious mechanical stimuli, and as high threshold (HT) neurons if they responded chiefly to noxious intensities of mechanical stimuli. Following intradermal injection of capsaicin, both WDR and HT STT cells showed substantially increased rates of discharge. In the case of WDR STT cells, this lasted for more than 15 minutes, mimicking the duration of pain in humans that follows comparable injections of capsaicin into the skin. However, most HT STT cells showed elevated firing rates for only 1-3 minutes. These observations suggest that WDR STT neurons contribute to the full course of capsaicin-induced pain, whereas most HT STT cells could only participate in the initial component of the pain.

When testing for hyperalgesia and allodynia began, it could be demonstrated that the threshold for activation of STT cells by heat stimuli was substantially reduced in the area immediately surrounding the injection site; presumably this change would be responsible for the primary heat hyperalgesia seen in human subjects (Simone et al., 1991). The effects of mechanical stimuli near the injection site varied; sometimes there was an enhanced response to application of a stiff von Frey filament, but often the response was diminished. These variable responses to mechanical stimuli may reflect both the analgesia to mechanical stimuli applied to a central area in which nociceptors were desensitized by capsaicin and the hyperalgesia in an adjacent area in which nociceptors were sensitized.

When responses were tested to stimuli applied in the area of skin that surrounded the injection site, it was found that STT cells became much more responsive to weak mechanical stimulation, as well as to application of a stiff von Frey filament (Simone et al., 1991). It was suggested that these enhanced responses correspond to the development of secondary allodynia and hyperalgesia. Interestingly, there was no increase in the responses to heat stimuli in the area of presumed secondary mechanical hyperalgesia. In fact, it has recently been shown that the responses to heat stimuli in this area of skin are reduced (Sluka et al., 1997).

Since no changes are seen in the responsiveness of primary afferent fibers supplying the skin in the area of secondary hyperalgesia and allodynia (Baumann et al., 1991; LaMotte et al., 1992), it was hypothesized that the hyperalgesia and allodynia associated with intradermal injection of capsaicin is due in part to sensitization of neurons in the central nervous system (Simone et al., 1991). To test this, a filament of dorsal root was cut and stimulated electrically using low intensity pulses before and after injection of capsaicin into the skin while recording the responses of STT cells (Simone et al., 1991). This ensured that the large myelinated afferents used to test the responsiveness of the STT cells were unaffected by peripheral events. After injection of capsaicin into the skin, the responses of the STT cells were increased at a time when secondary hyperalgesia and allodynia would be anticipated. Clearly, central sensitization must have occurred. A comparable experiment was done in human subjects by Torebjörk et al. (1992). A microneurography electrode was placed in a peripheral nerve at a site that when stimulated evoked a tactile sensation. Capsaicin was then injected a short distance away from the projected receptive field. When the area of secondary hyperalgesia encompassed the projected receptive field, stimulation in the nerve now provoked pain. The sensation reverted to a tactile one when the area of secondary hyperalgesia receded. Presumably, the capsaicin injection sensitized neurons in the central nervous system that signal pain to inputs from mechanoreceptors. This sensitization resulted in an enhanced activation of these neurons by the volleys in tactile afferent fibers evoked by the intraneural stimulating electrode. The result was a conversion of the purely tactile sensation to pain.

In later experiments, we confirmed that there was a central sensitization of STT cells following intradermal injection of capsaicin by demonstrating an increase both in the responses to mechanical stimulation of the skin and also to excitatory amino acids (EAAs) released iontophoretically from a multibarreled electrode placed near the STT cell (Dougherty & Willis, 1992). We found that central sensitization in monkeys, using the enhanced responses of WDR STT cells to weak mechanical stimuli and to EAAs as a test of sensitization, lasted about 2 hours, similar to the time course of allodynia in human subjects. Furthermore, we could mimic central sensitization by iontophoretically co-applying an EAA, N-methyl-d-aspartate (NMDA), and the neuropepide, substance P (SP), onto STT cells (Dougherty & Willis, 1991; Doughery et al., 1993). Responses to EAAs applied after the STT cells became sensitized were often enhanced for a period of several hours. However, sometimes the responses to one or more EAAs were depressed (Dougherty et al., 1993).

Later experiments provided evidence consistent with a causal role of EAAs and SP in the central sensitization of STT cells that follows intradermal injection of capsaicin. The central sensitization was prevented when either an NMDA receptor antagonist (Dougherty et al., 1992) or an antagonist of NK_1 (SP) receptors (Dougherty et al., 1994) was infused into the spinal cord dorsal horn by microdialysis.

Second messenger systems and central sensitization

The action of iontophoretically released EAAs, such as glutamate or even NMDA, on STT neurons is normally quite brief, a matter of a few seconds (Dougherty & Willis,

1992). However, central sensitization of the responses to EAAs or to peripheral stimulation lasts in the order of hours. How can this be?

NMDA receptors can activate signal transduction pathways because of the influx of Ca^{++} ions through open NMDA channels (MacDermott et al., 1986; Walaas & Greengard, 1991). Furthermore, NK_1 receptors are G-protein linked, giving an opportunity for SP to activate G-proteins and thus second messenger systems (Guard and Watson, 1991; Holland et al., 1993). We therefore postulated that central sensitization and the consequent secondary hyperalgesia and allodynia reflect the activation of signal transduction pathways in the spinal cord dorsal horn, perhaps in the STT cells themselves, but at least in the neural circuits impinging on STT cells. To test this idea, we began a series of experiments that employed activators and inhibitors of known steps in a number of signal transduction pathways. As indicated below, we now have evidence that several different signal transduction cascades are involved in central sensitization and that the details of the changes brought about in STT cells vary, depending on the particular signal transduction pathway that is engaged and on the particular types of neurons that are examined. The experiments that are described include not only ones on STT cells, but also a study of changes in behavioral responses of rats given intradermal injections of capsaicin. Inhibitors or activators of signal transduction pathways were infused into the spinal cord dorsal horn by microdialysis.

Behavioral Experiments

In rats, injection of capsaicin into the hindpaw results in a lowered threshold for withdrawal from von Frey filaments applied to an adjacent area of the foot, and an increased likelihood of withdrawal from the von Frey filaments (Fig. 1A; Sluka & Willis, 1997). However, there was no change in the paw withdrawal latency to noxious heat applied to the same area of skin. Thus, intradermal injection of capsaicin into the hindpaw in rats produced changes in behavioral responses suggesting that the rats had developed a pain state comparable to secondary mechanical allodynia in human subjects, and as in humans there was no secondary heat hyperalgesia following intradermal injection of capsaicin. Without drug treatment, the allodynia lasted for several hours (Fig. 1A). The degree of mechanical allodynia produced by capsaicin injection could be reduced by microdialysis administration of any of the following agents: a G-protein inhibitor (GDP-β-S), a non-selective inhibitor of protein kinases (H7), and selective inhibitors of protein kinase C (NPC15437; Fig. 1B), protein kinase A (H89; Fig. 1C) and protein kinase G (KT5823; Fig. 1D). The selectivity of H89 was tested by showing that it had no effect on hyperalgesia induced by 8-bromo-cGMP at a dose that reduced that caused by 8-bromo-cAMP. Similarly, KT5823 had no effect on the hyperalgesia produced by phorbol ester but reduced that produced by 8-bromo-cGMP. Finally, NPC15437 had no effect on the hyperalgesia produced by 8-bromo-cGMP but reduced that caused by phorbol ester.

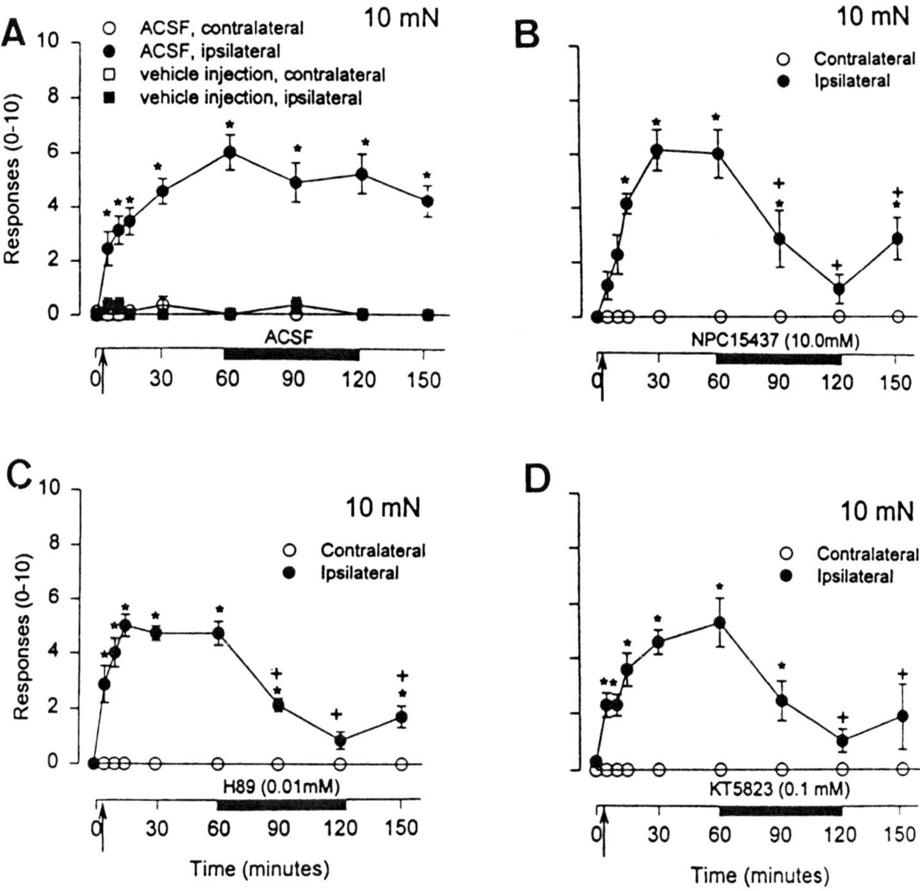

Figure 1. Behavioral experiments in rats. The graphs show the number of times that rats withdrew their paws in 10 trials of applications of a von Frey filament having a bending force of 10 mN to the plantar surface of the foot well away from the site of injection of capsaicin or vehicle. In the control experiments in A, there were no responses before and few responses following the injection of vehicle into either foot (filled and open squares). Capsaicin produced a long-lasting increase in the frequency of responses (mechanical allodynia) when injected into the foot (filled circles). Infusion of artificial cerebrospinal fluid (ACSF) into the spinal cord dorsal horn by microdialysis during the time indicated by the horizontal bar had no effect on the allodynia. B-D show the reductions in the allodynia that resulted from infusions of inhibitors of PKC (NPC 15437, 10 mM), PKA (H89, 0.01 mM) and PKG (KT5 823, 0.1 mM). (Modified from Sluka & Willis, 1997.)

Experiments Suggesting a Role of Protein Kinase C in Central Sensitization

Intradermal injections of capsaicin in anesthetized monkeys were also used to examine the role of signal transduction pathways in central sensitization of spinothalamic tract (STT) neurons (Lin et al., 1996; 1997; Sluka et al., 1997). Similar observations were made while recording from nociceptive dorsal horn neurons in rats (Peng et al., 1997).

Following a capsaicin injection, the responses of STT cells to brushing the skin with a camel hair brush (a tactile stimulus) and to application of a large arterial clip to a fold of skin (a marginally painful stimulus) were found to increase (Lin et al., 1996a; Sluka et al., 1997; cf. Dougherty et al., 1993; 1994). However, responses to pinching the skin with a small arterial clip (a distinctly painful stimulus) were unchanged (Lin et al., 1996; Sluka et al., 1997; cf. Dougherty et al., 1993; 1994), and the responses to noxious heat were reduced (Sluka et al., 1997). The increases in responses of STT cells to brushing the skin and to application of a large arterial clip to a fold of skin were interpreted as central sensitization. These events may reflect the changes in neural activity that underlies secondary mechanical allodynia and hyperalgesia. Administration of an inhibitor of protein kinase C (NPC15437) interfered with the ability of an intradermal injection of capsaicin to produce central sensitization. In the experiment illustrated in Fig. 2, the first injection of capsaicin produced sensitization of the STT cell, especially to BRUSH. After recovery, the protein kinase C inhibitor was administered. It had no effect on the responses of the cells, but it prevented the changes in responses to mechanical stimulation expected following the second injection of capsaicin.

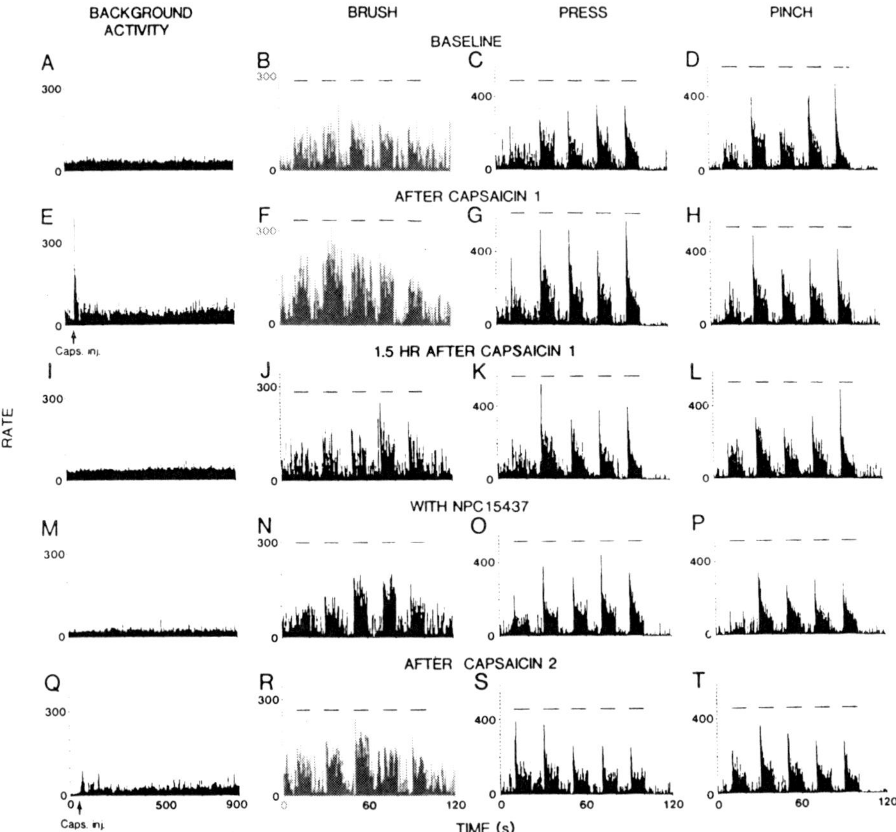

Figure 2. Activity of a wide dynamic range spinothalamic tract neuron before and after each of two intradermal injections of capsaicin. A-D are rate histograms showing the background activity of the cell and its responses to stimulation at 5 locations within its receptive field, using the following stimuli: BRUSH (brushing repeatedly with a camel hair brush); PRESS (application of a large arterial clip to a fold of skin, a marginally painful stimulus in human subjects); and PINCH (application of a small arterial clip to a fold of skin, a distinctly painful stimulus). E-H show that the first injection of capsaicin resulted in increases in background activity and in the responses to BRUSH and PRESS. I-L show that the activity had largely recovered by 1.5 h. M-P show that microdialysis infusion of the PKC inhibitor, NPC 15437, had no substantial effect of its own. However, Q-T demonstrate that a second injection of capsaicin now had little effect. (From Lin et al., 1996a.)

Infusion of the following inhibitors of signal transduction pathways into the spinal cord dorsal horn by microdialysis prevented central sensitization of STT cells by intradermal injections of capsaicin (Sluka et al., 1997): a G-protein inhibitor (GDP-β-S), a non-selective inhibitor of protein kinases (H7), and selective inhibitors of protein kinase C (NPC15437; see also Lin et al., 1996) and protein kinase A (H89). Interestingly, H89 also prevented the reduction in the responses to noxious heat.

The effects of intradermal capsaicin on the responses of STT cells could be mimicked by infusing the spinal cord dorsal horn by microdialysis with an active phorbol ester but not with an inactive phorbol ester (Fig. 3; Lin et al., 1996; cf., Palecek et al., 1994). This suggests that the effects of activation of protein kinase C are similar to those of an intradermal injection capsaicin and therefore would be consistent with the idea that the protein kinase C signal transduction cascade is activated by transmitters released in the dorsal horn following capsaicin administration.

Similar results were obtained in rats when recording from nociceptive dorsal horn neurons (Peng et al. 1997). Infusion of phorbol ester by microdialysis increased the responses of WDR neurons to brushing the skin, and this was blocked by coadministration of a selective inhibitor of protein kinase C (NPC15437).

Reduction in Inhibition during Central Sensitization

When stimuli are applied in the periaqueductal gray (PAG) in monkeys, STT cells are inhibited, presumably because of the activation of the descending analgesia system (Hayes et al., 1979; Gerhart et al., 1984). During the central sensitization that is observed following intradermal injection of capsaicin or microdialysis infusion of phorbol ester into the dorsal horn, PAG inhibition of STT cells is markedly reduced (Fig. 3; Lin et al., 1996a). Furthermore, the inhibition of STT cells produced by iontophoretic release of glycine and GABA is also reduced following intradermal capsaicin injection or infusion of phorbol ester into the dorsal horn (Fig. 4; Lin et al., 1996b). The reduction in PAG inhibition or in the inhibition produced by iontophoretic release of GABA or glycine following capsaicin injection can be prevented by microdialysis administration of a protein kinase C inhibitor (Fig. 4; NPC15437). These observations suggest that the increased responses of STT cells during central sensitization may reflect both an increase in the ability of EAAs to excite these neurons and a decrease in the ability of inhibitory amino acids to inhibit the same cells because of the action of protein kinase C.

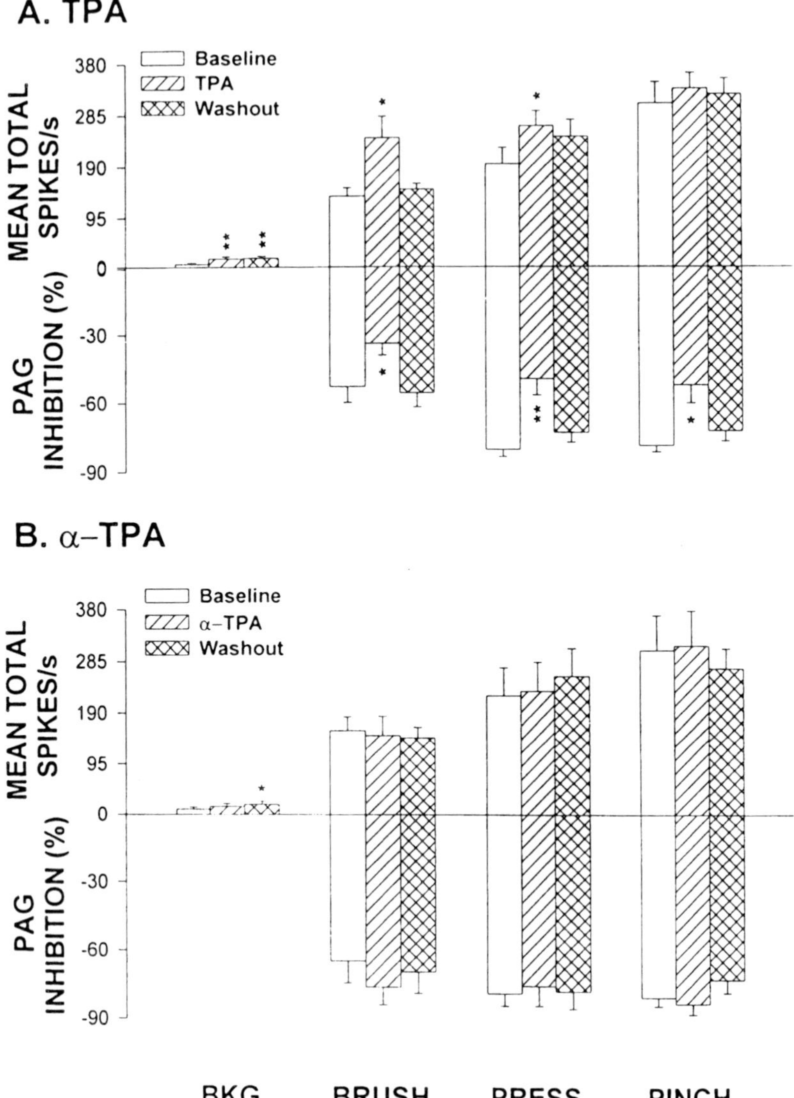

Figure 3. A and B show the effects of microdialysis infusion into the dorsal horn of an active phorbol ester, TPA, and the lack of effects of an inactive phorbol ester, (X-TPA, on the background activity (BKG) and the responses of a population of STT cells to BRUSH, PRESS and PINCH stimuli and on the inhibition of these responses that was produced by stimulation in the periaqueductal gray (PAG). The upward-going bars represent the background activity and responses of the neurons to mechanical stimuli. The downward-going bars show the percentage inhibition of responses when the PAG was stimulated. The open bars are the controls. The singly hatched bars are during infusion of phorbol ester. The doubly hatched bars are after washout of the drug. (From Lin et al., 1996a.)

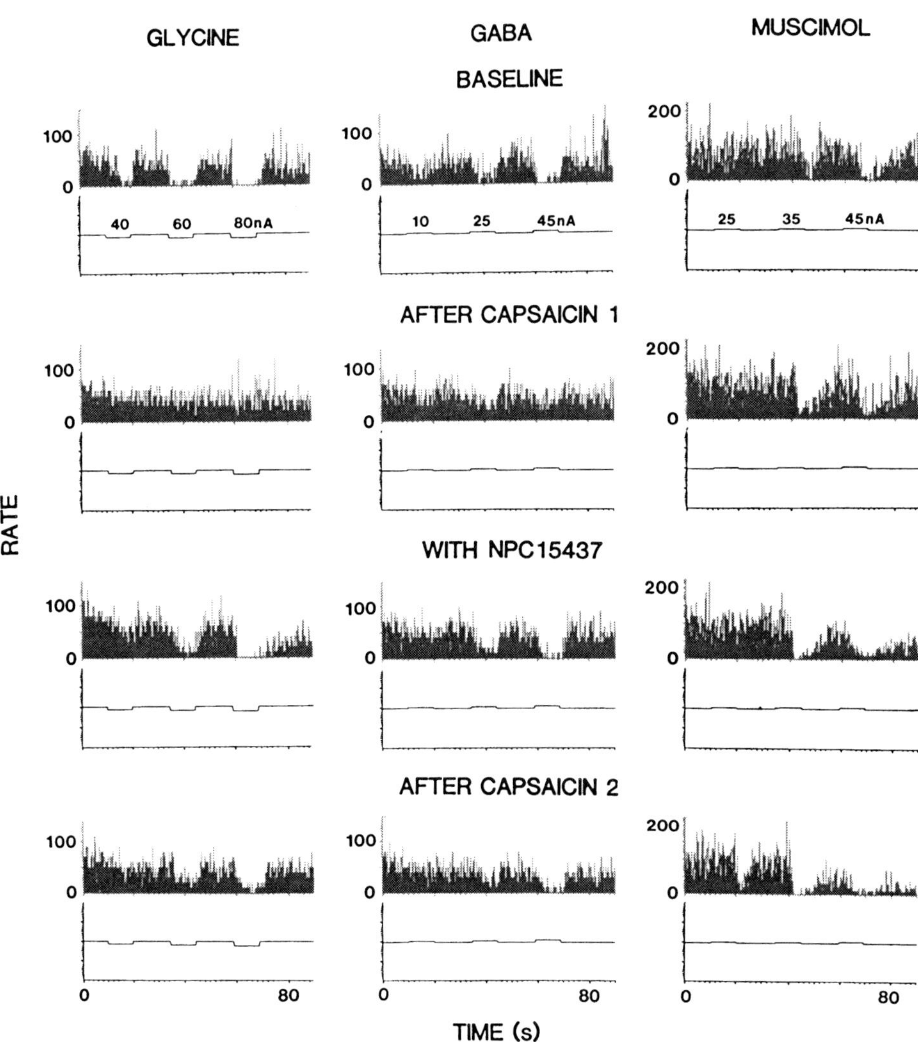

Figure 4. Effects of intradermal injection of capsaicin on the responses of an STT cell to iontophoretically applied glycine and GABA agonists. The upper row of rate histograms show the inhibition of the STT cell by several current doses of glycine, GABA and muscimol. The second row of histograms shows that the inhibition was reduced following capsaicin injection. The third row shows the inhibition after recovery and during the infusion of the PKC inhibitor, NPC 15437. The bottom row shows that a second injection of capsaicin now had no effect on the inhibition. (From Lin et al., 1996b.)

Role of the Protein Kinase G Pathway

We have recently found that the responses of WDR STT cells in the deep dorsal horn of the monkey spinal cord can be sensitized to both weak and strong mechanical stimuli by microdialysis infusion of 8-bromo-cyclic GMP, and that PAG inhibition is concurrently reduced (Lin et al., 1997). These effects can be prevented by pretreatment with a guanylate cyclase inhibitor. The sensitization produced by 8-bromo-cGMP differed from that produced by capsaicin or microdialysis infusion of phorbol ester in that the responses not only to BRUSH and PRESS but also those to PINCH stimuli were enhanced. Interestingly, STT cells in the superficial dorsal horn and HT STT cells in the deep dorsal horn showed reduced responses to mechanical stimulation of the skin after microdialysis administration of 8-bromo-cyclic GMP; for these neurons, PAG inhibition remained unaffected. Evidently, activation of a particular signal transduction pathway can have different effects on the responses to particular stimuli and on different types of STT cells.

Conclusions

In addition to overt pain, an injury can produce primary and secondary hyperalgesia and allodynia that long outlast the pain. The neural mechanisms that allow the persistence of hyperalgesia and allodynia include the activation of second messenger systems. When such systems are engaged in the axons of primary afferent nociceptors, the result can be primary hyperalgesia. Activation of signal transduction cascades in central neurons following synaptic release of such neurotransmitters as EAAs and SP appears to be responsible for central sensitization, which in turn can account for secondary hyperalgesia and allodynia. Signal transduction systems that have so far been suggested to be responsible for central sensitization include G-proteins and several protein kinase pathways, including protein kinase C, protein kinase G and protein kinase A. Not discussed here are the likely roles for other second messengers, such as nitric oxide and the prostaglandins.

Acknowledgements

The experiments described were conducted in the author's laboratory, and were supported by NIH grants NS09743 and NS11255. Thanks are expressed for the expert technical assistance of Kelli Gondesen and Griselda Gonzales.

References

Baumann TK, Simone DA, Shain CN and LaMotte RH (1991) Neurogenic hyperalgesia: the search for the primary cutaneous afferent fibers that contribute to capsaicin-induced pain and hyperalgesia. J Neurophysiol 66:212 -227.

Birrell GJ, McQueen DS, Iggo A and Grubb BD (1993) Prostanoid-induced potentiation of the excitatory and sensitizing effects of bradykinin on articular mechanonociceptors in the rat ankle joint. Neurosci 54:537-544.

Buck SH and Burks TF (1986) The neuropharmacology of capsaicin: review of some recent observations. Pharmacol Rev 38:179-226.

Davis KD, Meyer RA and Campbell JN (1993) Chemosensitivity and sensitization of nociceptive afferents that innervate the hairy skin of monkey. J Neurophysiol 69:1071 -1081.

Dougherty PM and Willis WD (1991) Enhancement of spinothalamic neuron responses to chemical and mechanical stimuli following combined micro-iontophoretic application of N-methyl -D-aspartic acid and substance P. Pain 47:85-93.

Dougherty PM and Willis WD (I 992) Enhanced responses of spinothalamic tract neurons to excitatory amino acids accompany capsaicin-induced sensitization in the monkey. J Neurosci 12:883-894.

Dougherty PM, Palecek J, Paleckova V, Sorkin LS and Willis WD (1992) The role of NMDA and non-NMDA excitatory amino acid receptors in the excitation of primate spinothalainic tract neurons by mechanical, chemical, thermal, and electrical stimuli. J Neurosci 12:3025 -3041.

Dougherty PM, Palecek J, Paleckova V and Willis WD (1994) Neurokinin 1 and 2 antagonists attenuate the responses and NKI antagonists prevent the sensitization of primate spinothalamic tract neurons after intradermal capsaicin. J Neurophysiol 72:1464 -1475.

Dougherty PM, Palecek J, Zorn S and Willis WD (1993) Combined application of excitatory amino acids and substance P produces long-lasting changes in responses of primate spinothalamic tract neurons. Brain Res. Rev. 18:227-246.

Dray A, Bettaney J, Forster P and Perkins MN (1988) Bradykinin-induced stimulation of afferent fibres is mediated through protein kinase C. Neurosci Lett 91:301 -307.

Gerhart KD, Yezierski RP, Wilcox TK and Willis WD (1984) Inhibition of primate spinothalamic tract neurons by stimulation in periaqueductal gray or adjacent midbrain reticular formation. J Neurophysiol 51:450 -466.

Guard S and Watson SP (1991) Tachykinin receptor types: classification and membrane signalling mechanisms. Neurochem Int 18:149 -165.

Häbler HJ, Jänig W and Koltzenburg M (1990) Activation of unmyelinated afferent fibres by mechanical stimuli and inflammation of the urinary bladder in the cat. J Physiol 425:545562.

Handwerker H O, Kilo S and Reeh PW (1991) Unresponsive afferent nerve fibres in the sural nerve of the rat. J Physiol 435:229-242.

Hardy JD, Wolff HG and Goodell H (1967) Pain Sensations and Reactions. Hafner Publishing Co., New York (reprinted from the 1952 edition, The Williams & Wilkins Co.).

Hayes RL, Price DD, Ruda MA and Dubner R (1979) Suppression of nociceptive responses in the primate by electrical stimulation of the brain or morphine administration: behavioral and electrophysiological comparisons. Brain Res 167:417 -421.

Holland LN, Goldstein BD and Aronostam RS (1993) Substance P receptor desensitization in the dorsal horn: possible involvement of receptor-G protein complexes. Brain Res 600:89-96.

LaMotte RH, Lundberg LER and Torebjörk HE (1992) Pain, hyperalgesia and activity in nociceptive C units in humans after intradermal injection of capsaicin. J Physiol 448:749-764.

LaMotte RH, Shain CN, Simone DA and Tsai EFP (1991) Neurogenic hyperalgesia· psychophysical studies of underlying mechanisms. J Neurophysiol 66:190 -21 1.

LaMotte RH, Thalhammer JG and Robinson CJ (1983) Peripheral neural correlates of magnitude of cutaneous pain and hyperalgesia: a comparison of neural events in monkey with sensory judgments in human. J Neurophysiol 50:1-26.

Lewis T (1942) Pain. The Macmillan press, London.

Lin Q, Peng YB and Willis WD (1996a) Possible role of protein kinase C in the sensitization of primate spinothalamic tract neurons. J Neurosci 16:3026 -3034.

Lin Q, Peng YB and Willis WD (1996b) Inhibition of primate spinothalamic tract neurons by spinal glycine and GABA is reduced during central sensitization. J Neurophysiol 76:1005 1014.

Lin Q, Peng YB, Wu J and Willis WD (1997) Involvement of CGMP in nociceptive processing by and sensitization of spinothalamic neurons in primates J Neurosci, In press.

MacDermott AB, Mayer ML, Westbrook GL, Smith SJ and Barker JL (1986) NMDA -receptor activation increases cytoplasmic calcium concentration in cultured spinal cord neurones. Nature 321:519 -522.

Merskey H and Bogduk N (1994) Classification of Chronic Pain; Descriptions of Chronic Pain Syndromes and Definitions of Pain Terms. 2nd ed. IASP Press, Seattle.

Meyer RA and Campbell JN (1981) Myelinated nociceptive afferents account for the hyperalgesia that follows a burn to the hand. Science 213:1527 -1529.

Ochoa J and Torebjörk HE (1989) Sensations evoked by intraneural microstimulation of C nociceptor fibres in human skin nerves. J Physiol 415:583-599.

Palecek J, Paleckova V, Dougherty PM and Willis WD (1994) The effect of phorbol esters on the responses of primate spinothalamic neurons to mechanical and thermal stimuli. J Neurophysiol 71:529-537.

Peng YB, Lin Q and Willis WD (1997) Involvement of protein kinase C in responses of ratdorsal horn neurons to mechanical stimuli and periaqueductal gray descending inhibition. Exp Brain Res, In press.

Schaible HG and Schmidt RF (1985) Effects of an experimental arthritis on the sensory properties of fine articular afferent units. J Neurophysiol 54:1109 -1122.

Schepelmann K, Messlinger K, Schaible HG and Schmidt RF (1992) Inflammatory mediators and nociception in the joint: excitation and sensitization of slowly conducting afferent fibers of cat's knee by prostaglandin '2. Neurosci 50:237-247.

Schepelmann K, Messlinger K and Schmidt RF (1993) The effects of phorbol ester on slowly conducting afferents of the cat's knee joint. Exp Brain Res 92:391 –398.

Simone DA, Baumann TK and LaMotte RH (1989) Dose-dependent pain and mechanical hyperalgesia in humans after intradermal injection of capsaicin. Pain 38:99 -107.

Simone DA, Sorkin LS, Oh U, Chung JM, Owens C, LaMotte RH and Willis WD (1991) Neurogenic hyperalgesia: central neural correlates in responses of spinothalamic tract neurons. J Neurophysiol 66:228-246.

Sluka KA and Willis WD (1997) The effects of G-protein and protein kinase inhibitors on the behavioral responses of rats to intradermal injection of capsaicin. Pain, In press.

Sluka KA, Rees H, Chen PS, Tsuruoka M and Willis WD (1997) Inhibitors of G-proteins and protein kinases reduce the sensitization to mechanical stimulation and the desensitization to heat of spinothalamic tract neurons induced by intradermal injection of capsaicin in the primate. Ex Brain Res, In press.

Torebjörk HE and Hallin RG (1973) Perceptual changes accompanying controlled preferential blocking of A and C fibre responses in intact human skin nerves. Exp Brain Res 16:321 -332.

Torebjörk HE, Lundberg LER and LaMotte RH (1992) Central changes in processing of mechanoreceptive input in capsaicin-induced secondary hyperalgesia in humans. J Physiol 448:765-780.

Walaas SI and Greengard P (1991) Protein phosphorylation and neuronal function. Pharmacological Reviews 43:299-349.

Willis WD (1985) The Pain System; The Neural Basis of Nociceptive Transmission in the Mammalian Nervous System. Karger, Basel.

Willis WD (ed.) (1992) Hyperalgesia and Allodynia. Raven Press, New York.

Willis WD and Coggeshall RE (1991) Sensory Mechanisms of the Spinal Cord. 2nd ed., Plenum Press, New York.

Pain Mechanisms and Management
S.N. Ayrapetyan and A.V. Apkarian (Eds.)
IOS Press, 1998

Dissociation between Peripheral and Central Components of the Endotoxin-Induced Hyperalgesia

N.E. Saadé[a,b], S.A. Kanaan[c], J.J. Haddad[c], S.F. Atweh[d],
S.J. Jabbur[b] and B. Safieh-Garabedian[c]
*Departments of [a]Human Morphology, [b]Physiology and
[d]Internal Medicine, Faculty of Medicine
Department of [c]Biology, Faculty of Arts and Sciences
American University of Beirut
Beirut, Lebanon*

Introduction

Tissue injury and/or inflammation are known to produce inflammatory pain and hyperalgesia which are triggered by a complex chemical machinery labeled by Dray as inflammatory soup (Dray, 1994). The resulting peripheral changes (production of cytokines, neurotrophins, eicosanoids, neuropeptides, NO_2 etc. leading to sensitization of nociceptors, Dray, 1994, Safieh-Garabedian et al, 1995, Treede and Magerl, 1995) can also lead to a sustained excitation of the central nervous system (starting at the dorsal horn level), that may also contribute to hyperalgesia at both central and peripheral levels (Schaible et al, 1987, Seltzer et al, 1995, Treede and Magerl, 1995, Willis, 1994).

We have recently described a new model of inflammatory pain induced by intraplantar (i.pl.) injection of endotoxin (ET) in the hindleg of rats and mice (Kanaan et al, 1996). ET injection produced local inflammation (redness, swelling, limping, etc.) in the injected leg, and mechanical and thermal hyperalgesia as assessed by paw pressure (PP), paw immersion (PI), hot plate (HP) and tail flick (TF) tests. Hyperalgesia, assessed by PP and PI tests, was observed in the injected leg (reduction to about 50% of the initial test latencies), did not spread to the non-injected legs and was thus considered as an indication for the localization of the inflammation. The decrease in the HP latency was attributed, at least in part, to the fact that the injected leg is in contact with the heated plate during the performance of this test, while the decrease in the TF latency was attributed to a unilateral spread of central hyperexcitable state. Consequently, the reduction of TF latency was considered as an indication of central hyperalgesia since neither the afferents nor the efferents of this reflex are involved in the inflammatory reaction. Further support to this hypothesis has been provided by two observations: First, $IL_1\beta$ and NGF levels increased only in the injected leg (Garabedian et al., submitted); Second, an increase in the *C-fos* protein expression was detected initially, in the spinal segments supplying the injected leg (Saadé et al., in preparation).

In the present study, we report the results of treatment with various drugs which act selectively either on the site of inflammation or on the dorsal horn neurons, in order to dissociate between the peripheral and the central components of the ET-induced hyperalgesia.

Methods

All experiments were performed on Sprague Dawley rats (weighing 150-200g), housed in standard colony conditions and in strict adherence to ethical guidelines for pain experimentation on animals (Zimmermann, 1983).

The animals were distributed into different experimental groups (n=5 each) according to the type of the treatment received, as detailed in Table 1. All rats were subjected to acute pain tests (PP, PI, HP, TF) during 3 days, in order to establish a baseline, before receiving i.pl. injection of ET ($1.25\mu g$, Difco Co., Detroit, Michigan, USA), except for one group injected with pyrogen-free ($50\mu l$) saline. Details concerning the procedures used for the pain tests and the ET injection have been previously described (Kanaan et al, 1996).

Table 1. List of the different experimental groups and their injections.

Group	Single	n	Repetitive	n
Saline (Sham)		5		
ET only	$1.25\mu g/kg$	5		
Xylocaine	0.5%	5		
	1%	5		
	2%	5		
Morphine	0.5mg/kg	5	$1\ \mu g/kg$	5
	1.0mg/kg	5		
Dexamethasone	$250\mu g/kg$	5	$200\mu g/kg$	5
Acetaminophen	7.5mg/kg	5	$12.5\mu g/kg$	5
	25 mg/kg	5		
NGF antiserum	$5\mu l/g$	5		
IL_1ra	$0.625\mu g$	5		

Xylocaine (Astra, Sweiden, 20mg/ml) was administered in $50\mu l$ injection i.pl. in the ET-injected leg. Morphine sulfate (10mg/ml) was injected i.p. at appropriate dosage in a total volume of $50\mu l$. Dexamethasone phosphate (lab. Renaudin France) was diluted in saline at selected doses in $50\mu l$ of saline. Acetaminophen (Poudre, Gift from Pharmaline Ind. Lebanon) was dissolved in 10ml phosphate buffer saline and injected i.p. at the indicated doses. Anti-NGF antibody (Gift from Prof. Clifford Woolf, University College, London) was injected i.p. 30min before ET injection. Recombinant human interleukin-1 receptor antagonist (IL_1ra) (NIBSC preparation 92/672) was injected i.p. in $100\mu l$ saline 30min before ET injection.   n = number

Drug Treatment

Two types of regimens were followed for drug administration. In the first, the drugs (acetaminophen, dexamethasone and morphine) were repetitively administered (i.p.) (in doses specified in Table 1) at 12h, 1h before and 2h30 min, 5h30 min and 8h30 min after the ET injection. In the second, the drugs were administered as one dose i.p. (except for xylocaine which was injected i.pl. in the ET-injected leg) at 8h30 min after the ET injection. Interleukin receptor antagonist (IL_1ra, $0.625\mu g$ in $100\mu l$ saline; i.p.) and anti-nerve growth factor (anti-NGF, 5µl/g; i.p.) were administered as one dose 30 min before the ET injection.

The effect of each drug was assessed by measuring the latency of each pain test at 9h after the ET injection, which is the time of maximum ET-induced hyperalgesia, as described previously (Kanaan et al, 1996, Safieh-Garabedian et al, 1996).

For each experimental group, the latency of each pain test was calculated as the average ± SEM of individual measurements and plotted as percent variation of the control value (obtained before the ET injection and from animals injected with saline). The degree of significance of the difference between the recorded value for each pain test and its control value was performed by ANOVA test, using the GraphPad software version 1.13.

Results

Injection of dexamethasone, a steroidal anti-inflammatory drug, known to inhibit the early phenomenon of inflammation and the synthesis of proinflammatory factors such as cytokines and eicosanoids (Schimer and Parker, 1996), elicited a stronger effect on the PP test. As shown in Fig. 1, a single dose of 250µg/kg exerted a significant reduction of PP hyperalgesia and milder effects on the TF and HP latencies. Injection of repetitive doses (200µg/kg) produced a total reversal of hyperalgesia assessed by the PP test and a significant reduction of the hyperalgesia assessed by the TF and HP tests.

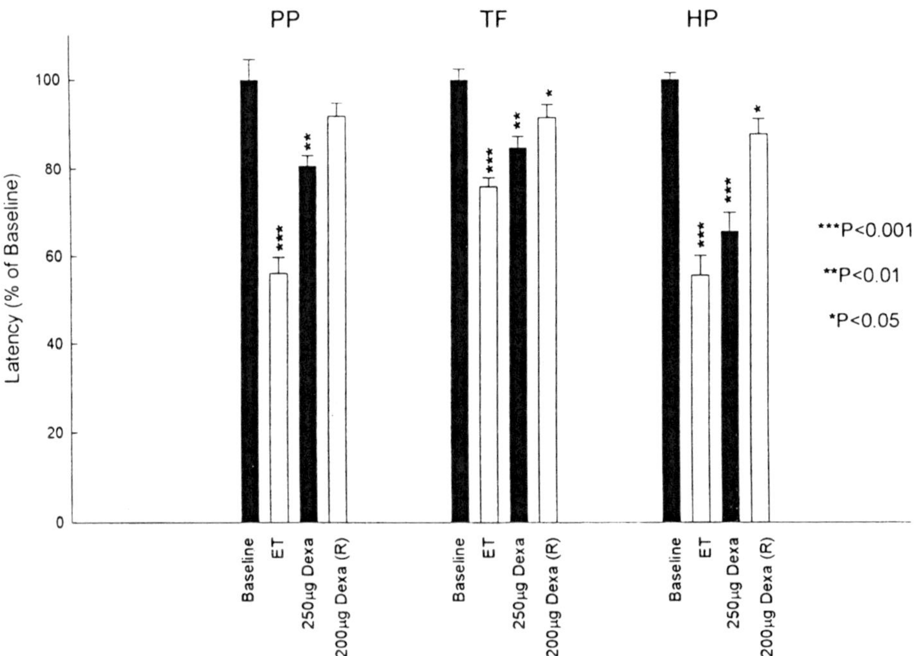

Figure 1. Effects of single or repetitive (R) injections of dexamethasone on the ET-induced hyperalgesia as assessed by the paw pressure (PP), the tail flick (TF) and the hot plate (HP) tests. The indicated doses are given as per kg. The significance of differences is calculated in reference to the baseline value for each pain test. All pain tests were performed 9h after the ET injection. Similar abbreviations and protocols are used in Figs. 2, 3 and 4.

Intraplantar injection of the local anesthestetic, xylocaine, showed, at all the doses, significant effects on the PP hyperalgesia and milder and less significant effects on the hyperalgesia assessed by the TF and the HP tests (Fig. 2).

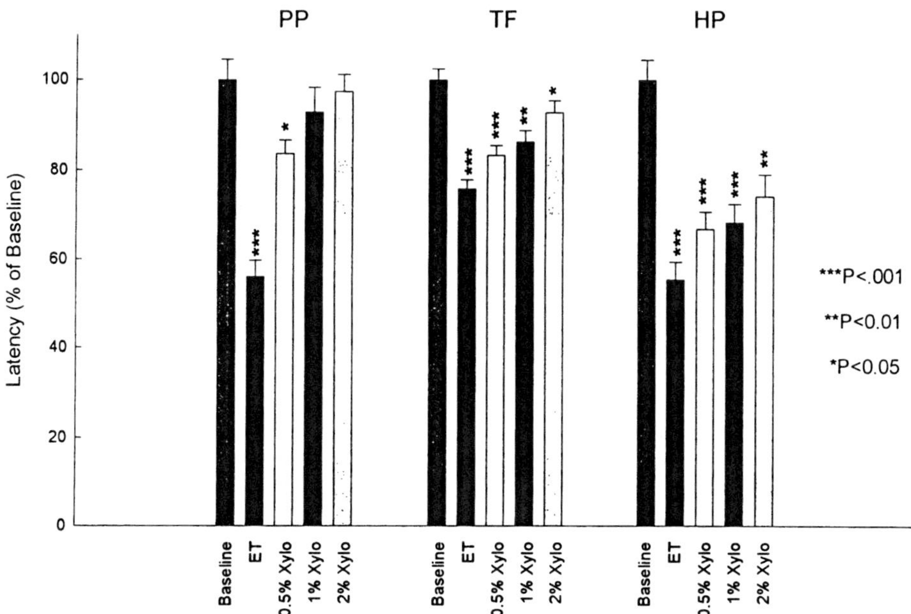

Figure 2. Effects of 3 doses of xylocaine on ET-induced hyperalgesia as assessed by the various pain tests. Xylocaine was administered at the indicated doses in one injection 8h.30min after the ET-injection.

Injection of acetaminophen (an inhibitor of prostaglandin formation, Ferreira et al, 1978) and considered as peripheral analgesic with mild central effects at low doses (Bianchi and Paneira, 1996, Ferreira et al, 1978, Hunskaar et al, 1985, Pelissier et al, 1995), exerted a maximal effect on the PP latency, while only repetitive injections or relatively high doses (25mg/kg) produced a significant reduction of the hyperalgesia assessed by the TF and the HP tests (Fig. 3).

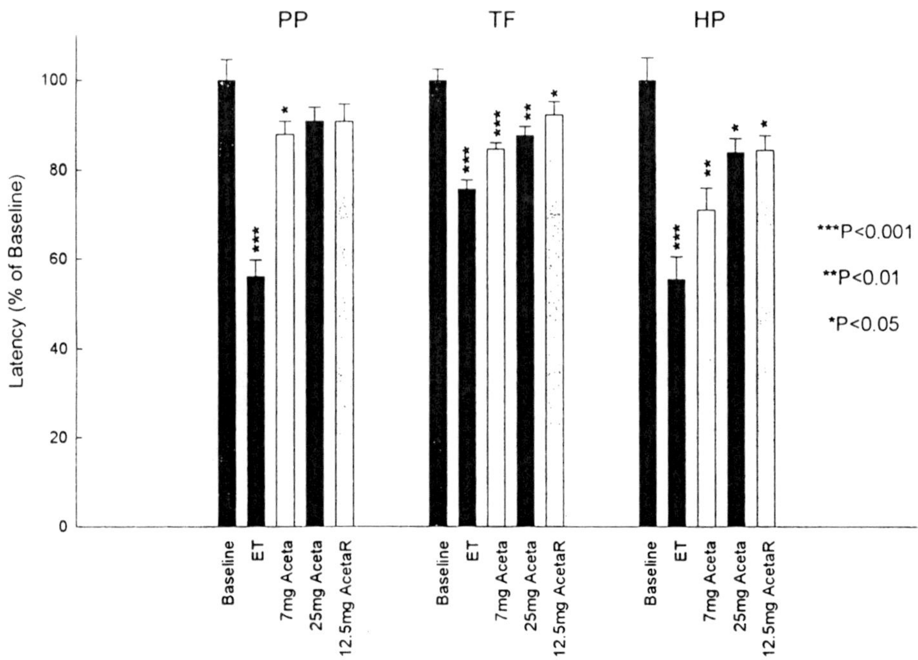

Figure 3. Effects of acetaminophen injections at three different doses, two single and one repetitive R, on the ET-induced hyperalgesia as assessed by the various pain tests.

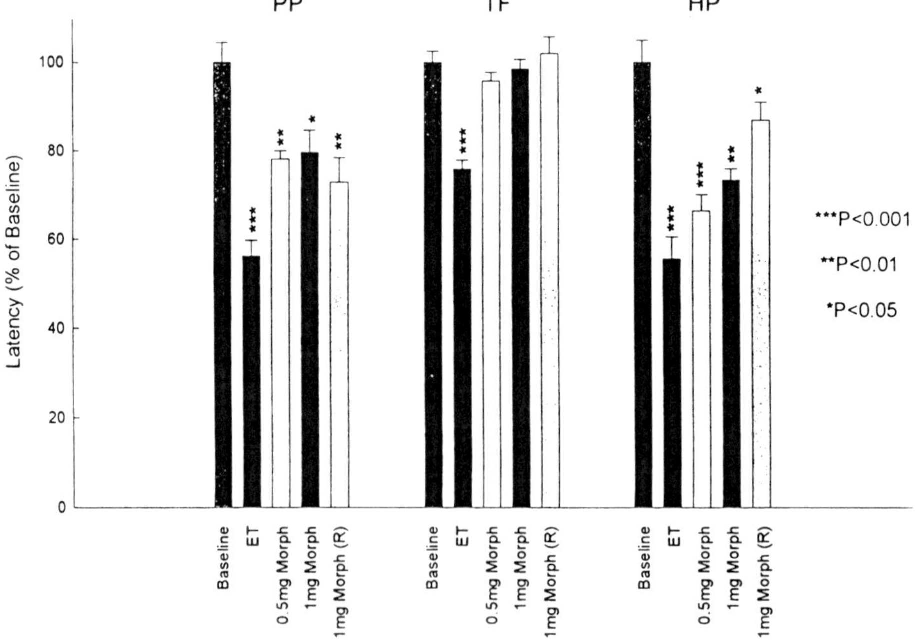

Figure 4. Effects of single repetitive (R) injections of morphine on the ET-induced hyperalgesia. Note that all injections were equally effective in reversing the TF latency to the baseline level.

Morphine injections (a centrally acting narcotic analgesic, (Hunskaar et al, 1985) at all doses, produced total reversal of the hyperalgesia assessed by the TF test and was less effective on the hyperalgesia assessed by the HP and the PP tests. The latter was least affected (Fig. 4).

Pretreatment with either anti-NGF antiserum or with IL_1ra produced further evidence about the dissociation between the hyperalgesias assessed by the different pain tests. Fig. 5 shows that anti-NGF injection reversed the mechanical hyperalgesia assessed on the injected leg, while the thermal hyperalgesia (PI, HP and TF tests) were either mildly or not affected at all. Furthermore, IL_1ra injection reversed the mechanical and the thermal hyperalgesias measured on the injected leg and reduced significantly the HP hyperalgesia but to a less extent the TF hyperalgesia (Fig. 6).

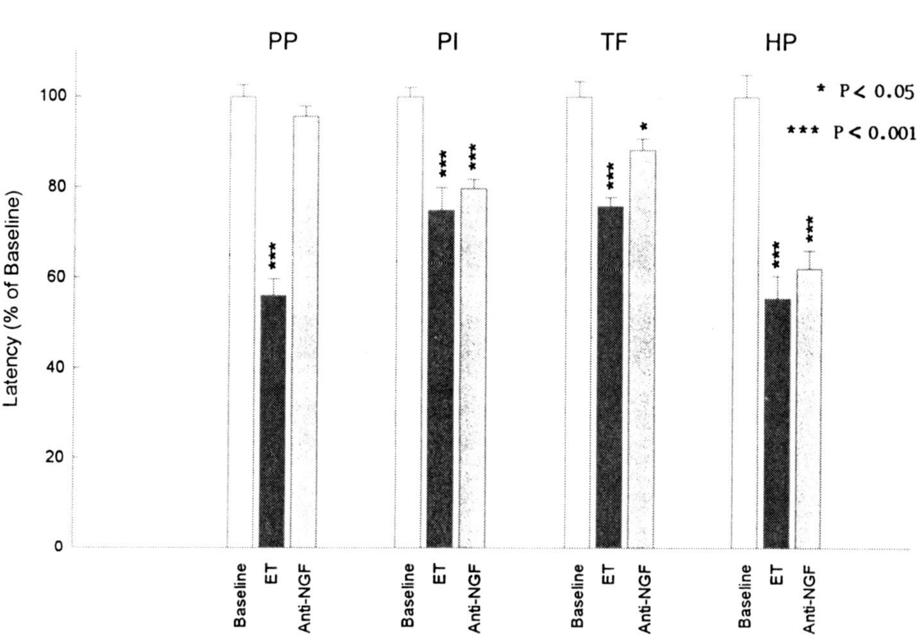

Figure 5. Effects of single injection of anti-NGF serum (5µl/g, i.p. 30min before ET injection) on the ET-induced hyperalgesia. Anti-NGF serum reversed the mechanical, while the thermal hyperalgesia was less affected.

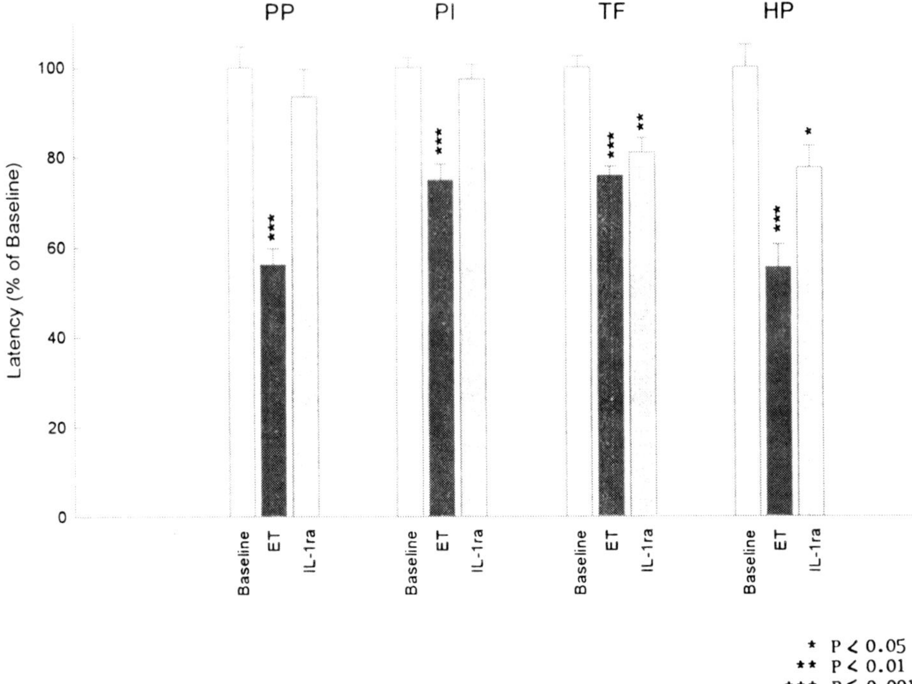

Figure 6. Reversal of the peripheral (mechanical and thermal) ET-induced hyperalgesia by IL_1ra antagonist injection (0.625µg in 100µl saline i.p., 30min before ET injection). The other pain tests were less affected by this injection.

Discussion

The results of this study reveal differential effects of the analgesic (acetaminophen and morphine), anti-inflammatory (dexamethasone) and anesthetic (xylocaine) drugs on the ET-induced hyperalgesia. This discrimination was more pronounced when using repetitive injections, starting before the induction of inflammation. Moreover, the selection of dosage for each drug is based on previously established data concerning its optimal effect (for morphine see Hunskaar et al, 1985, Okuyama ad Aihara, 1985; for acetaminophen see Honore et al, 1995, Hunskaar et al, 1985, Pelissier et al, 1995 and for dexamethasone see Safieh-Garabedian et al, 1996).

The selectivity of the effects of the drugs could not be attributed to a simple preferential action on the mechanical (PP) versus thermal (HP and TF) hyperalgesias, since these drugs exerted similar effects on the PI (thermal) and the PP (mechanical) tests when carried on the injected leg as summarized in Fig. 7. Consequently, the differential effects shown by the various drugs could be attributed to the preferential or selective effect of each drug either on the peripheral or on the central mechanisms of the ET-hyperalgesia.

As illustration, xylocaine (the local anesthetic) and dexamethasone (an inhibitor of cytokine production and COX-2 (Cronstein et al, 1992, Masferrer et al, 1990, Safieh-Garabedian, 1995) showed a maximum effect on the PP test (carried in the inflamed leg) and a minimum effect on the TF test (which reflects central hyperalgesic mechanisms).

Their relative efficacy on the HP hyperalgesia could be attributed to the involvement of the injected leg in the performance of this test. The effects of repetitive injections of dexamethasone reveal the importance of the preemptive treatment in preventing the induction of inflammation and the resulting hyperalgesia. Xylocaine was not assayed at repetitive doses in order to avoid repetitive irritation due to many injections in the inflamed leg.

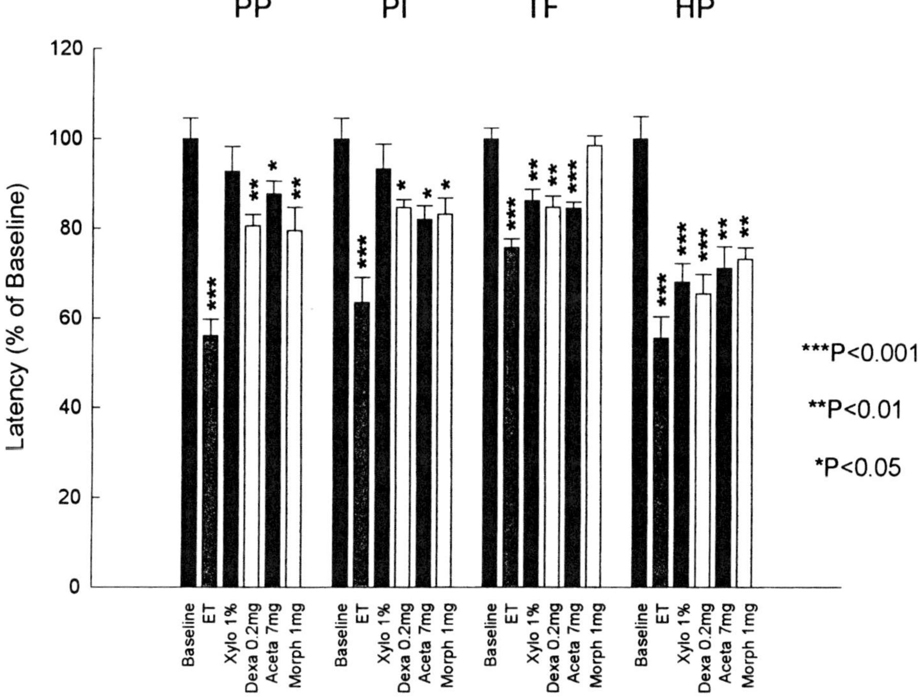

Figure 7. Comparison between the effects of single injection of each drug in our study on the various pain tests used to assess the ET-induced hyperalgesia. Each drug showed similar effects on mechanical and thermal hyperalgesia assessed on the ET-injected leg (PP and PI). Note that xylocaine, acetaminophen and dexamethasone were the most effective on peripheral hyperalgesia (PP and PI) while morphine was the most effective on central hyperalgesia (TF).

Similar effects to dexamethasone were shown by IL_1ra and anti-NGF which totally reversed the PP and the PI hyperalgesia (only IL_1ra) with mild effects on the other tests. This result is in line with our previous demonstration (Safieh-Garabedian et al., submitted) that ET injection induces significant increases of $IL_1\beta$ and NGF levels, which are reduced by dexamethasone, but without total reversal of the ET-induced Hyperalgesia. These results put together allow us to conclude that in this particular situation drug treatment can reverse the ET-induced peripheral hyperalgesia but not the central hyperalgesia.

Treatment with morphine (which affects preferentially the activities of dorsal horn neurons at the dosage used (Hunskaar et al, 1985, Okuyama and Aihara, 1985) reversed totally the TF hyperalgesia with mild effects on the PP and the HP hyperalgesias. The selectivity of these effects was substantiated further with repetitive injections whereby the HP hyperalgesia was more affected, while the effect on the PP hyperalgesia was not enhanced. These observations give further evidence about the possible dissociation between central and peripheral ET-induced hyperalgesias through the appropriate drug treatment.

Acetaminophen injection showed equal effects on all the pain tests used (an effect which was enhanced by repetitive injections). This result is in line with the recently accumulating evidence about the efficacy of acetaminophen on central and peripheral hyperalgesias (Bianchi and Paneira, 1996, Ferreira et al, 1978, Honore et al, 1995, Pelissier et al, 1995).

Finally, our results allow us to draw the following conclusions:

First, local injections of ET can induce thermal and mechanical hyperalgesias and peripheral and central hyperalgesias, which probably involve separate neurohumoral mechanisms.

Second, TF hyperalgesia, observed after i.pl. injection of ET, reflects a central hyperexcitable state induced by remote peripheral inflammation. This demonstrates a possible dissociation between peripheral and central components of the inflammation-induced hyperalgesia.

Third, each of the different drugs had more pronounced effects on the ET-induced hyperalgesia, when administered before and repetitively after the induction of the ET-inflammation. This demonstrates clearly the value of preemptive treatment (either with analgesics or with anti-inflammatory drugs) in the prevention and/or alleviation of inflammatory pain (Clifford, 1994).

Acknowledgements

The authors thank Raffy Jalakhian, Nada Lutfi, Reem Abou Zein and Riad Maalouf for their technical assistance in this study. This research was funded in part by Diana Tamari Sabbagh Fund and University Research Board.

Plenary discussion

Apkarian V.: Is the endotoxic model sympathetically mediated or dependent? What are the effects of blocking the sympathetics on the model?

Saadé N.: We did not try yet the effects of either surgical or chemical sympathectomy, but we assume a sympathetic involvement in the endotoxin induced hyperalgesia, which could be a peripheral correlate or reflection of the central hyperalgesic state induced by the endotoxin injection.

Reeh W.: To my knowledge, all acute "hyperalgesic" effects of NGF and related neurotrophins are secondary to cell degranulation, i.e. they are not direct to nociceptive nerve endings. The anti-hyperalgesic effects of anti-NGF you showed, could they be related to prevention of mast cell degranulation?

Saadé N.: In our histological study of the inflammatory reaction to endotoxin injection we detected a typical mast cell degranulation. This allows the speculation that the effects of anti-NGF serum could be related to a possible upregulation of NGF secondary to mast cell regulation, but this does not exclude the existence of other possible mechanisms.

References

Bianchi M and Panerai AE (1996) The dose-related effects of paracetamol on hyperalgesia and nociception in the rat, Br J Pharmacol 117:130-132.

Clifford JW (1994) A new strategy for the treatment of inflammatory pain prevention or elimination of central sensitization, Drugs 47 (Suppl. 5):1-9.

Cronstein BN, Kimmel SC, Levin RI, Martiniuk F and Weissmann G (1992) A mechanism for the antiinflammatory effects of corticosteroids: the glucocorticoid receptor regulates leukocytes adhesion to endothelial cells and expression of endothelial-leukocyte adhesion molecule 1 and intracellular adhesion molecule 1, Proc Natl Acad Sci USA 89:9991-9995.

Dray A (1994) Tasting the inflammatory soup: the role of peripheral neurons, Pain Rev 1:154-171.

Ferreira SH, Lorenzetti BB and Corrêa FMA (1978) Central and peripheral anti-algesic acation of aspirin-like drugs, Eur J Pharmacol 53:39-48.

Honoré P, Buritova J and Besson JM (1995) Aspirin and acetaminophen reduced both FOS expression in rat lumbar spinal cord and inflammatory signs produced by carrageenin inflammation, Pain 63:365-375.

Hunskaar S (1987) Similar effects of acetylsalicylic acid and morphine on immediate responses to acute noxious stimulation. Pharmacol Toxicol 60:167-170.

Hunskaar S, Fasmer OB and Hole K (1985) Acetylsalicylic acid, paracetamol and morphine inhibit behavioral responses to intrathecally administered substance P or capsaicin, Life Sci 37:1835-1841.

Kanaan SA, Saadé NE, Haddad JJ, Abdelnoor AM, Atweh SF, Jabbur SJ and Safieh-Garabedian B (1996) Endotoxin-induced local inflammation and hyperalgesia in rats and mice: A new model for inflammatory pain, Pain, in press.

Masferrer JL, Zweifel BS, Seibert K and Needleman P (1990) Selective regulation of cellular cyclooxygenase by dexamethasone and endotoxin in mice, J Clin. Invest 86:1375-1379.

Okuyama S and Aihara H (1985) The site of action of morphine and indomethacin differs with electrical stimulation of cutaneous or tibial nerves in normal and adjuvant arthritic rats, Arch Inter Pharmacodyn Thér 276:133-141.

Pelissier T, Alloui A, Paeile C and Eschalier A (1995) Evidence of a central antinociceptive effect of paracetamol involving spinal 5HT3 receptors, Pharmacol. Neurotoxicol 6:1546-1548.

Safieh-Garabedian B, Jalakhian RH, Saadé NE, Haddad JJ, Jabbur SJ and Kanaan SA (1996) Thymulin reduces hyperalgesia induced by peripheral endotoxin injection in rats and mice, Brain Res 717:179-183.

Safieh-Garabedian B, Poole S, Allchorne A, Winter J and Woolf CJ (1995) Contribution of interleukin-1β to the inflammation-induced increase in nerve growth factor levels and inflammatory hyperalgesia, Br J Pharmacol 115:1265-1275.

Schaible HG, Schmidt RF and Willis WD (1987) Enhancement of the responses of ascending tract cells in the cat spinal cord by acute inflammation of the knee joint, Exp. Brain Res 66:489-499.

Schimer BP and Parker KL (1996) Adrenocorticotropic hormone; adrenocortical steroids and their synthetic anlogs; inhibitors of the synthesis and actions of adrenocortical hormones. In: The Pharmacological Basis of Therapeutics, McGraw-Hill, New York (AG Gilman eds) pp. 1449-1485.

Seltzer Z, Beilin B, Ginzburg R, Paran Y and Shimko T (1991) The role of injury discharge in the induction of neuropathic pain behavior in rats, Pain 46:327-336.

Treede RD and Magerl W (1995) Modern concepts of pain and hyperalgesia: beyond the polymodal C-nociceptor, NIPS 10:216-228.

Willis WD (1994) Central plastic responses to pain. In Progress in Brain Research and Management, (GF Gebhart DL Hammond and TS Jensen eds), Vol. 2, IASP, Seattle pp. 301-324.

Zimmermann M (1983) Ethical guidelines for investigations of experimental pain in conscious animals, Pain 16:109-110.

Thymulin at High Doses Reduces Endotoxin-Induced Hyperalgesia by Reducing Interleukin-1β and Nerve Growth Factor Levels in the Hind Paw of Rats

B. Safieh-Garabedian[a], R. H. Jalakhian[a], S. J. Jabbur[b], N. E. Saadé[b]
and S. A. Kanaan[a]
[a]Department of Biology
Faculty of Arts and Sciences and [b]Departments of Human Morphology and Physiology
Faculty of Medicine, American University of Beirut
Beirut, Lebanon

Abstract. Rats with intraplantar injection of endotoxin (1.25μg) in the hind paw, developed localized inflammatory hyperalgesia as assessed by paw pressure test (mechanical), and hot plate and tail flick tests (thermal). Also in these animals there was a significant elevation in the level of the inflammatory mediators IL-1β and NGF, in the skin of the injected paw. Intraperitoneal thymulin treatment at supraphysiological doses (1μg), resulted in a significant reversal in the endotoxin-induced hyperalgesia, as assessed by the different pain tests. Thymulin administration also, significantly reduced the endotoxin-induced elevation in IL-1β and NGF levels in the injected hind paw.

Introduction

The thymus gland produces several peptide hormones that play an important role at different stages in T cell differentiation (Bach 1983; Kendall 1991). One such hormone, thymulin (Bach et al 1976), known to be involved in immunomodulation (Safieh-Garabedian et al 1992), is a highly conserved nonapeptide produced within the thymus gland by two discrete populations of epithelial cells located in subcapsular/perivascular cortex and medulla, respectively (Dardenne et al 1977; Kendall et al 1991). Recent work has indicated that thymulin has modulatory effect on cytokine release by human peripheral mononuclear cells (Safieh-Garabedian 1993). We have, more recently, developed a new model of localized inflammatory hyperalgesia in rats and mice, using peripheral endotoxin (ET) injections. The resulting hyperalgesia is assessed by mechanical (paw pressure) and thermal (hot plate and tail flick) pain tests (Kanaan et al 1996). In this ET model, we have demonstrated that thymulin at supraphysiological doses significantly reduces ET-induced hyperalgesia (Safieh-Garabedian et al 1996).

Recently, several investigators, have described an important role for the pro-inflammatory cytokine interleukin-1β (IL-1β) (Ferreira et al 1988; Watkins et al 1995) and the neurotrophic factor NGF (Donnerer et al 1992; Lewin et al 1993; Woolf et al 1994), in the generation of inflammatory hyperalgesia. In the present study we have investigated whether thymulin reduces hyperalgesia by reducing the level of the known mediators, like IL-1β and NGF in the ET injected hind paw skin of rats.

Methods

Animals

Adult male Sprague-Dawley rats (Charles River, Celco, Como, Italy) were used in all the experiments (5-6 per group). The animals (150-200g) were housed under optimum conditions of light (12h light and 12h dark) and temperature (22 ± 2°C), with food and water provided *ad libitum*. All experiments were carried out with strict adherence to ethical guidelines (Zimmerman, 1983).

Behavioral measurements

Thermal and mechanical pain tests were performed for 3 consecutive days prior to any injections to establish a constant baseline. The paw pressure test (PP) was used to assess mechanical hyperalgesia, and the hot plate (HP), paw immersion (PI), and tail immersion tests (TF) were performed for the assessment of thermal hyperalgesia, as described in detail previously (Kanaan et al., 1996). Briefly, for the HP test, animals were individually placed on a hot surface plate (52.8°C-53.4°C) and the latency of the first sign of paw licking or jumping to avoid the heating pain was taken as an index of the pain threshold. For the TF test, the tail of each animal was immersed into a beaker of distilled water (T = 50.5°C) and the withdrawal latency for tail flicking was recorded and scores were based on 3 tests with a 5-min interval between consecutive tests. For the PI test, the injected paw was dipped in a beaker of distilled water (T = 48°C) and the latency was recorded as the immersed paw is withdrawn from the hot water. Mechanical hyperalgesia was measured by the paw pressure test (PP), by applying a constant pressure of 0.20 kg/cm^2 alternately to the left and right hind paws with a 5-min interval between consecutive applications. The pressure was discontinued when the animals displayed a typical pain reaction characterized by a vigorous flexion reflex (for more details see Kanaan et al., 1996).

Experimental protocols

Different groups of rats received either intraplantar (i.pl.) injections of ET (1.25µg/50µl saline) prepared from *Salmonella typhi* (Difco laboratories, Michigan, USA) or ET plus Intraperitoneal (i.p.) injections (1µg) of thymulin (Sigma Chemical Co., St. Louis, Missouri, USA) in 100µl physiological saline, 30 min before and 2.5h after the ET injection. A group of rats, acting as controls, received together with the ET-injection 100µl saline, whereas another group received 1µg thymulin injection only. Pain tests (described above) were performed on each experimental animal at 9h, which has been shown to be the peak of the ET-induced hyperalgesia (Kanaan et al 1996). Skin tissues were removed at 4h. Animals were terminally anaesthetized (sodium pentobarbital; 50mg/kg) and the entire hind paw skin (from left and right feet) was removed. The tissue samples were weighed, snap frozen on dry ice and stored at -70°C to be processed for IL-1β and NGF determinations.

IL-1β and NGF assays

Skin tissue was homogenized in phosphate buffered saline (PBS; pH=7.4) containing 0.4M NaCl, 0.05% Tween-20, 0.5% bovine serum albumin, 0.1mM phenylmethylsulfonyl fluoride, 0.1mM benzethonium chloride, 10mM EDTA and 20KI/ml aprotinin. The homogenates were centrifuged at 12,000 g for 60 min at 4°C. Both NGF and IL-1β content in the supernatants were measured by two-site Enzyme-Linked Immunosorbent Assay (ELISA) as detailed previously (Safieh-Garabedian et al 1995).

Statistical Analysis

Results are given as mean ± standard error of mean (SE). The degree of significance of differences between experimental groups was performed by the ANOVA test, using the Graph Pad Software version 1.13 and Prism version 1. All graphical plots were constructed using Jandel Sigma Plot version 3.0 for Windows '95.

Results

ET (1.25μg) injections (i.pl.) resulted in a significant decrease in mechanical hyperalgesia (47.27 ± 6.50 %; P<0.001) as assessed by the PP test and thermal hyperalgesia (54.10 ± 6.90 %; P<0.01) and (75.30 ± 3.82 %; P<0.05) as assessed by the HP and TF tests, respectively, and compared to saline controls. When thymulin (1μg), was administered (i.p.) together with the ET, there was a significant recovery in mechanical hyperalgesia as determined by the PP latency (77.27 ± 2.94 %; P<0.01), thermal hyperalgesia as determined by the HP test (71.77 ± 5.84 %; P<0.05), and complete recovery in the TF test (82.49 ± 3.95 %). Results given in Fig. 1. Thymulin (1μg) injection alone, had no significant effect on any of the pain tests utilized (data not shown).

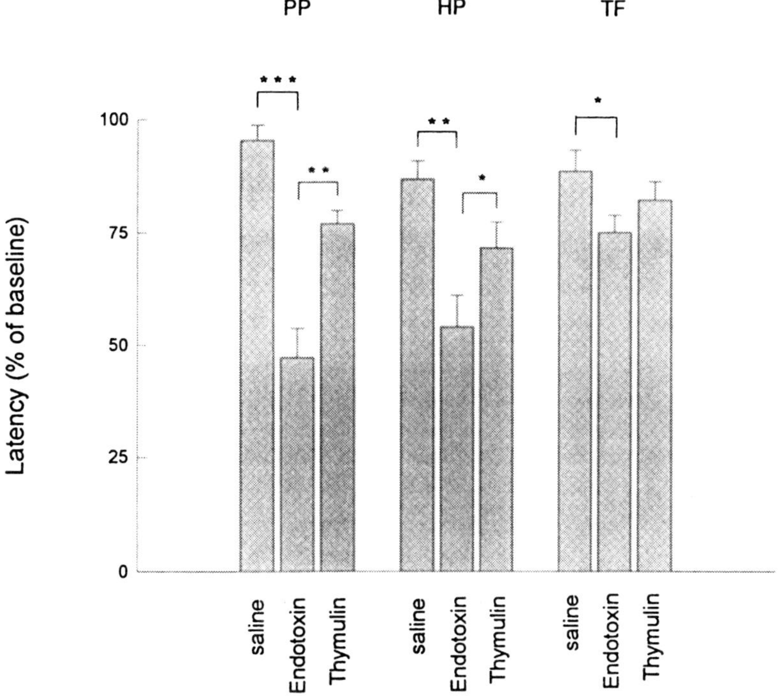

Figure 1. Histograms showing the effect of thymulin (1 μg) injection (i.p.) on ET-induced (1.25 μg; i.pl. injection in the hind paw of rats) mechanical (PP) and thermal (HP and TF) hyperalgesia obtained at 9h. (* P<0.05, ** P<0.01, *** P<0.001)

ET injection (1.25 µg) resulted in a significant (P<0.001) elevation in the level of IL-1β in the hind paw skin of rats (3372 ± 911 pg/hind paw) at 4h, when values were compared with saline injected animals (300 ± 100 pg/hind paw). This increase was significantly (P<0.001) reduced (619.78 ± 196 pg/hind paw) by thymulin (1 µg) injection 30 min before the ET administration (Fig. 2).

ET injection (1.25 µg) resulted in a significant (P<0.001) elevation in the level of NGF in the hindpaw skin of rats (23.00 ± 6.78 ng/hind paw) at 4h, when values were compared with saline injected animals (5.20 ± 0.57 ng/hind paw). This increase was significantly (P<0.001) reduced (7.99 ± 0.60 ng/hind paw) by thymulin (1 µg) administration 30 min before the ET injection (Fig. 3).

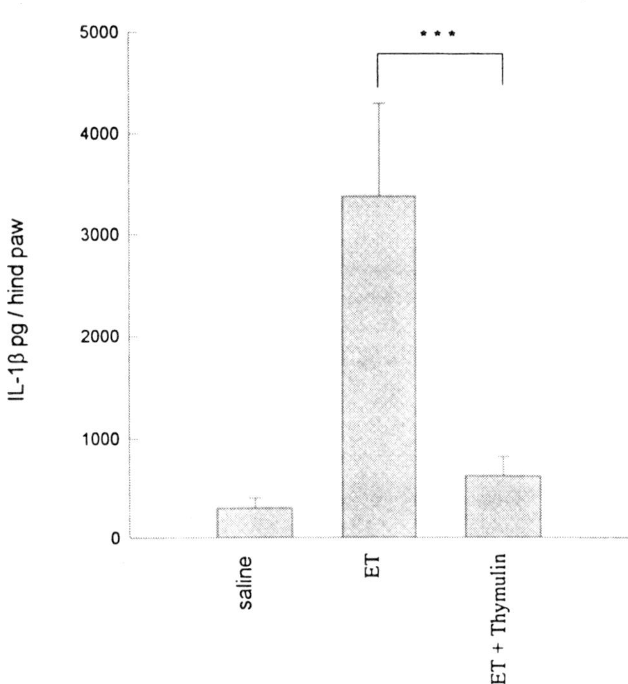

Figure 2. The effect of thymulin (1µg) injection (i.p.) on ET-induced (1.25µg) elevation of IL-1β level in the injected hind paw of the rat obtained at 4h. The values obtained in the non-injected paw were not significantly different than those for the saline injected paw (data not shown). *** P<0.001

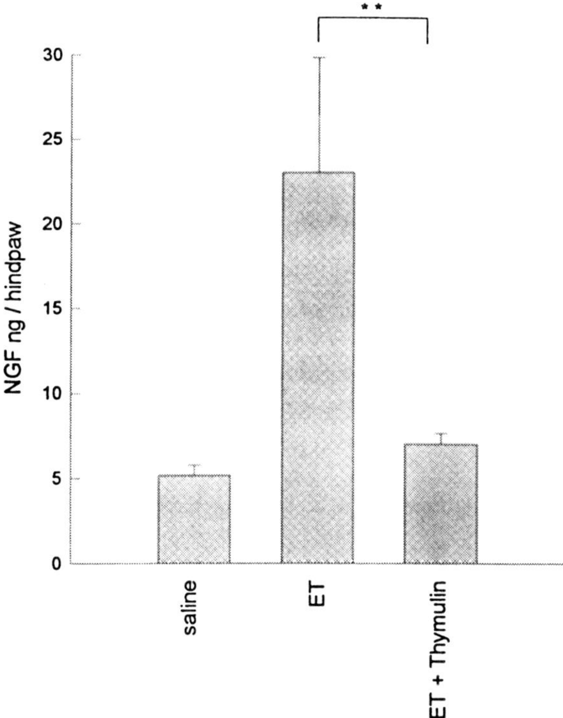

Figure 3. The effect of thymulin (1μg) injection (i.p.) on ET-induced (1.25μg) elevation of NGF level in the injected hind paw of the rat obtained at 4h. The values obtained in the non-injected paw were not significantly different than those for the saline injected paw (data not shown). ** P<0.01

Discussion

Our results clearly indicate that ET (1.25μg) injections (i.pl.) in the hind paw of rats result in a significant increase in sensitivity to pain as assessed by the PP test (mechanical hyperalgesia) and the HP and TF tests (thermal hyperalgesia) at 9h after the injection. This increase in sensitivity was reduced significantly (PP and HP tests) by thymulin, whereas in the case of the TF test there was complete recovery. This effect was obtained at supraphysiological doses of thymulin only, as characterized in more detail previously (Safieh-Garabedian et al 1996). Thymulin on the other hand, at low concentrations induces hyperalgesia in rats, an effect which might be mediated via prostaglandin-E_2 (Safieh-Garabedian et al in press). Intraplantar injections of ET also resulted in a significant elevation in IL-1β and NGF levels in the injected hind paw of rats at 4h, and no such elevations were observed in the non-injected leg. Similar elevations were also observed in rats injected with complete Freund's adjuvant (Donnerer et al 1992; Woolf et al 1994; Safieh-Garabedian et al 1995). The pleiotropic cytokine IL-1βappears to be involved in all inflammatory responses (Dinarello 1991). It has been shown that either local or systemic injection of this cytokine causes hyperalgesia (Ferreira et al 1988; Watkins et al 1994). Furthermore, IL-1β induces the production of NGF in a number of cell types in culture (Lindholm et al 1987; Matsuoka et al 1991), and contributes to the inflammation-induced increase of NGF levels in the skin of rats, which is reduced significantly by administering the receptor antagonist (IL-1ra) (Safieh-Garabedian et al 1995). In this study, thymulin significantly reduced the levels of IL-1β and NGF in the injected hind paw of the rats, and this reduction in NGF could be subsequent to a reduction in the level of IL-1β, for reasons explained above. In a previous work, it has been shown that thymulin at high doses inhibits IL-1β production in peripheral blood mononuclear cells (Safieh-Garabedian et al 1993).

In conclusion, the results of this study indicate that the mechanism by which thymulin reduces hyperalgesia could be via the reduction of the levels of two important mediators of inflammation namely, IL-1β and NGF.

Acknowledgements

The authors thank John Haddad, Nada Lutfi and Riad Maalouf for their technical assistance in this study. This research was funded in part by the University Research Board and Diana Tamari Sabbagh Fund.

Plenary discussion

Basbaum A.: What is the source of IL-1 in this model? How does thymulin block it? Is there evidence for a sympathetic source of IL-1? M. Schuthzberg, I believe, showed IL-1 immunoreactivity in sympathetics.

Safieh-Garabedian B.: I can't answer at the moment whether there is a sympathetic source for IL-1β.

Besson J.-M.: Did you try the effect of thymidin in other inflammatory tests, e.g. formalin. carragenin, etc?

Safieh-Garabedian B.: No, thymulin has not yet been tested in another model.

Amassian V.: Did you measure the temperature of your animals after the local endotoxin injection?

Safieh-Garabedian B.: Yes. No significant changes in temperature were found.

Amassian V.: Following up on a question of Prof. Basbaum, is it possible that the local injection increased contralateral parietal lobe activity, which led to altered sensitivity to sensory stimulation and changes analogous to those found with magnetic stimulation?

Safieh-Garabedian B.: It is difficult to give a definite answer to this question. However, local injection of endotoxin can induce hyperalgesia in pain tests organized mainly at the spinal level, i.e. the tail flick test.

References

Bach JF (1983) Thymulin (FTS-Zn). Clinics Immunol Allergy 3:133-157.

Bach JF, Dardenne M, Pléau JM and Rosa J (1976) Biochemical characterization of a serum thymic factor. Nature 266:55-56.

Dardenne M, Pléau JM, Nabarra B, Lefranchie P, Derrien M, Choay J and Bach JF (1977) Structural isolation of circulating thymic factor. A peptide isolated from pig serum. 1. Isolation and purification. J. Biol. Chem 252:8040-8044.

Dinarello C A (1991) Interleukin-1 and interleukin-1 antagonism. Blood. 77:1627-1652.

Donnerer J, Schuligoi R and Stein C (1992) Increased content and transport of substance P and calcitonin gene-related peptide in sensory nerves innervating inflammed tissue: evidence for a regulatory function of nerve growth factor in vivo Neurosci 13:2136-2148.

Ferreira SH, Lorenzetti BB, Bristow AF and Poole S (1988) Interleukin-1β as a potent hyperalgesic agent antagonized by a tripeptide analogue. Nature 334:698-700.

Kanaan S, Saadé NE, Haddad JJ, Abdelnoor AM, Jabbur SJ and Safieh-Garabedian B (1996) Endotoxin-induced local inflammation and hyperalgesia in rats and mice: A new model for inflammatory pain. Pain, in press.

Kendall MD (1991) Functional anatomy of the thymic microenvironment. J Anat 177:1-29.

Kendall MD, Safieh-Garabedian B, Sareen A, Venn G, Matheson L and Ritter M (1991) Thymulin-secreting cells in humans. In: Lymphatic Tissues and In Vivo Immune Responses Marcel Dekker, (B Imhof, S Berrih-Akinn and S Ezine eds.) New York pp. 41-43.

Lewin GR, Ritter AM and Mendell LM (1993) Nerve growth factor-induced hyperalgesia in the neonatal and adult rat. J Neurosci 13:2136-2148.

Lindholm D, Neumann R, Meyer M and Thoenen H (1987) Interleukin-1 regulates synthesis of nerve growth factor in non-neuronal cells of sciatic nerve. Nature 330:658-659.

Matsuoka I, Meyer M and Thoenen H (1991) Cell type specificity regulation of nerve growth factor (NGF) synthesis in non-neuronal cells: comparison of Schwann cells with other cell types. J Neurosci 11:3165-3177.

Safieh-Garabedian B, Kendall MD, Khamashta MA and Hughes GRV (1992) Thymulin and its role in immunomodulation. J Autoimmunol 5:547-555.

Safieh-Garabedian B, Ahmed K, Khamashta MA and Hughes GRV (1993) Thymulin modulates cytokine release by peripheral blood mononuclear cells: a comparison between healthy volunteers and patients with systemic lupus erythematosus. Int Arch Allergy Immunol 101:126-131.

Safieh-Garabedian B, Poole S, Allchorne A, Winter J and Woolf CJ (1995) Contribution of interleukin-1β to the inflammation-induced increase in nerve growth factor levels and inflammatory hyperalgesia. Brit J Pharmacol. 115:1265-1275.

Safieh-Garabedian B, Jalakhian RH, Saadé NE, Haddad JJ, Jabbur SJ and Kanaan SA (1996). Thymulin reduces hyperalgesia induced by peripheral endotoxin injection in rats and mice. Brain Res 717:179-183.

Safieh-Garabedian B, Kanaan SA, Jalakhian R, Poole S, Jabbur SJ and Saadé NE Hyperalgesia induced by low doses of thymulin injections: Possible involvement of Prostaglandin-E$_2$. J Neuroimmunol, in press.

Watkins LR, Wiertelak EP, Goehler L, Smith KP, Martin D and Maier SF (1994) Characterisation of cytokine-induced hyperalgesia. Brain Res 654:15-26.

Watkins LR, Maier SF and Goehler LE (1995) Immune activation: the role of pro-inflammatory cytokines in inflammation, illness responses and pathological pain states. Pain 63:289-302.

Woolf CJ, Safieh-Garabedian B, Ma Q-P, Crilly P and Winter J (1994) Nerve growth factor contributes to the generation of inflammatory sensory hypersensitivity. Neurosci 62:327-331.

Zimmermann M (1983). Ethical guidelines for investigations of experimental pain in conscious animals. Pain 16:109-110.

Pain Mechanisms and Management
S.N. Ayrapetyan and A.V. Apkarian (Eds.)
IOS Press, 1998

The Effect of Diet on Neuropathic Pain Expression in Rats

Y. Shir[1], A. Ratner[2], S. N. Raja[3], J. N. Campbell[3] and Z. Seltzer[2,4]

[1]*Department of Anesthesiology and Pain Relief Service, Hadassah University Hospital,*
[2]*Physiology Branch, Faculty of Dental Medicine,*
Hebrew University, Jerusalem, Israel
[3]*Johns Hopkins Medical Institutions,*
Baltimore, Md., USA
[4]*Department of Physiology, Faculty of Medicine,*
Hebrew University, Jerusalem, Israel

Abstract. Since the introduction of models of neuropathic pain following partial nerve injury, it became evident that the same preparation may produce variable sensory disorders across different laboratories. Even when the same model has been used in the same lab, some experimenters, including ourselves, observed a variable expression of sensory disorders at different times, although the rat strain, vendor, gender, age and weight, surgical approach and sensory testing procedures were not changed. Based on a large series of experiments we report here that this variability can be attributed, at least in part, to differences in the diet the animals consumed. The effect of food composition on the expression of neuropathic pain was tested following: (1) Partial hindpaw denervation, produced by ligating 1/3-1/2 of the sciatic nerve (PSL model; Seltzer et al. '90). This model produces mechanical allodynia and thermal hyperalgesia at the hindpaw. (2) Total hindpaw denervation, produced by sciatic and saphenous neurectomy and expressed by self mutilation (autotomy) of the hindpaw. For 14-21 days prior to nerve injury and up to 60 days thereafter, rats were fed with diets from various vendors, differing in their content and type of protein. In the PSL model we found that rats fed on diets containing soy expressed weaker sensory disorders than rats fed on diets based on casein or bread and cucumbers. In contrast, following total denervation the casein-based diet strikingly suppressed autotomy levels compared to rats fed on soy or bread and cucumbers. We conclude that: (1) diet significantly affects neuropathic pain in rats, (2) these effects are model-specific. Modulation of diet in humans may emerge as a novel mode of prophylaxis or even therapy of neuropathic pain. We draw attention of colleagues in the field of neuropathic pain research to the possibility that although animal food vendors may supply a rat chow that meets the formulary standards in terms of the proportion of fat/carbohydrates/proteins *etc*, they may vary the types of protein included, without notification. As shown here, this may greatly affect experimental outcome in a model under study.

Introduction

Over the last decade several animal preparations have been introduced, aimed at modeling neuropathic pain of humans following nerve injury (Zeltser and Seltzer, 1994; Seltzer, 1995). In the original descriptions of these models robust sensory disorders were reported (Bennett and Xie, 1988; Seltzer et al., 1990; Kim and Chung, 1992; Na et al., 1994). One of these models, a unilateral tight ligation of 1/2-1/3 of the sciatic nerve in rats

(Partial Sciatic Ligation - the 'PSL' model) was produced by us (Seltzer et al., 1990). Starting hours after the PSL injury and for several months thereafter, these rats expressed signs of spontaneous pain and mechanical and thermal allodynia and hyperalgesia in the partially denervated foot. We showed that much like the Sympathetically-Maintained Pain syndrome in humans (SMP), these disorders depend on the sympathetic outflow for their production and maintenance, and disappear following postoperative (PO) chemical sympathectomy (Shir and Seltzer, 1990a).

The sensory disorders of the PSL model were consistently produced in a number of studies carried out in our lab at the Hebrew University (HUJI) during the time period 1986-1990 (Shir and Seltzer, 1988;1990a-c; Seltzer et al., 1990; Seltzer and Shir, 1991; Shir et al., 1992). Since its publication, other labs have been using the PSL model, some of which use different methods than ours for testing the sensory disorders. This could account for the lesser robustness they reported compared to our original observations (Dougherty et al., 1992; Behbehany and Dollberg-Stolik, 1994; Cui et al., 1996; Kim et al., 1997). Other researches reported robust sensory disorders in the PSL model although they also used testing methods different than ours (Tracey et al., 1995; Takaishi et al., 1996). Some labs encountered total failure in trying to replicate the PSL or other models of partial nerve injury. Thus, variable testing methods cannot explain the differences in expression of the PSL model across labs.

Starting in 1991 and for several years thereafter, we encountered a sudden difficulty in replicating the pain disorders of the original PSL model. A similar sudden weakening of the PSL model was also noted by at least two other labs. Believing that identification of the variable(s) affecting expression of these models is important at the basic and clinical levels, we conducted a series of experiments modifying the surgical procedures, age/weight of the animals, strain of rats and animal vendor. However, none of these modifications reinstituted the robust expression of the original PSL model.

Surmising that food could be the common denominator affecting the expression of the sensory disorders of the PSL model (and perhaps also other models), we conducted another series of experiments in which we modified the composition of the food the rats were fed. In addition, in order to examine whether food affects neuropathic pain of other etiologies, we tested its effect on autotomy (self-mutilation), a behavior induced in rats by total hindpaw denervation (Wall et al., 1979a; Wall et al., 1979b). The data described here have been presented in abstract forms elsewhere (Shir et al., 1996a,b).

Materials and methods

This study followed University and national regulations for humane experimentation on animals, and the guidelines of the International Association for the Study of Pain.

Animals

We report here the results of 15 experimental groups, comprising adult male rats (Table 1; n=8-16 rats/group). In experiments on the PSL model we used rats of the Wistar strain (groups RMH-1,-2) and Sabra strain (groups AMBAR, KOF-1,-2,-3, CAS-1, SOY-1, CB-1,-2). For the autotomy experiments we used rats of the HA selection line (groups KOF-4 and CB-3), and Sabra strain rats (groups SOY-2, KOF-5 and CAS-2). HA rats were selected genetically from the Sabra strain for the expression of high levels of autotomy behavior following total hindpaw denervation by sciatic and saphenous neurectomy (Devor and Raber, 1990). HA rats were provided as a gift from Marshall Devor.

Rats weighed 300-350 g at the time of operation. They were kept in standard colony conditions (3-4 per metal cage with a floor covered with pine-wood shavings and saw dust). Water and food were supplied *ad libitum.* The temperature was kept at 22-24°C. Day/night cycle was lights on at 07:00 and off at 19:00.

Table 1.

Neuropathic pain model	Group	Variables tested	
		Diet/vendor	Rat strain
PSL	AMBAR 1	510, AMBAR	Sabra
PSL	RMH 1	RMH, Agway	Wistar
PSL	RMH 2	RMH, Agway	Wistar
PSL	KOF 1	19510, Kofholk	Sabra
PSL	KOF 2	19510, Kofholk	Sabra
PSL	KOF 3	19510, Kofholk	Sabra
PSL	CB 1	cucumbers & bread	Sabra
PSL	CB 2	cucumbers & bread	Sabra
PSL	SOY 1	soy-based, Weizmann	Sabra
PSL	CAS 1	casein-based, Weizmann	Sabra
Autotomy	KOF 4	19510, Kofholk	HA
Autotomy	KOF 5	19510, Kofholk	Sabra
Autotomy	CB 3	cucumbers & bread	HA
Autotomy	SOY 2	soy-based, Weizmann	Sabra
Autotomy	CAS 2	casein-based, Weizmann	Sabra

Surgery

The PSL Model (for details see Seltzer et al., 1990): Under inhalation anesthesia and aseptic conditions the right sciatic nerve was exposed at a high-thigh level, just distal to the posterior biceps semitendinosus nerve from the common sciatic nerve. Using a mini-needle the dorsal 1/3-1/2 of the nerve thickness was trapped and tightly ligated with an 8-0 silk suture. The wound was then closed with 2 muscle sutures (4-0 silk or cotton) and 3-4 skin staples. This procedure was used in our original reports (Shir and Seltzer, 1988; 1990a-c; Seltzer et al., 1990; Seltzer and Shir, 1991; Shir et al., 1992) and in most experimental groups of the present report (Table 1).

The autotomy model (Wall et al, 1979a,b): Under inhalation anesthesia and aseptic conditions the saphenous and sciatic nerves were transected in two locations along the nerve, the proximal cut preceding the distal cut. This formed a gap several millimeters wide between the stumps, producing a nerve-end neuroma at the proximal stump and a total denervation of the paw. The wound was closed as described above.

Behavioral tests

The responses of intact and operated rats to the following sensory stimuli were determined bilaterally. However, for brevity, here we report the results of the operated side only. Group averages appear ± the standard error of the mean.

1. The PSL model (Seltzer et al., 1990):   Using the following tests the operated animals were examined several times up to 5 weeks PO, and their responses were compared to preoperative baseline values.

A. Mechanical allodynia: Withdrawal threshold to touch was measured with a set of von Frey hairs ranging from 0.25 to 20.0 g. The rat was placed in a chamber with a mesh metal floor, covered by an opaque plastic dome 20X30 cm, 10 cm high. Reaching the plantar surface of the paw from underneath, each hair was indented in the midplantar skin until it bowed. This was repeated 5 times at a frequency of about two stimuli per second. At suprathreshold intensities rats responded by elevating the paw, sometimes accompanied by a flick. If subthreshold, the stimulus intensity was increased by using the next hair in the series. The presence of mechanical allodynia was concluded from a significant PO reduction in the withdrawal threshold to touch compared to the preoperative baseline values.

B. Thermal hyperalgesia: This was determined by beaming infrared pulses of noxious, but not tissue damaging intensity, at the midplantar area of each foot, alternating between the two hindpaws. The infrared pulses were produced from a CO_2 laser (120 msec, 5 W, 150 mCal, 1.5 mm in diameter). The CO_2 laser was guided by a visible He/Ne aiming beam which illuminated the target with a red spot. The time that lapsed between lifting the paw until replacing it on the floor ('Response duration') was recorded with a stop watch. Two minutes were allowed between pulses to avoid sensitization. A significant increase in the response duration of operated animals compared to the baseline values of intact animals was regarded as thermal hyperalgesia.

2. Scoring autotomy behavior: Autotomy was scored twice weekly by the same two observers for up to 9 weeks. The scorers were unaware of the type of food supplied to the rats under observation. We used a slightly modified scoring scale devised by Wall et al. 1979a,b. In this cumulative score 1 point was assigned for the injury of two or more nails and an additional point to each half toe, to a maximum of 11. Rats reaching maximal permitted scores were euthanized promptly and this score was plotted with the group average.

The incidence of rats expressing high autotomy levels (scores $\geq$ 6) at the end of the observation period was compared using the X^2 test of the frequency data. Average onset day of autotomy was defined as the group average of the first day in which autotomy was observed in each rat in the group. Rats that did not self-injure the paw by the last day of the experiment ('d') were assigned an onset day of 'd+1'. Student's t-test was used for statistical evaluation. Values of $p<0.05$ were regarded as significant.

Rat chow formulas
        Rats were fed with the following formulas Table 1):

'**AMBAR 510**' (Ambar, Inc., Emek Chefer, Israel): This diet was a commercially available balanced diet composed of mixed vegetable (mainly soy), fish proteins (11%) and casein (approximately 10%), carbohydrates (67.3 %), fat (3.4%), fiber (3.2), ash (4.9%) and enriched by vitamins and trace elements. This diet had been the routine rat chow provided at HUJI until 1991, during the time period when robust and sTable expression of the PSL model was evident (plots denoted by 'Original' in the Figures).

'RMH' - product RMH-1000 (Agway, Inc., Syracuse, USA) is a commercially available balanced diet composed of mixed vegetable, fish and meat proteins (14.5%), carbohydrates (67.5%), fat (6.5%), fiber (4%), ash (7.5%) and enriched by vitamins and trace elements. RMH has been the routine rat chow provided at JHU. It was also used in some experiments at HUJI. Experimental groups RMH-1,-2 were fed with this diet.

'KOF' - Product 19510 (Kofholk, Inc., Tel Aviv, Israel) is a commercially available balanced diet composed of mixed vegetable (mainly soy), fish and casein proteins (21%), carbohydrates (67.3 %), fat (3.4%), fiber (3.2), ash (4.9%) and enriched by vitamins and trace elements. This diet has been the routine rat chow provided at HUJI since 1991, coinciding the period when we first encountered the weakening of the PSL model. Although the percentage of its ingredients has been relatively constant over the years since 1991, we found that the type of protein (vegetable, fish or casein) markedly changed by the vendor from batch to batch according to availability and costs of ingredients. Groups KOF 1-5 were fed with this diet.

'CB' is made of fresh cucumbers and white bread from local stores. We used this diet since its ingredients were known, remained unchanged throughout the experiment and could be repeatedly used in future experiments when needed. Although deficient in some essential food components, this diet supplies enough calories. We were assured by animal dietitians that this temporary imbalance would be compensated by endogenous storage and would not affect the rats' health for the duration of the experiment. Groups CB 1-3 were fed with this diet.

'SOY': A semi-purified formulation (Weizmann Institute, Israel), containing pulp soy as the sole source of protein (20%), carbohydrates (65%), fat (soy oil 5%), fiber (5%) ash (3.5%), vitamins and trace elements. It has been reported that some proteins in animal food originating from plants, mainly soy, contain phytoestrogens, i.e., compounds that possess estrogenic activity (Whitten and Naftolin, 1991). Estrogen is a known modulator of GABAa receptors (Perez et al., 1988), enhancing the antinociceptive effect of GABA (Yaksh and Malmberg, 1994). Since RMH and the 19510 diets, like most commercially available rat chows, contain variable concentrations of soy, we tested whether levels of neuropathic pain behavior in the PSL and autotomy models could be affected by the presence of soy-derived phytoestrogens in the diet. Groups SOY-1,-2 were fed with this diet.

'CAS': A semi-purified formulation based on casein as the sole protein source (Weizmann Institute, Israel). This diet contained 20% casein, produced by precipitation of crude cow milk (MD Food Ingredients, Videback, Denmark), carbohydrates (65%), fat (corn oil, 5%), fiber (5%) ash (3.5%), vitamins and trace elements. This soy-free formulation served as a control diet in groups CAS-1,-2. Formulation of diets (4) and (5) was based on Whitten and Naftolin, 1992.

Results

The effects of diet on the PSL model

Most experiments were designed to compare the sensory disorders of 2-3 rat groups consuming different diets. Some diets were associated with only very weak neuropathic pain disorders or none at all. Since our main goal in these experiments was to identify the variable responsible for weakening the PSL model, the behavioral follow up was terminated as soon as it became clear that the variable under study was irrelevant, sometimes within a week PO. When we observed robust mechanical allodynia and thermal hyperalgesia, the behavioral follow up was extended to a few weeks PO. For comparison, we included in some of the Figures data from our original PSL reports, when Sabra rats consumed the Ambar 510 diet (Shir and Seltzer, 1988; 1990a-c; Seltzer et al., 1990; Seltzer and Shir, 1991; Shir et al., 1992). In Figures 1-3 groups were clustered according to the type of diet rather than by orders of experiments.

RMH: Wistar rats were fed with the RMH diet throughout their lifetime and PO. Compared to our original results using Sabra rats fed during 1988-1991 on Ambar 510 (Original; Fig. 1a,b), partial nerve injury in the RMH-1 group (and again in the replication experiment on the RMH-2 group) produced only weak mechanical allodynia (Fig. 1a) and thermal hyperalgesia (Fig. 1b).

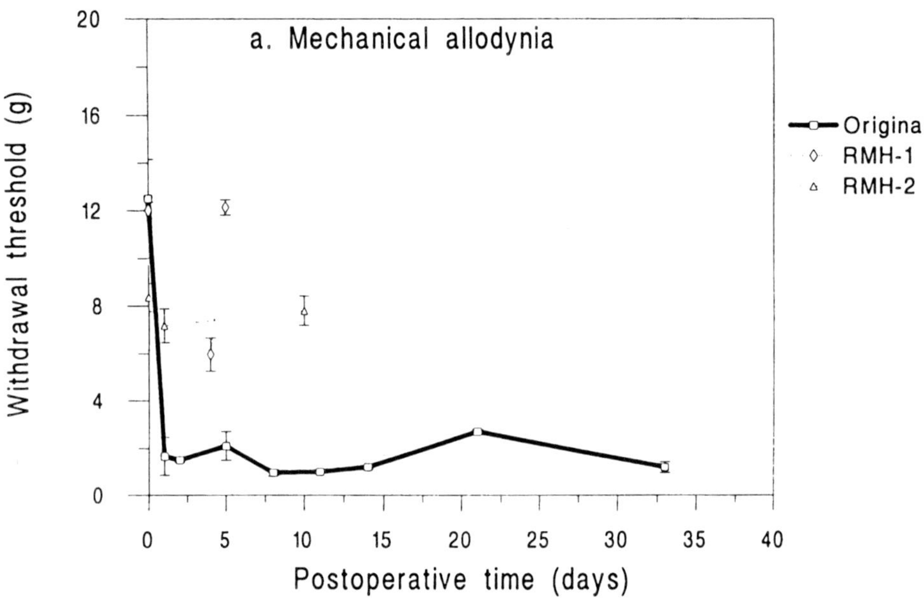

Figure 1. The sensory disorders produced by partial sciatic injury in the PSL model in Wistar rats (RMH-1,-2). Plots marked by the thick line denote archival results from our original report on the PSL in Sabra rats fed on the Ambar 510 diet (Seltzer et al., 1990). **Fig. 1a:** Mechanical allodynia is determined from a significant reduction in the withdrawal threshold to repetitive touch applied with von Frey hair at the denervated hindpaw. Consumption of the RMH diet was associated with very weak and transient allodynia compared to that reported originally.

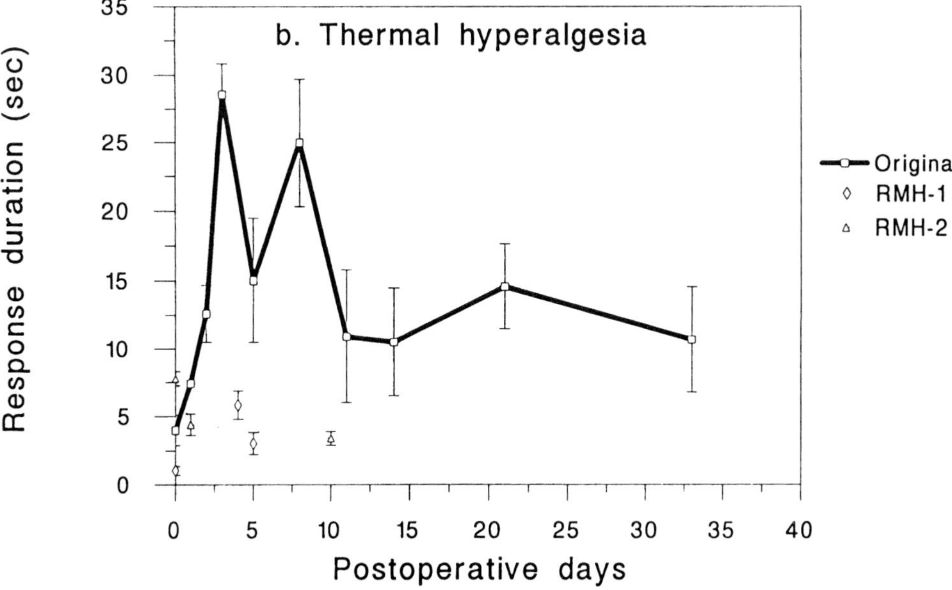

Fig. 1b: Thermal hyperalgesia is determined from a significant increase in response duration to a suprathreshold laser heat pulse directed at the hindpaw. The RMH fed rat groups produced weak hyperalgesia compared to the original groups.

KOF: Feeding Sabra rats with the KOF diet throughout their lifetime and for 22 days PO yielded only weak sensory disorders (KOF-1; Figs. 2a,b). The same results were observed in the replication experiments on the KOF-2 and -3 groups, where the latter were compared to CB-1 and -2).

a. Mechanical allodynia

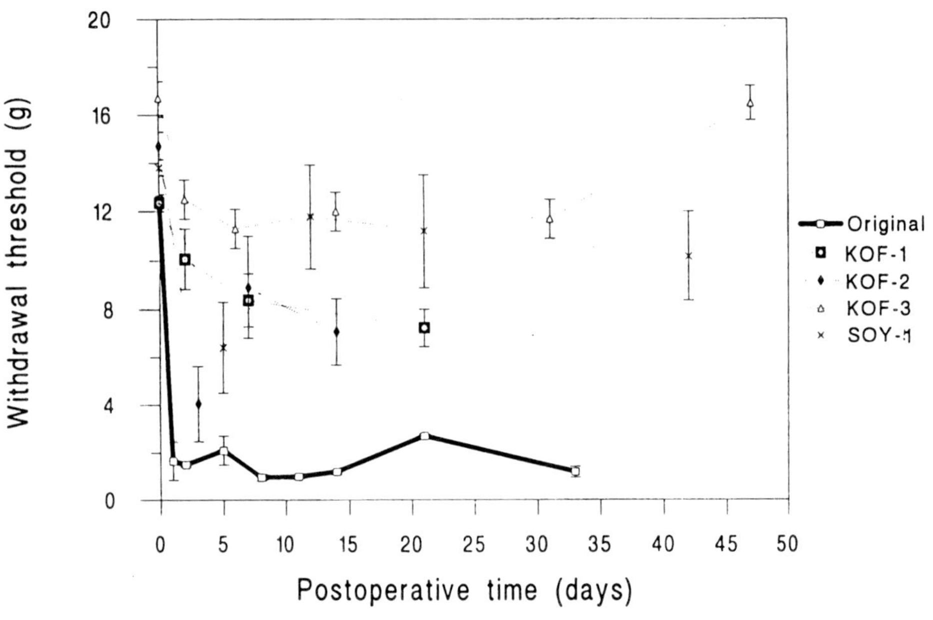

b. Thermal hyperalgesia

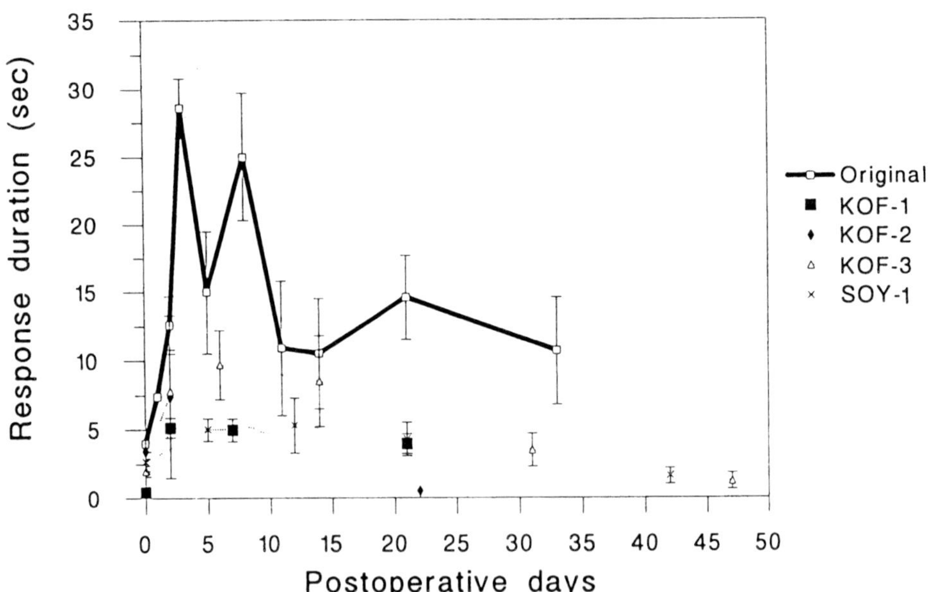

Figure 2. Mechanical allodynia (in Fig. 2a) and thermal hyperalgesia (Fig. 2b) produced by partial sciatic injury in the PSL model in Sabra rats fed on soy-containing diets (KOF 1-3 and the SOY-1 group; denoted by thin lines). The sensory disorders of the original PSL model are plotted in thick lines. Note that the mechanical allodynia to von Frey hair stimulation (Fig. 2a) and thermal hyperalgesia (Fig. 2b) was weaker and short lasting in these groups as compared to the original reports.

SOY: Feeding Sabra rats for 18 days preoperatively and 42 days PO with this alternative diet which contains soy as the sole protein source (SOY-1 group), produced weak sensory disorders (Figs 2a,b), similar to rats fed on the other soy-containing diet (the RMH- and KOF-fed groups).

CB: Sabra rats fed on cucumbers and bread for 18 days preoperatively and 21 days PO (CB-1 group) expressed robust mechanical allodynia (Fig. 3a) and thermal hyperalgesia (Fig. 3b), approaching those seen in our original reports. The replication experiment in group CB-2 showed the same results. These experiments were carried out simultaneously with the KOF-2 and -3 groups.

a. Mechanical allodynia

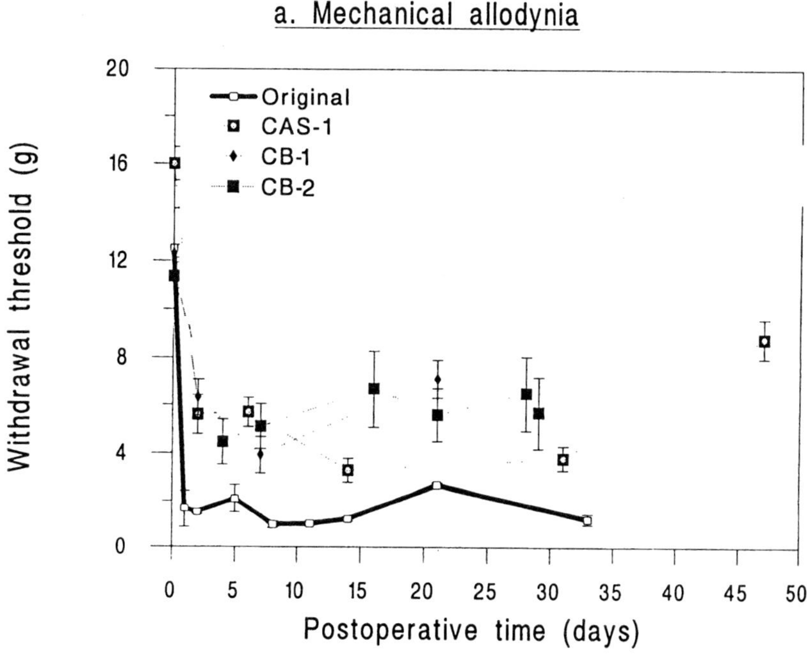

Figure 3. Mechanical allodynia (in Fig. 3a) and thermal hyperalgesia (Fig. 3b) produced in Sabra rats by partial sciatic injury in the PSL model. In thin lines are plotted the sensory disorders of CAS-1 rats, fed on the casein-based diet, and CB -1,-2 groups, consuming cucumbers and bread. The sensory disorders of Sabra rats fed on Ambar 510 diet in the original PSL model are plotted in thick lines. **Fig. 3a:** Note that robust mechanical allodynia to von Frey hair stimulation developed in all tested groups. This sensory disorder did not normalize for at least a month PO.

b. Thermal hyperalgesia

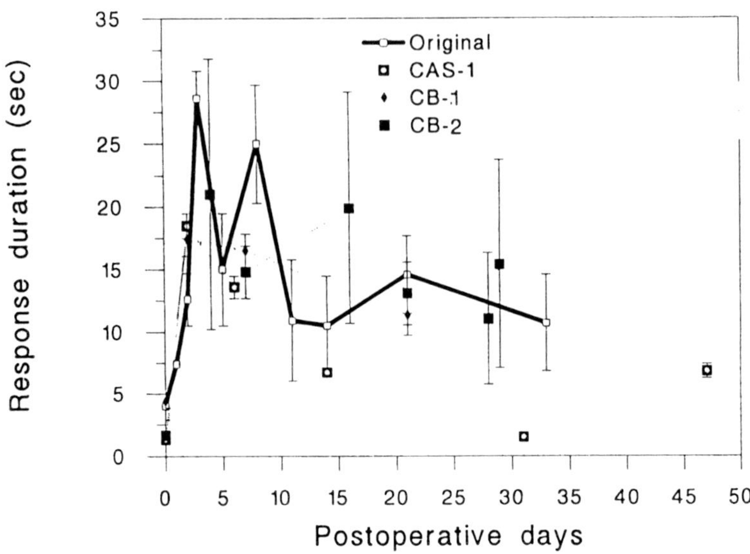

Fig. 3b: Compared to the thermal hyperalgesia to a strong laser heat pulse that was reported by us originally, robust hyperalgesia developed in the CAS-1 group, but deteriorated thereafter. In the CB -1,-2 groups the thermal hyperalgesia fully replicated the original observations.

CAS: Sabra rats fed for 18 days preoperatively and 42 days PO on the casein-based diet (CAS-1) expressed robust mechanical allodynia, like that seen in the CB groups (Fig. 3a). However, while the thermal hyperalgesia during the first week resembled that of the CB groups and the results of the original reports, it weakened rapidly thereafter (Fig 3b).

The effects of diet on autotomy

KOF *vs.* CB: In this experiment HA rats fed on the KOF diet throughout their lifetime (KOF-4) were compared to HA rats fed on cucumbers and bread (CB-3) diet for 18 days preoperatively and for 25 days PO (Fig. 4a). Figure 4b shows that consuming cucumbers and bread shortened significantly the onset day of autotomy (3.7±0.4 vs. 10.1±1.5, for CB-3 and KOF-4, respectively; p<0.01, t-test). Autotomy levels at the end of the observation period (d25) were not different between the two groups (p=0.1; X^2 test; Fig. 4a).

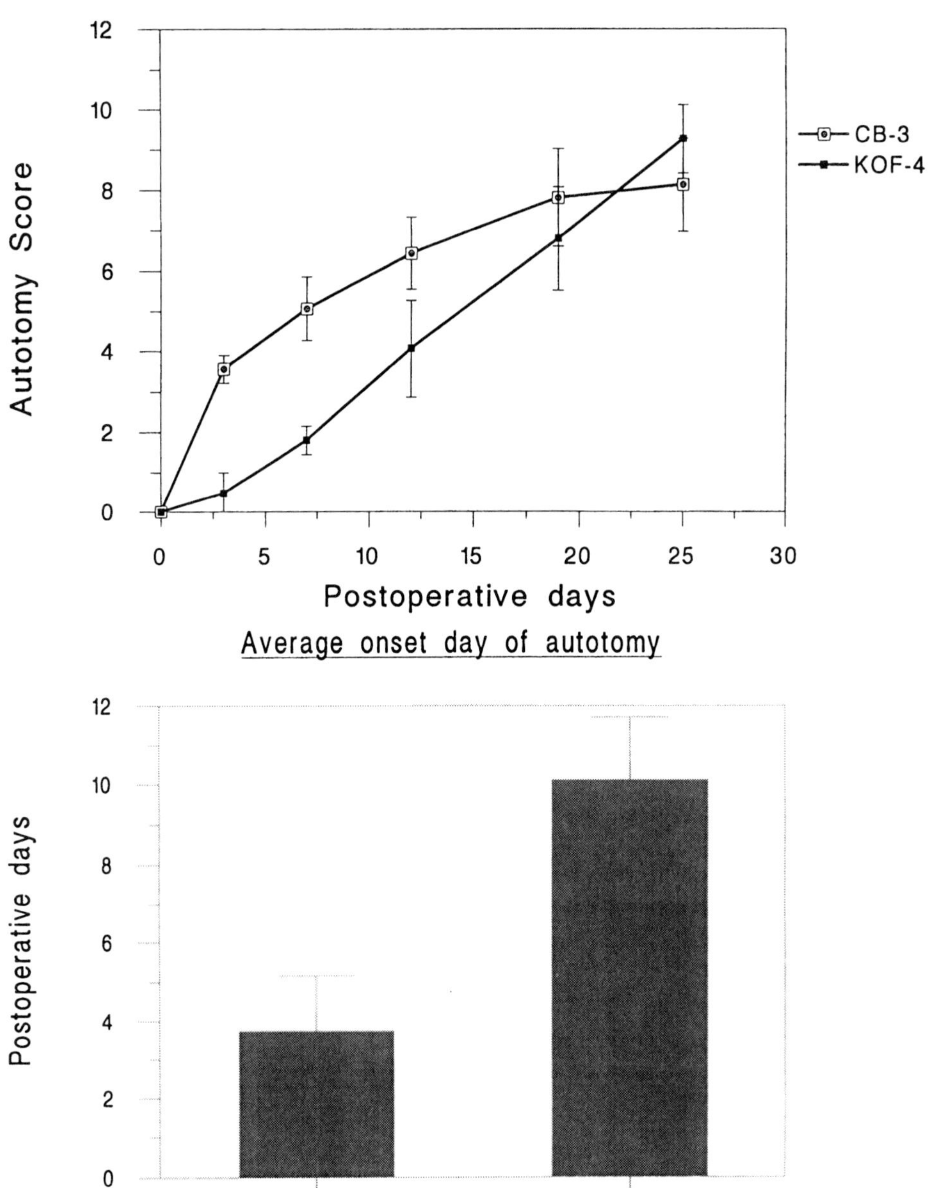

Figure 4. Comparison of autotomy in HA rats fed with the 19510 (KOF-4) or cucumbers and bread (CB-3) diets. **Fig. 4a:** The average increase in the cumulative autotomy scores (±SEM) during the PO time. **Fig. 4b:** Average onset day of autotomy in the KOF-4 group was significantly delayed compared to that of the CB-3 group (p<0.01; t-test).

KOF and SOY vs. CAS: In this experiment Sabra rats were fed with the KOF diet throughout their lifetime (KOF-5), or the alternative soy-based diet (SOY-2) or a casein-based diet (CAS-2) for 21 days preoperatively and for 48 days PO. The course of autotomy of the two soy groups was very similar. The incidence of high autotomy scores in these groups was not different significantly (p=0.8, X^2 test; Fig. 5a). Therefore, the data of the KOF-5 and SOY-2 groups were pooled and compared to the CAS-2 group.

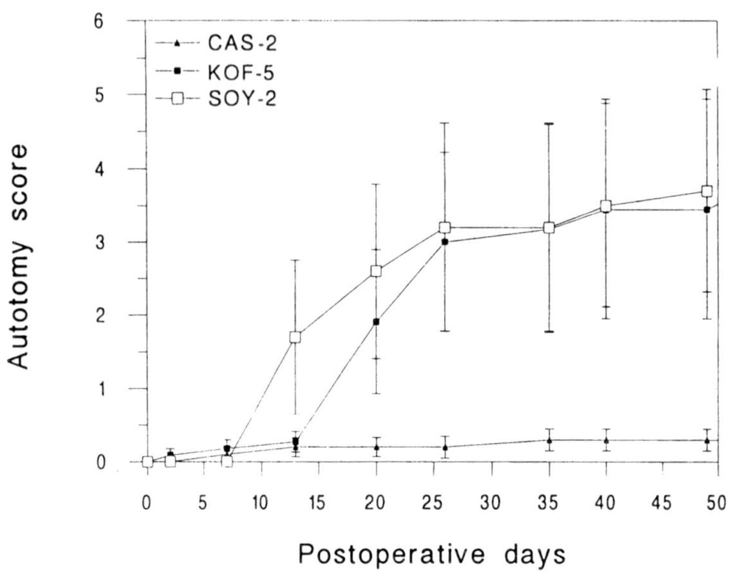

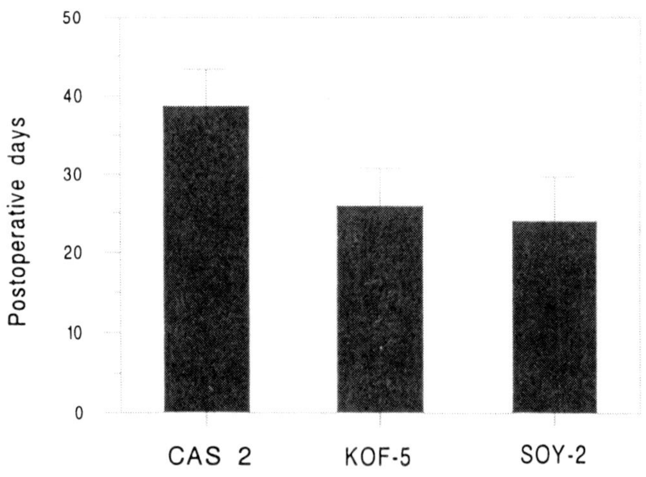

Figure 5. Comparison of autotomy in Sabra rats fed with the casein-based diet (CAS-2), 19510 diet (KOF-5) or the alternative soy-based diet (SOY-2). **Fig. 5a:** The course of autotomy following total hindpaw denervation. Note that the course of autotomy in the two soy containing diet groups was similar. Incidence of high autotomy (scores $\geq$ 6) at d48 PO was not different between the KOF-5 and SOY-2 groups (p=0.8; X^2 test). However, a striking suppresion of autotomy was observed in the CAS-2 group compared to rats fed on the soy-containing diets. **Fig. 5b:** Average onset day of autotomy. Onset of autotomy of the CAS-2 group was significantly delayed when compared to the pooled KOF/SOY groups (p<0.0002; t-test).

Consuming the casein-based diet strikingly suppressed autotomy compared to rats fed on the soy-containing diets. A significant difference in the incidence of high autotomy scores was found at the end of the observation period (d48 PO) between the pooled KOF/SOY group and the CAS-2 group (p=0.02, X^2 test; Fig. 5a). The average onset day of autotomy in the CAS-2 group was significantly delayed when compared to the pooled KOF/SOY group (day 38.8±4.5 vs. 25.0±5.3, respectively; p<0.0002; t-test; Fig. 5b).

Note that the average onset day of Sabra rats is significantly delayed compared to HA rats. This is typical of the HA line (Devor and Raber, 1990).

Discussion

This study indicates that diet, consumed prior to the nerve injury and throughout the PO behavioral observation period, is a fundamental variable in the expression of neuropathic pain in rats. Moreover, the two neuropathic pain models used in this study were affected differently by diet. Notably, the casein-based diet produced robust sensory disorders in the PSL model but suppressed the autotomy model. Because the PSL and the autotomy models differ both in type of nerve injury and in behavioral expression, the dietary effects observed here are model-specific.

In the PSL model we encountered very weak levels of mechanical allodynia and thermal hyperalgesia in all groups fed on the RMH, 19510 and the soy-based diet where soy served as the sole protein source. The common denominator of these food types, as in most other commercially available rat diets, is the inclusion of a substantial proportion of soy protein. As mentioned above, soy and also alfalfa and other proteins in rat chow originating from plants, contain phytoestrogens. These are nonsteroidal flavonoids that exert powerful estrogenic effects on the CNS, gonads and other tissues (Whitten and Naftolin, 1991). Estrogen is a known agonist (Perez et al., 1988) of the antinociceptive neurotransmitter GABA (Yaksh and Malmberg, 1994), acting at the benzodiazepine binding site on the GABAa receptor (Wilson, 1996). Based on these data we speculate that the weakening of the PSL model encountered by us and others, and the suppression of the PSL model in the present study were caused by diets rich in phytoestrogens.

In contrast to the PSL model, the autotomy model was not suppressed by the soy-containing diets, possibly indicating a differential role of GABAa-mediated mechanisms in these two models. The lack of suppression of autotomy in Sabra rats continuously treated with diazepam is compatible with this hypothesis (Seltzer et al., 1989).

HA and LA rats were selected genetically for differential expression of autotomy following hindpaw peripheral neurectomy (Devor and Raber, 1990). These rat lines also differ in the levels of sensory disorders in the PSL model (Seltzer and Shir, 1991; Shir et al., 1992) and the Kim and Chung (1992) neuropathic pain model (Devor et al., personal communication). These findings lend further support to the suggestion that autotomy is related to pain, and indicate that autotomy following total denervation and models of neuropathic pain following partial denervation share genetic determinants. Therefore, it is likely that these models also share at least some underlying pathophysiological mechanisms. It could be argued that diet would affect the expression of the PSL and autotomy models by modulating mechanisms common to both. However, our results do not support this suggestion, since some types of diet were associated with high levels of autotomy while suppressing the PSL model, and *vice versa*.

The effects exerted by diet on these models range widely, from totally preventing the expression of the pain-related behavior in some diets, to enabling its fullest expression in others. In the autotomy model, the casein-based diet in Sabra rats suppressed the autotomy levels nearly totally. In contrast, high levels of autotomy were seen in HA and Sabra rats fed on the 19510 diet, and in rats fed on bread and cucumbers. Thus, 19510 may be regarded as the diet of choice for experiments requiring high autotomy levels. In other experiments carried out in our lab since 1991 on HA and Sabra rats fed on 19510 we observed a similar course of autotomy to that reported here. Likewise, the same course of autotomy was observed in many experiments carried out by the group of Marshall Devor in Jerusalem, using HA and Sabra rats fed on the 19510 diet (personal communication). This demonstrates that when the same food formula is provided by the same vendor, the expression of pain behavior in a given model can be sTable and repeaTable over years. Moreover, when all variables including type of diet are carefully controlled, levels of autotomy are not lab-specific. The same conclusion may be drawn for the PSL model. Over the years since 1991 the levels of the PSL sensory disorders were similar in many groups fed on the same diet (e.g., the 19510 or RMH diets), even though the experiments were carried out up to 5 years apart, in our two labs in HUJI and JHU.

Effects of diet on brain and behavior have been documented extensively. For example, consuming a palaTable food is analgesic in acute pain tests, an effect mediated by the endogenous opioid system (Ren et al., 1997; Zhang et al., 1997). We showed that rats consuming a saccharin solution at a highly preferred concentration, expressed significantly lower levels of autotomy than a control group consuming tap water (Seltzer et al., 1987). Thus, it could be argued that diets which suppressed the expression of the PSL and autotomy behaviors in the current study were highly palaTable. Since the effects of diet were model-specific and sometimes contrasting, their putative analgesic effects (or their absence) point at the possible role played by endogenous pain-suppressing agents such as opioids in the mechanisms underlying these models.

Alternatively, it is possible that specific constituents of the food were analgesic, regardless of their palatability. Such ingredients could exert a direct analgesic effect, e.g., taurine. Taurine is an inhibitory neurotransmitter with documented antinociceptive effects in acute pain tests (Serrano et al., 1990). Recently we found that dietary supplementation of 1% taurine in the drinking solution significantly suppressed autotomy levels in HA rats following peripheral hindpaw neurectomy (Belfer et al., 1996). It is also possible that some ingredients in food would suppress neuropathic pain by constituting a precursor for an analgesic agent (e.g. tryptophan). Indeed, consumption of a high tryptophan diet in rats suppressed autotomy levels following hindpaw denervation (Abbott and Young, 1991). Since tryptophan is the precursor of serotonin, autotomy suppression may have been caused by increasing serotonergic pain modulatory pathways in the brain and spinal cord. CNS levels of antinociceptive biogenic amines correlated with the levels of autotomy (reviewed by Coderre et al, 1986; Seltzer et al., 1989, 1990). The content of these agents in the diets tested here and CNS of rats fed on these diets is currently under investigation. Finally, rats consuming soy bean oil, at a level 5 times higher than the daily fat requirements, had significantly increased thresholds in acute pain tests. This analgesic effect could not be attributed to an increase in caloric intake or body weight (Yehuda et al., 1986).

Although we were able to substantially overcome the sudden difficulties in replicating the pain disorders of the original PSL model by dietary manipulations, some of its features could still not be replicated fully. For instance, the robust mirror image mechanical and thermal allodynia in the PSL model, reported by us originally (Seltzer et al., 1990), totally disappeared when the sensory disorders on the ipsilateral side weakened. Partial recovery of the mirror image phenomena was noted with some diets. The robustness of the mirror image disorders seems to be correlated to those on the ipsilateral side. Weaker disorders on the ipsilateral side were accompanied by even weaker, delayed or absent mirror image disorders (Dougherty et al., 1992; Behbehany and Dollberg-Stolik, 1994; Cui et al., 1996; Kim et al., 1997), and *vice versa* (Tracey et al., 1995; Takaishi, 1996). It is possible that the duration of the preoperative feeding period with diets producing robust PSL expression levels, was too short for priming the CNS to the expression of mirror image disorders. We are currently investigating whether feeding rats since birth, or even *in utero,* can affect the nervous system for life, thus priming it for a full expression of neuropathic pain, or alternatively, preventing its expression.

We conclude that diet significantly affects the development of neuropathic pain in rats. These effects are model-specific. Modulation of diet in humans may emerge as a novel mode of prophylaxis or even therapy of neuropathic pain. We draw attention of colleagues in the field of neuropathic pain research to the possibility that although animal food vendors may supply a rat chow that meets the formulary standards in terms of the proportion of fat/carbohydrates/proteins *etc,* they may vary the types of protein included, without notification. As shown here, this may greatly affect experimental outcome in a model under study.

Acknowledgements

We are grateful to Marshall Devor for his comments on this manuscript and the generous supply of HA rats, and to Gary Bennett for his comments and advice. This study was supported by the USA-Israel Binational Science Foundation, and by the Hebrew University Center for Research on Pain.

References

Abbott FV, Young SN (1991) The effect of tryptophan supplementation on autotomy induced by nerve lesions in rats. Pharmacol Biochem Behav 40:301-304.

Behbehani MM, Dollberg-Stolik O (1994) Partial sciatic nerve ligation results in an enlargement of the receptive fields and enhancement of the response of dorsal horn neurons to noxious stimulation by an adenosine agonist. Pain 58:421-428.

Belfer I, Davidson E, Ratner A, Shir Y, Beery E, Seltzer Z (1996) Dietary supplementation of the inhibitory amino acid taurine suppresses autotomy in rats genetically selected for high levels of neuropathic pain behavior. Abstracts - 8th World Congress on Pain, IASP Publications, Seattle, p. 470.

Coderre TJ, Grimes RW, Melzack R (1986) Deafferentation and chronic pain in animals: an evaluation of evidence suggesting autotomy is related to pain. Pain 26:61-84.

Cui JG, Linderoth B, Meyerson BA (1996) Effects of spinal cord stimulation on touch evoked allodynia involve GABAergic mechanisms. An experimental study in the mononeuropathic rat. Pain 66:287-295.

Devor M, Raber P (1990) Heritability of symptoms in an experimental model of neuropathic pain. Pain 42:51-68.

Dougherty PM, Garrison CJ, Carlton SM (1992) Differential influence of local anesthetic upon two models of experimentally induced peripheral mononeuropathy in the rat. Brain Res 570:109-115.

Ginzburg R, Seltzer Z (1990) Subdural spinal cord transplantation of adrenal medulla suppresses chronic pain behavior in rats. Brain Res 523:147-150.

Kim SH, Chung JM (1992) An experimental model for peripheral neuropathy produced by segmental spinal nerve ligation in rat. Pain 50:355-363.

Kim KJ, Yoon YW, Chung JM (1997) Comparison of three rodent neuropathic pain models. Exp Br Res 113:200-206.

Na HS, Han JS, Ko KH, Hong SK (1994) A behavioral model for peripheral neuropathy produced in rat's tail by inferior caudal trunk injury. Neurosci Lett 177:50-52.

Perez J, Zucchi I, Maggi A (1988) Estrogen modulation of the gamma-aminobutyric acid receptor complex in the central nervous system of rat. J Pharmacol Exp Ther 244:1005-1010.

Ren K, Blass EM, Zhou Q, Dubner R (1997) Suckling and sucrose ingestion suppress persistent hyperalgesia and spinal Fos expression after forepaw infammation in infant rats. Proc Natl Acad Sci USA 94:1471-1475.

Seltzer Z, Raz I, Brandt R, Boim R (1987) Autotomy is prevented by hyperglycemia and reduced by consuming sweet solutions. Pain 4:S202.

Seltzer Z, Tal M, Sharav Y (1989) Suppression of autotomy following peripheral nerve injury in rats by amitriptylline, diazepam and saline. Pain 37:245-252.

Seltzer Z, Dubner R, Shir Y (1990) A novel behavioral model of neuropathic pain disorders produced in rats by partial sciatic nerve injruury. Pain 43:245-250.

Seltzer Z, Shir Y (1991) Sympathetically-maintained causalgiform disorders in a model of neuropathic pain: A review. J Basic Clin Physiol Pharmacol 2:18-56.

Seltzer Z (1995) The relevance of animal neuropathy models for chronic pain in humans. Semin Neurosci 7:211-219.

Serrano JS, Serrano MI, Guerrero MR, Ruiz R, Polo J (1990) Antinociceptive effect of taurine and its inhibition by naloxone. Gen Pharmacol 21:333-336.

Shir Y, Seltzer Z (1988) Lack of sensitization of primary afferent receptors by prostaglandins in a rat model of causalgic chronic pains. Agents and Actions, 25:252-254.

Shir Y, Seltzer Z (1990a) Effects of sympathectomy in a model of causalgiform pain produced by partial sciatic nerve injury in rats. Pain 45:309-320.

Shir Y, Seltzer Z (1990b) Large diameter A-fibers mediate mechanical hyperalgesia and C-fibers mediate thermal hyperalgesia in a new model of causalgiform pain disorders in rats. Neurosci Lett 115:62-67.

Shir Y, Seltzer Z (1990c) Blocking the injury discharge during partial sciatic nerve injury does not prevent the appearance of causalgiform pain disorders in the rat. Pain (Suppl.) 5:S175.

Shir Y, Devor M, Seltzer Z (1992) Genetic and strain differences in the expression of causalgiform pain disorders in rats. Abst of the Amer Pain Society Mtg.

Shir Y, Ratner A, Raja SN, Campbell JN, Seltzer Z (1996a) The effect of diet on neuropathic pain following partial nerve injury in rat. Abstracts - 8th World Congress on Pain, IASP Publications, Seattle, p. 352.

Shir Y, Ratner A, Seltzer Z (1996b) Effects of diet on autotomy behavior in rats following peripheral neurectomy. Abstracts - 8th World Congress on Pain, IASP Publications, Seattle, p. 352.

Takaishi K, Eisele JHJr, Carstens E (1996) Behavioral and electrophysiological assessment ogf hyperalgesia and changes in dorsal horn responses following partial sciatic nerve ligation in rats. Pain 66:277-306.

Tracey DJ, Cunningham JE, Romm MA (1995) Peripheral hyperalgesia in experimental neuropathy: mediation by α_2 adrenoreceptors on postganglionic sympathetic terminals. Pain 60:317-327.

Wall PD, Devor M, Inbal R, Scadding JW, Schonfeld D, Seltzer Z, Tomkiewicz MM (1979a) Autotomy following peripheral nerve lesions: experimental anesthesia dolorosa. Pain 7:103-113.

Wall PD, Scadding JW, Tomkiewitz MM (1979b) The production and prevention of experimental anaesthesia dolorosa. Pain 6:175-185.

Whitten PL, Naftolin F (1991) Dietary plant estrogens: a biologically active background for estrogen action. In: Hochberg R, Naftolin F (eds.), The New Biology of Steroid Hormones, Raven, New York, pp. 155-167.

Whitten PL, Naftolin F (1992) Effects of phytoestrogen diet on estrogen-dependent reptroductive processes in immature female rats. Steroids 57:56-61.

Wilson MA (1996) GABA physiology: modulation by benzodiazepines and hormones. Crit Rev Neurobiol 10:1-37.

Yaksh TL, Malmberg AB (1994) Central pharmacology of nociceptive transmission. In: R Melzack and PD Wall (Eds.), Textbook of Pain, 3rd Ed., Churchill-Livingstone, Edinborough, pp. 165-200.

Yehuda S, Leprohon-Greenwood CE, Dixon LM, Coscina DV (1986) Effects of dietary fat on pain threshold, thermoregulation and motor activity in rats. Pharmacol Biochem Behav 24:1775-1777.

Zeltser R, Seltzer Z (1994) A practical guide for the use of animal models for neuropathic pain. In: J Boivie, P Hansson, U Lindblom, (eds.), Touch, Temperature and Pain, IASP publications, Seattle, 1994, pp. 337-379.

Zhang T, Reid K, Acuff CG, Jin CB, Rockhold RW (1997) Cardiovascular and analgesic effects of a highly palaTable diet in spontaneously hypertensive and Wistar-Kyoto rats. Pharmacol Biochem Behav 48:57-61.

Supraspinal Physiology

Manifestations and Mechanisms of Pain

Karen J. Berkley
Program in Neuroscience, Florida State University
Tallahassee, FL, USA

In 1992, at the age of 81, my father was in an automobile collision in which his left ankle was badly broken. My father, an architect who throughout his life had studiously avoided discussing anything biological, but knowing of my interest in pain, announced excitedly to me several days later that, much to his astonishment, he had been in "no pain!" when the accident happened, despite the fact that it was obvious at the time that his foot had been rendered suitable only for walking backwards. His pain, he said, did not arrive until well after he felt safe in the hospital.

My father is not alone in his experience. For example, in a recent poll of eight students in a seminar on pain that I teach, four recounted similar occurences in which significant injury failed to evoke pain until several hours afterwards. Many of us have heard descriptions of the initially pain-free encounter that David Livingstone, the Scottish explorer and missionary, had with a tiger in Africa, or have read P.D. Wall's lively discussions of the initial flight or fight of a wounded deer or dog and his own initially pain-free encounter with shrapnel during a political riot (Wall, 1979), or have appreciated the clever study by Melzack et al. (1982) showing that the experience of pain in 37% of badly-injured patients arriving at a hospital emergency room was delayed for 1-9 hrs after the injury. Thus, clinical studies, as well as vivid anecdotal descriptions, testify to the fact that, under any given set of pathophysiological circumstances, the creation of the motivating experience of pain by the nervous system depends upon the individual's need for and access to a safe, healing environment.

Citizens of the two countries in which this conference took place have lived and continue to live in a climate of danger and uncertain societal well being. Thus, given the discussion above, it seems likely that, under similar pathophysiological conditions, the nervous system's creation of pain would be different for Armenians and Nagorno-Karabaghians when compared with those of us who live in secure, affluent environments with ready access to healthcare and safety.

In order to develop better treatment strategies for pain under these various and varying situational conditions, we need improvements in our understanding of the central neural mechanisms involved in creating it. Currently, the most popular conceptualization of central neural pain mechanisms can be diagrammed as shown in Fig. 1A. This fasicular view specifies that there exists a complex pathway from the spinal cord through brainstem to cortex whose neurons process nociceptive stimuli and whose function is the creation of pain. Various descending inputs from the brain to this pathway where it arises in the spinal cord can modulate its activity and thus modulate the creation of pain. This pathway is separate from another whose function is the perception of touch.

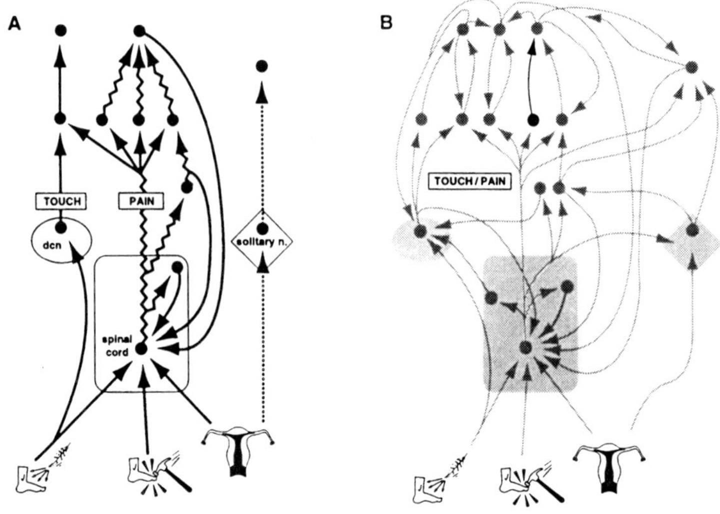

Figure 1. These diagrams present conceptualizations of how the transmission of stimulus information from bodily receptors in skin, muscles and viscera to and through various central neural pathways might give rise to perceptions of pain and touch. A represents the currently popular fascicular view in which the different pathways of information flow are invested with different perceptual functions. B represents a holistic, distributed ensemble view in which the many perceptions of pain and touch arise from the overall balance of activity that results as cooperatively-controlled stimulus information flows through all three primary afferent recipient areas (the solitary and dorsal column nuclei and the spinal cord dorsal horn) into a dynamic brain. (Adapted from Berkley and Hubscher, 1995a.) See text for further details.

While this conceptualization has helped improve our treatments for pain by encouraging us to take advantage of various methods designed to modulate sensory input to the spinal cord, such approaches are at best awkward when psychosocial situational and societal factors, such as those in the examples above, are brought into play. Given the dominance of these factors for the pain experience, perhaps our current conceptualization needs modification.

In considering such changes, it is helpful to return to basic principles and restate current thinking in more detail. Thus, it is well known that information about various bodily events is conveyed by primary afferent fibers to various brain targets via neurons in the solitary nucleus, dorsal column nuclei and spinal cord. Because primary input to the solitary nucleus is derived from afferent fibers in the vagus nerve that supply visceral organs, the route through the solitary nucleus has been commonly considered to be the entry port to a central pathway for visceral functions (Fig. 1A). Because the primary input to the dorsal column nuclei is derived mainly from afferent fibers in somatic nerves that supply cutaneous receptors responsive to gentle tactile stimuli, the route through the dorsal column nuclei has been commonly considered to be the entry port for a central pathway associated with touch and spatiotactile functions (Fig. 1A). And fii...ly, because the primary input to the spinal cord is from visceral and gentle tactile cutaneous fibers, as well as from fibers that supply receptors responsive to noxious stimuli, the spinal cord grey matter has been considered as an entry port for second pathways for visceral function and for touch, as well as for a major pathway for pain (Fig. 1A; as discussed above).

Two features of this conceptualization open for discussion are (a) the investment of these pathways with perceptual functions and (b) the separateness of the pathways. With regard to (a), investment of pathways with percepts, one might question the appropriateness of assigning a perceptual function to a system whose fibers in actuality are coding information about stimulus events. Thus, one might ask, "Is there indeed any such thing as a 'pain fiber' ?" Some might argue that any afferent fiber that responds to a noxious stimulus is a "pain fiber" because noxious stimuli are painful. But, is it the percept of "pain" that is embedded in the coding process of that fiber's activity or is it the nature of the stimulus event that is coded? That the latter answer is the most appropriate seems obvious. In addition, we all know not only that not all noxious stimuli are painful, but also that stimuli that provoke pain do not have to be noxious. Thus, it seems almost silly to invest an entire single pathway through the central nervous system with a perceptual function, when in fact its function is to process information about certain stimulus events.

With regard to (b), separateness, it is now common knowledge (Willis and Coggeshall, 1991; Berkley, 1993) that, anatomically, multiple routes exist by which neurons in the solitary nucleus, the dorsal column nuclei and the spinal cord gray matter influence each other's activity. For starters, there are direct pathways between the spinal cord and solitary nucleus, and the spinal cord and dorsal column nuclei (both directions). Furthermore, neurons in all three ports of entry share some common targets (e.g., parabrachial nucleus, inferior olive, lateral thalamus, medial thalamus), which in turn interconnect and either directly or indirectly feed information backwards to the three different ports.

Electrophysiological data support these interactions in at least two ways. First, neurons in the dorsal column and solitary nuclei and spinal dorsal horn in fact respond convergently to each others assigned stimuli. For example, neurons in the dorsal column nuclei have recently been found to respond convergently, not only to gentle cutaneous stimuli, but also to gentle and noxious visceral stimuli (Rigamonti and Hancock, 1978; Berkley and Hubscher, 1995a; 1995b; Hirshberg et al., 1996). Similarly, neurons in the solitary nucleus respond not only to gentle visceral stimuli, but also to noxious cutaneous stimuli (Person, 1989). Moreover, while such convergent responsiveness has long been known for neurons in primary somatosensory cortex (Amassian, 1951), recent studies strengthen the distributed nature of the information processing (Apkarian et al., 1995; Apkarian, this volume, 1997) within the thalamus and cortex. And finally, responses of neurons in both the solitary and dorsal column nuclei are altered by vagotomy (Gahery and Vigier, 1974; Hubscher and Berkley, 1995). Secondly, response properties of neurons, while specific at any one moment of testing, are not necessarily specific over time because they are subject to constant modifications via the convergent and divergent connective features discussed above. This fact is well known for spinal neurons (Willis and Coggeshall, 1991), but is less well acknowledged for the dorsal column and solitary nuclei, although it clearly exists in both places (Berkley and Hubscher, 1995a;1995b; Hubscher and Berkley, 1995).

How might these considerations change our conceptualization of pain mechanisms to one that provides a more graceful way to incorporate the situational factors discussed in the first paragraphs of this chapter? If we agree from the discussions above that the job of the different pathways is to cooperate in the convergent processing of information about various bodily stimuli, then it becomes reasonable to accept a conceptualization in which bodily perceptions such as pain arise not out of the activity in a single pathway of information flow, but rather out of a cooperatively-controlled balance of the information flowing through all systems. In other words, as diagrammed in Fig. 1B, pain (and other bodily) perceptions occur as a consequence of distributed ensembles of central neuronal activity that result from a balance of cooperatively-controlled information about bodily stimuli (skin, muscles, viscera) flowing through all three entry ports (i.e., spinal cord, dorsal column nuclei, solitary nucleus) into an active and dynamic brain.

While the conceptualization in Fig. 1B is not as simple as the one in Fig 1A, it shifts the creation of pain as being determined less by the nature of the incoming stimulus than by the nature of the brain activity into which the incoming stimulus information finds itself arriving. Incorporating the concepts of ensemble and distributed processing now common in the study of other neural systems (e.g., Deadwyler and Hampson, 1997), this view clearly embraces the situational and social factors discussed in the first part of this chapter. Furthermore, the conceptualization in Fig. 1B encourages us to change our approach towards our investigation of pain mechanisms. Rather than seeking an understanding of how the processing of noxious stimuli by neurons in the spinal cord are modulated (as would be suggested by Fig. 1A), Fig 1B encourages us instead to search for an understanding of the rules by which the cooperative processing of bodily information distributed through the various central pathways is governed.

Plenary discussion

Morpurgo C.: A comment: Considering the dramatic influences the inhibitory interneurons have on the motor, sensory and visceral reflexes, why don't we pay more attention to what can control pain by acting on these interneurons instead of going on with surgical or pharmacological deafferentation studies?

Jabbur S.:A comment: In a previous study reported at a satellite symposium of the International Congress of Physiology in Australia (edited by Rowe 1983), we came to the same conclusion using the technique of interaction of isolated and separated dorsal column and anterolateral column inputs to thalamic ventral posterior lateral nucleus and primary somatosensory cortex neurons. Any sensory stimulus probably activates all the known somatic sensory tracts, and results in interactions between activities in these tracts at all central levels all the way to the cerebral cortex resulting in perception. Moreover, there are also intermodality interactions as illustrated in the demonstrations of visual and auditory influences on cuneate and gracile neurons driven by somatic and auditory stimuli.

References

Amassian VE (1951) Fiber groups and spinal pathways of cortically represented visceral afferents. J Neurophysiol, 14 445-460.

Apkarian AV, Bruggemann J, Shi T and Airapetian LR (1995) A thalamic model for true and referred visceral pain. In: Visceral Pain, Progress in Pain Research and Management (GF Gebhart ed), Vol.5. Seattle: IASP Press, pp. 217-260.

Apkarian AV (1997) Physiology of pain. In this volume.

Berkley KJ (1993) On the significance of viscerosomatic convergence. APS J, 2 239-247.

Berkley KJ and Hubscher CH (1995a) Are there separate central nervous system pathways for touch and pain? Nature Med, 1 766-773.

Berkley KJ and Hubscher CH (1995b) Visceral and somatic sensory tracts through the neuroaxis and their relation to pain: lessons from the rat female reproductive system. In: Visceral Pain, Progress in Pain Research and Management (GF Gebhart ed), Vol.5. Seattle: IASP Press, pp. 195-216.

Deadwyler SA and Hampson RE (1997) The significance of neural ensemble codes during behavior and cognition. Annu Rev Neurosci, 20 217-244.

Gahery Y and Vigier D (1974) Inhibitory effects in the cuneat nucleus produced by vago-aortic afferent fibers. Brain Res, 75 241-246.

Hirshberg RM, Al-Chaer ED, Lawand NB, Westlund KN and Willis WD (1996) Is there a pathway in the posterior funiculus that signals visceral pain? Pain, 67 291-305.

Hubscher CH and Berkley KJ (1995) Spinal and vagal influences on the responses of rat solitary nucleus neurons to stimulation of uterus, cervix and vagina. Brain Res, 702 251-254.

Melzack R, Wall PD and Ty TC (1982) Acute pain in an emergency clinic: latency of onset and descriptor patterns related to different injuries. Pain, 14 33-43.

Person RJ (1989) Somatic and vagal afferent convergence on solitary tract neurons in cat: electrophysiological characteristics. Neuroscience, 30 283-295.

Rigamonti DD and Hancock MB (1978) Viscerosomatic convergence in the dorsal column nuclei of the cat. Exp Neurol, 61 337-348.

Wall PD (1979) On the relation of injury to pain. The John J. Bonica Lecture. Pain, 6 253-264.

Willis WD and Coggeshall RE (1991) Sensory Mechanisms of the Spinal Cord, 2nd edn., Plenum Press, New York.

Pain Mechanisms and Management
S.N. Ayrapetyan and A.V. Apkarian (Eds.)
IOS Press, 1998

A Possible Involvement of Meso-Striato-Limbic Structures in Pain Modulation

S.J. Jabbur[a], S.F. Atweh[b], B. Safieh-Garabedian[c], S.A. Kanaan[c] and N.E. Saadé[a,d]
Departments of [a]Physiology, [d]Human Morphology and
[b]Internal Medicine, Faculty of Medicine
Department of [c]Biology, Faculty of Arts and Sciences
American University of Beirut
Beirut, Lebanon

Much more is known about the peripheral nerves and central ascending pathways and nuclei involved in carrying and modulating nociceptive information up to the thalamic level than about the further elaboration of this information processing at the highest central nervous system levels in the telencephalon. The latter includes cerebral cortical areas, the basal ganglia, and various associated structures within the limbic system. The functional significance of nociceptive information processing within these telencephalic areas assumes importance in view of the fact that the sensation of pain, which usually accompanies actual or impending tissue damage, is a multifaceted experience (Melzack and Casey, 1968). It includes the interrelated sensory-discriminative (concerned with location, intensity, quality and duration of nociceptive stimuli), affective-motivational (concerned with emotional, aversive and autonomic responses) and cognitive-evaluative (voluntary control over the first two dimensions thus involving learning and memory) dimensions (Melzack and Casey, 1968) and leads, ultimately, to a variety of possible motor responses (e.g. flexion withdrawal reflexes, startle and orientation behaviors, and more complex postural adjustments and voluntary acts) which aim at reducing the painful sensations and recuperating the damage to the injured body (Melzack and Wall, 1965).

Most of the earlier research on nociceptive pathways has concentrated on the sensory-discriminative aspect of pain. However, during the past two decades, accumulating experimental and carefully documented clinical evidence indicates that the cerebral cortex, the basal ganglia and closely interrelated areas in the limbic system are well suited to involvement in the affective-motivational and cognitive-evaluative dimensions of pain, and the more crucial modulation of ascending nociceptive inormation and its integration into a coordinated sensori-motor response.

Although the role of the cerebral cortex in pain sensation is less well understood than in any other sensory modality, a number of animal and human studies provide evidence for the involvement of the cerebral cortex in the processing of nociceptive information and the perception of pain (for a review, see Kenshalo And Willis, 1991). Also, in contrast to the better documented role of the basal ganglia in motor functions, a number of animal and human studies indicate that the basal ganglia are involved in the processing of nociceptive and non-nociceptive somatosensory information (for a review, see Chudler and Dong, 1995). Before discussing some of these earlier studies, we propose to present a set of observations on the effects of various kinds of surgical or chemical cerebral lesions in rats in tests of acute and chronic pains.

Methods

The data reported from our laboratory were obtained from Sprague-Dawley rats of both sexes with strict adherence to the ethical standards for investigating pain in experimental animals (Zimmermann. 1983). All surgical procedures were performed under deep anesthesia and followed by prophylactic injection of penicillin and decadron. During the observation period, the animals were maintained under standard colony conditions (4-5 rats/cage) with 12 hr dark/light cycle and free access to food and water.

Various groups of rats (n=6-21 in each) were each subjected to one or two types of cerebral lesions (by gentle suction or chemical application), and to tests of either acute pain and/or chronic pain. Part of the data, referred to in this presentation, has just been published and can be referred to for more details on methods (Saade et al, 1996a, Saade et al, 1996b).

Cerebral lesions

After fixation of the head of the anesthetized rat in a stereotaxic frame, one of the following types of cerebral lesions was performed: (1) *hemidecortication*, by suction of all parts of the cerebral cortex on one side, (2) *hemispherectomy*, by suction of the rostral part of the cerebral hemisphere, including the olfactory bulb, the white matter and part of the neostriatum in addition to the total decortication, also on one side, (3) *unilateral striatal lesion*, by stereotaxic injection of either kainic acid (KA) which is excitoxic to cell bodies in the striatum, or/and 6-hydroxydopamine (6-OHDA) which is toxic to dopaminergic cell bodies or terminals or (4) *unilateral lesion to substantia nigra (SN)* and *neighboring ventral tegmental area (VTA)*, by stereotaxic injection of 6-OHDA or KA. Results of pain tests are compared to sham operated animals which had all the surgical procedures, except for the ablation part, or chemical injection of solvent in saline into the striatum or SN (and VTA), but without KA or 6-OHDA. At the end of the experiments, the extents and locations of the cerebral lesions were determined histologically.

Pain tests

Three types of acute pain tests were routinely used. The *tail flick test (TFT)* and the *hot plate test (HPT)* were used to assess thermal nociceptive thresholds. The *paw pressure test (PPT)* was used to assess the mechanical nociceptive threshold and the laterality of effects following striatal or nigral lesions, since TFT and HPT receive bilateral supraspinal influences (for more details, see Kanaan et al, 1996). Occasionally, the *paw immersion test (PIT)*, similar to the TFT, was used on both legs in order to distinguish thermal from mechanical hyperalgesia. The acute pain tests were administered to each animal one week before, and for a minimum of two weeks after the central lesion or sham injection. Each animal acted as its own control and the possibility of spontaneous variations of acute pain tests with time was ruled out after comparing the test results in experimental and sham control groups before and after surgery (or injection).

Autotomy, following cutting, ligating and sectioning of both saphenous and sciatic nerves, was used as a model for *chronic deafferentation pain* (Wall et al, 1979). Each rat was examined daily for at least 7 weeks and for ethical reasons, Wall's (Wall et al, 1988) new autotomy score (ranging from 1-10) was employed. Four criteria were used to quantitate autotomy: time of onset, time to reach full score (or first sign of bleeding), maximum score reached and percentage of rats exhibiting autotomy in each group (Saade et al, 1990). Autotomy criteria in rats with denervation only were similar to those with sham lesions and collectively both groups acted as controls. Autotomy criteria following denervation of either ipsilateral or contralateral leg performed 1-2 weeks after the cerebral lesion were compared to those of controls.

Data analysis
    The results obtained from each animal and for each type of pain test were averaged for each time interval in each experimental group and the effects of cerebral or sham lesions were presented either as tables showing the effects on each criterion of autotomy or each pain test, or as graphs showing the average autotomy scores or acute pain test thresholds for each group as a function of time. The degree of significance of experimental from control values was assessed by the ANOVA test using GraphPad software version 3.15.

Results

Effects of Hemidecortication and Hemispherectomy on Autotomy
    Among our earliest findings was that decortication delayed significantly autotomy in the contralaterally denervated leg and reduced slightly its incidence while hemispherectomy abolished autotomy in the contralaterally denervated leg and delayed its onset and reduced its incidence (from 100% to 60%) in the ipsilaterally denervated leg (Table 1).

Table 1. Autotomy characteristics observed in hemidecorticate and hemispherectomized rats (following either contralateral or ipsilateral leg denervation)

Experiment	n	Onset of autotomy (Days±SEM)	% showing autotomy
Control	6	7.8±2.8	100
Sham	6	10.3±3	100
Hemidecortication	11	25.6±2.1**	90.9
Hemispherectomy contralateral leg denervation	16	0	0
Hemispherectomy ipsilateral leg denervation	5	34.±6.1*	60

Abbreviation:
n: number
SEM: standard error of the mean
*   P<0.002
** P<0.0001   as compared to control
(Data given in Tables 1 and 2 are based on experiments reported by Saadé et al. (66,69).

After failing to observe autotomy 7 weeks following contralateral denervation, the hemispherectomized rats were subjected to a denervation of the ipsilateral leg. This resulted in autotomy in 62% of the rats, which was bilateral in 37% of the rats and exclusively ipsilateral or contralateral in 25% of the rats (Table 2). The autotomy criteria were similar to those in control and sham rats.

The fact that the hemispherectomy included the rostral parts of the striatum extended our research into the effects of basal ganglia lesions.

Table 2. Autotomy characteristics in hemispherectomized rats subjected to ipsilateral leg denervation 7 weeks following contralateral leg denervation

Self attack to	**n**	**Onset of autotomy (Days±SEM)**	**% showing autotomy**
Ipsilateral leg only	3	24±8.9	18.75
Contralateral leg only	1	23±0	6.25
Both legs: - ipsilateral - contralateral	6	8.5±0.7 8.3±0.6	37

Effects of Unilateral Basal Ganglia Lesions on Autotomy and Acute Pain Tests

Unilateral lesion (with KA) in the striatum produced similar results to the effects of hemispherectomy on contralateral denervation and also on ipsilateral denervation in those rats that did not exhibit autotomy for a 7 week period following contralateral denervation, with the only difference with hemispherectomy that striatal lesions failed to influence autotomy in the ipsilateral-denervated leg. Furthermore, striatal lesion with KA increased the latencies of the HPT and TFT and the threshold of the PPT in the contralateral leg (Fig. 1).

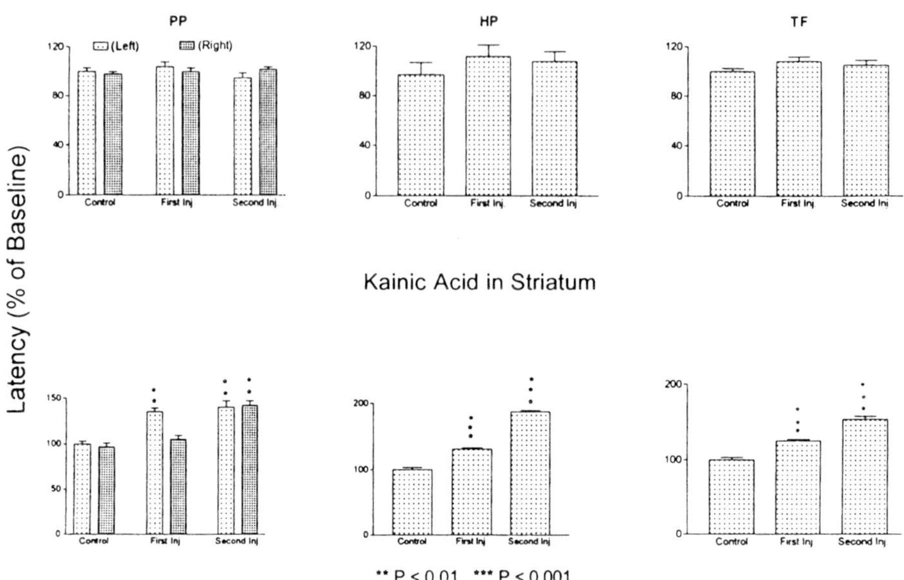

Figure 1. Increases in the latencies of the various nociceptive reflexes following first and second injections of kainic acid (KA) in the striatum. KA injection dose was 0.5 µl (0.01M) dissolved in saline. Each value represents the average of 3 measurements performed on individual rats in each group before injections (baseline, and served as control) and one week after each injection. Values presented as % of the baseline control or saline (sham) values. Note the increases in the HP and TF tests latencies after 1st injection (right striatum) and further increases after the second injection (left striatum) of KA, and the increase in the PP test in the contralateral leg after the first injection--but no further increases after the second injection. PP test, paw pressure test; HP, hot plate test; TF, tail flick test. Similar abbreviations will be used in the succeeding figures.

The importance of dopaminergic input to the striatum and other forebrain structures led to the next series of observations on the effects of more selective and specific lesions in the basal ganglia and SN (and VTA) on autotomy following leg denervation and on tests of acute pain.

1. Striatal lesion with either 6-OHDA or 6-OHDA+KA

Injection of 6-OHDA (toxic to dopaminergic neurons and their terminals) into the striatum had the opposite effect to that of KA in that it accelerated autotomy (Table 3) and decreased the latencies of all the nociceptive reflexes (Fig. 2). Acceleration of autotomy was evident from the decreases in the time of onset and the time of reaching maximum score, as compared to values in sham rats. Autotomy and the acute pain tests were made on two different rat groups. Simultaneous injection of 6-OHDA plus KA into another rat group produced changes in AT criteria that were not significantly different from those produced with 6-OHDA alone.

Table 3. Autotomy characteristics in rats subjected to injections of 6-OHDA
in the striatum and in the SN-VTA area

	n	AT onset (Days±SEM)	% showing AT
Sham	6	10.8±2.3	100
6-OHDA in striatum and contralateral leg denervation	6	32±0.32*	100
6-OHDA in SN and VTA and contralateral leg denervation	6	3.3±0.52*	100

* P<0.007 as compared to sham group

Abbreviations:
6-OHDA = hydroxydopamine and as described in table 1.

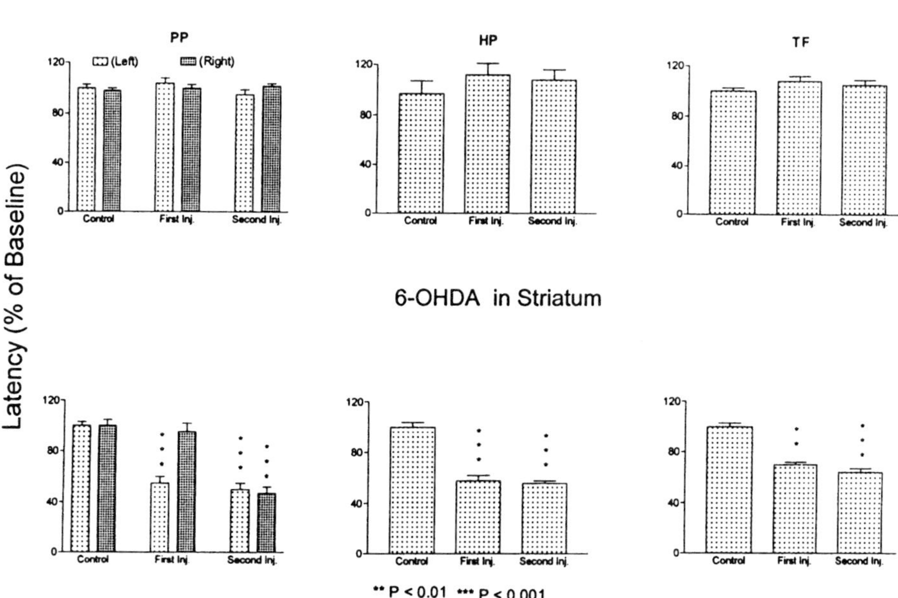

Figure 2. Decreases in the latencies of the various nociceptive reflexes following first and second injections of 6-hydroxydopamine (6-OHDA) in the right and left striatum, respectively: 6-OHDA dose was 3.5 µl (6µg/µl) dissolved in 0.1% ascorbic acid. Results are opposite to those presented in Fig. 1, except that the second injection of 6-OHDA had no additive effect on the PP and the TF tests.

2. SN and VTA lesion with 6-OHDA

Unilateral injection of 6-OHDA into the SN and VTA in another group of rats produced significant decreases in the latencies of the HPT and TFT and also of the PPT and PIT in the contralateral leg, with no changes in the latencies of the PPT and PIT in the ipsilateral leg (Fig. 3). Furthermore, denervation of the contralateral leg 2 weeks after the 6-OHDA injection in the same rat group accelerated autotomy (Table 3).

In another group of rats, the injection of 6-OHDA into the SN and VTA on one side, which led to the expected changes in latencies of the HPT and TFT and also of PPT in the contralateral leg was followed 3 weeks later by a second injection in the SN and VTA on the other side. This led to further, and significant, decrease in the TFT latency without any further decreases in the HPT latencies. Latencies of the PPT in the leg contralateral to the new injection site decreased to the same level as the other leg following the first injection.

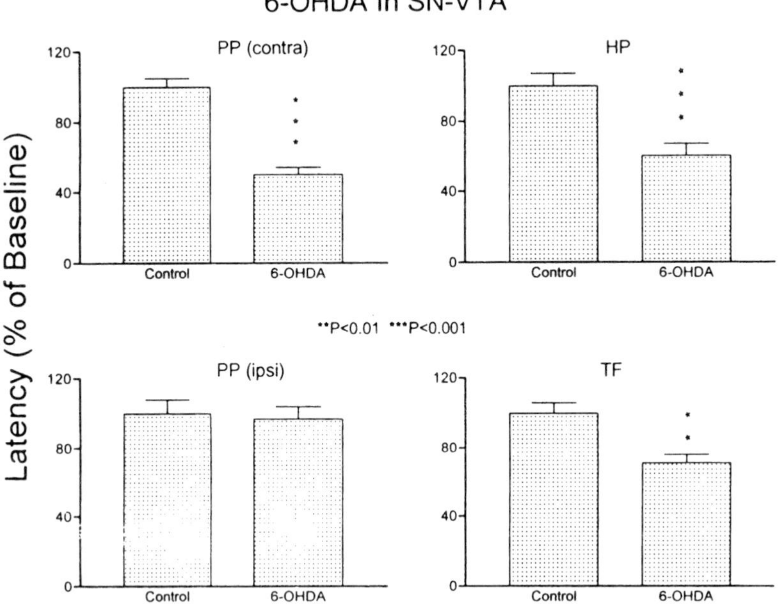

Figure 3. Decreases in the latencies of the various nociceptive reflexes following injection of 6-OHDA in SN-VTA. Note the decreases in the HP and TF tests and PP test (in the contralateral leg).

3. SN and VTA lesion with KA

Unilateral injection of KA in the SN and VTA in another group of rats failed to produce any significant change in the nociceptive reflexes nor in AT behavior which was triggered by contralateral leg denervation two weeks following the KA injection.

Discussion

Until recently, there had been little consensus about the involvement of the cerebral cortex in pain processing, a conclusion based largely on observations on patients with cortical injury during the early part of this century (Head and Holmes, 1911) and on electrical cortical stimulation in alert humans by Wilder Penfield and associates (Penfield and Boldrey, 1937). The accumulating experimental and clinical data, however, now indicate that several cortical areas can be involved in the processing of nociceptive information and pain perception. Several studies have shown responses to mechanical, thermal or electrical nociceptive stimuli in primary (SI) or secondary (SII) somatosensory cortical areas of rats, cats and monkeys using the evoked potential techniques or single unit recordings (for a review see Chudler at al, 1990, Kenshalo and Willis, 1991). Using sophisticated noxious stimuli, more recent studies have shown that the electro-physiological properties of SI cortical neurons (albeit, a small minority) in anesthetized monkeys are related to pain localization and the discrimination of pain intensity (Chudler at al, 1990, Kenshalo et al, 1988, Kenshalo and Isensee, 1983, Kenshalo and Willis, 1991). Similar electrophysiological studies in awake behaving monkeys have also described nociceptive neurons in other areas in the posterior parietal cortex including SII, area 7b (which occupies the opercular region and the inferior parietal lobule) and insular areas (Dong et al, 1994), and changes in the contralateral cutaneous pain sensibility to thermal nociceptive stimuli after compression of area 7b (Dong et al, 1996). These experimental animal studies complement the recently accumulating clinical observations that relate changes in pain sensibility to injury in the same areas in the posterior parietal cortex (for a review, see Greenspan and Winfield, 1992, Kenshalo and Willis, 1991) and experimental human studies that relate painful stimulation to changes in local cerebral blood flow and/or metabolism (using positron-emission tomographic and/or magnetic resonance imaging techniques) in various cortical areas including SI, SII and insula in the parietal lobe and, anterior cingulate gyrus and orbitofrontal cortex in the frontal lobe (Casey et al, 1994, Coghill et al, 1994, Derbyshire et al, 1994, Talbot et al, 1991).

Autotomy following peripheral neurectomy in rats continues to serve as an animal model for chronic deafferentation pain (Blumenkopf and Lipman, 1991), despite some lingering doubt about the validity of the model (Dong, 1989, Rodin and Kruger, 1984). Although the initial research on autotomy concentrated on its peripheral mechanisms (Wall et al, 1979), central mechanisms initiated by the denervation have also been shown to be involved, as evidenced by abnormal bursts of activity at spinal, thalamic and cortical levels (Albe-Fessard et al, 1984, Lombard et al, 1979a, Lombard et al, 1979b, Ovelmen-Levitt et al, 1991, Wall and Devor, 1981) and more recently, by modulatory influences on autotomy of selective lesions to ascending and descending spinal tracts (Saade et al, 1990, Saade et al, 1993, Wall et al, 1988) and previous exposure to injury (Saade et al, 1993). The set of experiments described here on the effects of forebrain lesions on autotomy, compared to those on acute pain tests, lend further support to the utility and validity of the autotomy model.

Among the first major findings in our studies on rats were the observations that total hemidecortication delayed autotomy (without preventing its occurrence), while hemispherectomy (which includes, in addition to the total decortication, removal of parts of the limbic system, striatum and interconnections between cortical and subcortical structures) prevented completely its occurrence in the denervated contralateral leg, and delayed and reduced its incidence in the denervated ipsilateral leg. The bilaterality of hemispherectomy effects is in line with previous studies suggesting bilateral projection of the nociceptive input (Albe-Fessard, 1984, Ovelmen- Levitt, 1991, Rampin and Morain, 1987, Wall et al, 1988). Furthermore, our findings appear to be in line with previous studies showing absence of effect on autotomy following more localized lesion to SI (Wall et al, 1988), and delay and reduction of autotomy following anesthetic block of the cingulum (Vaccarino and Melzack, 1991). The latter is part of a widespread limbic circuit which provides reciprocal connections between the hippocampus, the mammillary bodies, the anterior thalamic nuclei and the cingulate cortex (Domesick, 1970) and has been postulated to be integral to the processing of emotions (Papez, 1937). The effect on autotomy of hemispherectomy were much more pronounced than cingulotomy and the total inhibition appears to be related to injury of important subcortical structures which include the striatum.

Compared to the huge lesion of a hemispherectomy, a more confined chemical lesion to the striatum (also on one side) produced comparable and similar effects on autotomy, except for failing to influence the denervated ipsilateral leg. Thus, hemispherectomy and striatal lesion prevented the occurrence of autotomy following contralateral leg denervation and in the majority (60-70%) of rats following either type of cerebral lesion, a denervation of the ipsilateral leg, seven weeks after denervation of contralateral leg, now led to autotomy of either or both legs. This important finding argues strongly against attributing autotomy to motor weakness, sensorimotor incoordination, neglect, sensory inattention or an attempt to get rid of an insensate appendage (Rodin and Kruger, 1984), and suggested, as reasonable explanation, the release of central generator mechanisms by the summation of the nociceptive inputs coming from both denervated legs (Saade et al, 1996b). This explanation is supported by two previous studies from our laboratory which gave evidence for bilateral rostral nociceptive transmission in the anterolateral columns (Saade et al, 1990) and for the ability of the nervous system to store nociceptive information from previous exposure to injury (Saade et al, 1993).

The striatum is part of the basal ganglia which are among the most important central nervous system structures concerned with motor processes in general, but more specifically with planning and execution of learned motor behaviors and with the control of context-dependent and voluntary movements (for a review, see Hikosaka, 1994). From the animal survival point of view, special significance is assumed by those movements that aim at protecting the living organism from impending or actual tissue damage to the body, and at planning motor reactions to nociceptive stimuli. This makes it reasonable to expect an important role for the basal ganglia in nociception and pain. Chudler and Dong (1995) have recently evaluated, in an excellent review, the possible roles of the basal ganglia in the various dimensions of a painful experience (alluded to in the Introduction), and presented several lines of evidence for such involvements. First, electrophysiological studies with single units have demonstrated the existence of neurons with large receptive fields in the globus pallidus-striatum (Bernard et al, 1992, Chudler et al, 1993) and in the substantia nigra (Barasi, 1979, Gao etal, 1990, Schultz and Romo, 1987, Tsai et al, 1980) which either increase or decrease their discharge frequency following noxious stimuli. Second, measurements of regional blood flow in humans with PET scans (Coghill et al, 1994, Jones et al, 1991, Talbot at al, 1991) and local glucose utilization with 2-DG autoradiography in rats (Mao et al, 1993) have demonstrated preferential activity increases in the striatum following noxious stimuli. Third, despite the overwhelming motor disabilities in basal ganglia disease, somatosensory abnormalities (including changes in pain sensation), have, since a long time, been also known to occur (Snider et al, 1976). Abnormalities in pain perception, which are neither associated with, nor are part of the motor defects, have been shown to be present in Parkinson's disease (Koller, 1984, Quinn et al, 1986, Sage et al, 1990, Snider et al, 1976), Huntington's disease (Albin and Young, 1988), basal ganglia hemorrhage (Lee and Wang, 1991), and extrapyramidal syndrome, following intake of neuroleptic drugs for psychiatric disorders (Decina et al, 1992). The most studied of these abnormalities has been the pains accompanying Parkinson's disease which have been reported to occur in about 30% of the patients, and to be described as usually intermittent and difficult to localize but occasionally bilateral (Snider et al, 1976). Conflicting increases or decreases in pain tolerance and pain thresholds have been reported in different studies on Parkinsonian patients (Guieu et al, 1992, Urakami et al, 1990), and a number of neurotransmitters and neuromodulators have been shown to be associated with the basal ganglia (for a review, see Chudler and Dong, 1995, Graybiel, 1990) and these include dopamine, noradrenaline, GABA and acetylcholine, any of which could be implicated in the pain symptoms and the changes in pain perception in Parkinson's disease. In view of the established importance of dopamine in the pathophysiology of Parkinson's disease, our attention was directed to study its effects on pain tests in rats.

In our study, chemical lesions (with 6-OHDA) of either striatal dopaminergic terminals or dopaminergic neurons in SN and VTA accelerated and intensified autotomy and decreased the latencies of all the tested nociceptive reflexes. These effects were diametrically opposite to those of striatal lesion with KA, and the latter did not annul the effects of 6-OHDA when added to it in the injection. These findings indicate the undue importance of dopaminergic output to the basal ganglia and are in line with the few previous studies, despite differences in methodology, on the effects of lesions to dopaminergic neurons on acute pain tests (Carey, 1986, Morgan and Franklin, 1990, Rosland et al, 1992). Furthermore, our findings correlated well with studies showing nociceptive inhibitory effects from activation of striatal dopamine receptors (Lin et al, 1981) or from SN stimulation as illustrated by the depression of dorsal horn WDR neurons (Barnes et al, 1979, Fleetwood-Walker et al, 1988), parafascicular neurons (Li et al, 1992), polysynaptic reflexes (Jurna et al, 1978) and the HP and TF tests (Jurna et al, 1978).

The acceleration and intensification of autotomy after lesion of the dopaminergic neurons (in SN and VTA) or their terminals (in the striatum) are comparable to the explosive autotomy previously described (Saade et al, 1993), and substantiate further the notion that although explosive autotomy is triggered by peripheral neurectomy, it is maintained, to a large extent, by central generating mechanisms, in this instance specifically released by dopaminergic denervation. This hypothesis could provide an experimental neural substrate for the dysaesthesias and pains in Parkinson's disease patients (Koller, 1984, Quinn et al, 1986, Sage et al, 1990, Snider et al, 1976). Moreover, self-injurious behavior (SIB) has been described in mice (Dunnett et al, 1989), rats (Baumeister and Frye, 1986) and monkeys (Goldstein et al, 1986) following manipulations of the brain catecholaminergic system, and has been associated with disruptions of the monoaminergic (mainly dopaminergic) system in some metabolic diseases (Baumeister and Rollings, 1974, Bryson et al, 1971, Winchel and Stanley, 1991) and in schizophrenic patients (Dworkin, 1994, Winn, 1994). Although SIB has been commonly attributed to insensitivity to pain, evidence from recent clinical and experimental studies (Bhatia and Marsden, 1994, Decina et al, 1992) indicate that it is more likely due to a disruption in the processing of nociceptive information at the level of the basal ganglia and the prefrontal lobe leading to a disturbance in pain sensation which could range from analgesia to hyperalgesia and could, therefore, include spontaneous pains. Indeed this close relationship within the forebrain has recently prompted some investigators to include basal ganglia disease under the more global concept of the frontal lobe syndrome (Degos et al, 1993, Laplane et al, 1989).

Extensive neuroanatomical data describing the neural circuits which could be involved in the processing of nociceptive information by the basal ganglia have been recently reviewed (Chudler and Dong, 1995, see also Alexander and Crutcher, 1990, Gerfen, 1992, Parent and Hazrati, 1993). Chudler and Dong (1995) have broadly divided these neural pathways into four subsystems, according to each of four sources of afferent nociceptive inputs: first, cerebral cortex; second, parabrachial area and amygdala; third, thalamus and tectum; and fourth, dorsal raphe nucleus. Also, several efferent pathways from the striatum and/or the SN project back to the same area of the afferent source, thus resulting in neuronal feedforward and feedback loops which could provide the neural substrate for the various dimensions of a painful experience (particularly the affective-motivational and the cognitive-evaluative), the modulation of a painful experience, the regulation of ascending nociceptive information and, last but not least, the provision of a pathway to the highest motor centers which control the motor responses to nociceptive stimuli.

Finally, it is worth noting that the SN, which is the main concern of this study, plays a key role in each of the four groups of neuronal circuits in the basal ganglia just described. SN neurons have been reported to be influenced, directly or indirectly, by nociceptive inputs from the parabrachial area, the superior colliculus, the amygdala, the hypothalamus, and various limbic cortical areas, and to send dopaminergic efferents to the striatum, nucleus accumbens, the hypothalamus, the amygdala, the raphe nuclei, the locus coeruleus, and various limbic cortical areas (including the prefrontal cortex) [for reviews, see Chudler and Dong, 1995, Fallon and Loughlin, 1985, Kemel et al, 1988, Thierry et al, 1983]. Also, a major non-dopaminergic (mainly GABAergic) efferent component of the SN projects to various thalamic nuclei and brainstem areas (Di Chiara et al, 1979, Fallon and Loughlin, 1985, Kemel et al, 1988, Kilpatrick et al, 1980). These dopaminergic and non-dopaminergic efferents suggest a dual organization of the SN-VTA efferents which could account for the differences obtained in our study between the lack of significant effects on nociceptive reflexes and autotomy following non-selective lesion with KA, and the acceleration of nociceptive reflexes and autotomy following selective dopaminergic lesion with 6-OHDA. This duality of SN-VTA efferents is further supported by the study reporting changes in nociceptive reflexes and SIB following intranigral injections with GABA and GABAergic agonists (Baumeister and Frye, 1986).

Based on the results described here, we conclude that the processing of nociceptive information involves the following forebrain structures:

(1)   the striatum and other areas in the cerebral hemispheres, as evidenced by the decreased pain reactivity following hemispherectomy (and to a lesser extent hemidecortication) or unilateral striatal lesion;

(2)   the dopaminergic neurons in the SN (and VTA) and their output to the striatum, as evidenced by the increased pain reactivity following selective lesion (with 6-OHDA) of dopaminergic neurons in the SN (and VTA) or their terminals in the striatum;

(3)   the non-dopaminergic output neurons in the SN (and VTA) as evidenced by the lack of effects on pain reactivity following non-selective lesion (with KA) of neurons in the SN (and VTA), as compared to the effects of the more selective lesion to dopaminergic neurons in the same region.

These results and conclusions provide further evidence to the sizable experimental and clinical literature (alluded to in the Discussion) on the involvement of the basal ganglia and their reciprocal interconnections with various areas in the cerebral cortex (mainly the septal area, the cingulate gyrus and the prefrontal cortex) in the processing of nociceptive information. Any imbalance in the activities of such multiple parallel loops (which involve complex excitatory and inhibitory interconnections that rely on various types of neurotransmitters, including dopamine) can lead to changes in the processing of nociceptive information which can ultimately lead to changes in the perception of pain. Following various lesions to the forebrain, therefore, it is not surprising to expect changes in pain behavior that can range from indifference to pain, in one extreme, to central spontaneous pain, in the other.

Acknowledgements

The authors wish to Suhad Shbeir, Riad Maalouf and Nada Lutfi for their technical assistance in this study. This research was funded in part by the Diana Tamari Sabbagh Fund and the University Research Board.

Plenary discussion

Berkley K.: Male or female rats?

Jabbur S.: Both sexes were used.

Berkley K.: Was there a stereotypic behavior following dopaminergic lesions?

Jabbur S.: Dopamine lesions produced some hyperactivity but these motor manifestations disappeared within one week after the lesion.

Amassian V.: Would you comment on the contrast between two sets of observations? First, operations at the thalamic level - stereotaxic intralaminar N. lesion or the cortical level- bilateral congulotomy have to be bilateral to be effective. However, entopeduncular lesion in the cat, the homologue of the internal palladium, if unilateral abolish contralateral inhibition of contact placing into water by cats (Amassian and Weitenbaker). Does this reflect a difference between the circuitry for pain perception and learning to make or not make a particular motor response to an aversive stimulus?

Jabbur S.: In the brain centers that receive bilateral and convergent inputs, it is not uncommon to observe that uniateral lesion of these centers do not elicit specific deficits. The same is not true for brain centers that exclusively receive unilateral input and project efferent outputs influencing one side of the body..These types of centers could also be labelled as "diffuse" or "specific", respectively and both types are involved in sensori- motor integration. When it comes to central processing of nociceptive information and pain it is quite difficult if not impossible to make a distinction between these two types of centers. Indeed, the accumulating experimental and clinical data indicate that there is no pathway which is specific and exclusive to the processing of nociceptive information and pain. This somewhat contrasts to all other sensory modalities.

References

Albe-Fessard D, Condes-Lara M, Sanderson P and Levante (1984) A Tentative explanation of the special role played by the areas of the paleospinothalamic projection in patients with deafferentations syndromes. In:Advances in Pain Research and Therapy, Vol. 6, Neural Mechanisms of Pain. (L Kruger and JC Liebeskind eds.) Raven Press, New York pp. 167-182.

Albe-Fessard D and Lombard MC (1983) Use of an animal model to evaluate the origin of and protection against deafferentation pain. In: Advances in Pain Research and Therapy, Vol. 5, Proc. III World Congress on Pain (JJ Bonica, U Lindblom and A. Iggo eds.) (JJ Bonica, U Lindblom and A. Iggo eds.) Raven Press, New York pp. 691-700.

Albin RL and Young AB (1988) Somatosensory phenomena in Huntington's disease, Mov Disord 3: 343-346.

Alexander GE and Crutcher MD (1990) Functional architecture of basal ganglia circuits: neural substrates of parallel processing, Trends Neurosci 13:266-271.

Barasi S (1979) Responses of substantia nigra neurons to noxious stimulation, Brain Res 171:121-130.

Barnes CD, Fung SJ and Adams WL (1979) Inhibitory effects of substantia nigra on impulse transmission from nociceptors, Pain 6:207-215.

Baumeister AA and Frye GD (1986) Involvement of the midbrain reticular formation in self-injurious behavior, stereotyped behavior, and analgesia induced by intranigral microinjection of muscimol, Brain Res 369:231-242.

Baumeister AA and Rollings JP (1974) Self-injurious behavior, Int. Rev. Res. Ment. Retard 8:1-34.

Bernard JF, Huang GF and Besson JM (!992) Nucleus centralis of the amygdala and the globus pallidus ventralis: electrophysiological evidence for an involvement in pain processes, J Neurophysiol 68:551-569.

Bhatia KP and Marsden CD (1994) The behavioural and motor consequences of focal lesions of the basal ganglia in man, Brain 117:859-876.

Blumenkopf B and Lipman J (1991) Studies in autotomy: its pathophysiology and usefulness as a model of chronic pain, Pain 45:203-209.

Bryson Y, Sakati N, Nyhan WL and Fish CH (1971) Self-mutilative behavior in the Cornelia de Lange syndrome, Am J Ment Defic 76:319-324.

Carey RJ (1986) Acute ipsilateral hyperalgesia and chronic contralateral hypoalgesia after unilateral 6-hydroxydopamine lesions of the substantia nigra, Exp Neurol 91:277-284.

Casey KL, Minoshima S, Berger KL, Koeppe RA, Morrow TJ and Frey KA (1994) Positron emission tomographic analysis of cerebral structures activated specifically by repetitive noxious heat stimuli, J Neurophysiol 71:802-807.

Chudler EH, Anton F, Dubner R and Kenshalo DR Jr (1990) Responses of nociceptive SI neurons in monkeys and pain sensation in humans elicited by noxious thermal stimulation: effect of interstimulus interval, J Neurophysiol 63:559-569.

Chudler EH and Dong WK (1995) The role of the basal ganglia in nociception and pain, Pain 60:3-38.

Chudler EH, Sugiyama K and Dong WK (1993) Nociceptive responses in neurons in the neostriatum and globus pallidus of the rat, J Neurophysiol 69:1890-1903.

Coghill RC, Talbot JD, Evans AC, Meyer E, Gjedde A, Bushnell MC and Duncan GH (1994) Distributed processing of pain and vibration in the human brain, J Neurosci 14:4095-4108.

Decina P, Mukherjee S, Caracci G and Harrison K (1992) Painful sensory symptoms in neuroleptic-induced extrapyramidal syndromes, Am J Psychiatry 149:1075-1080.

Degos J-D, da Fonseca N, Gray F and Cesaro P (1993) Severe frontal syndrome associated with infarcts of the left anterior cingulate gyrus and the head of the right caudate nucleus, Brain 116:1541-1548.

Derbyshire, S.W.G., Jones, A.K.P., Devani, P., Friston, K.J., Feinmann, C., Harris, M., Pearce, S., Watson, J.D.G. and Frackowiak, R.S.J. (1994) Cerebral responses to pain in patients with atypical facial pain measured by positron emission tomography, J. Neurol. Neurosurg. Psychiatry 57:1166-1172.

Di Chiara G, Porceddu ML, Morelli M, Mulas ML and Gessa GL (1979) Evidence for a GABAergic projection from the substantia nigra to the ventromedial thalamus and to the superior colliculus of the rat, Brain Res 176:273-284.

Domesick VB (1970) The fasciculus cinguli in the rat, Brain Res 20:293-320.

Dong WK (1989) Is autotomy a valid measure of chronic pain? In: Issues in Pain Measurement (CR Chapman and JD Loeser eds.) Raven Press, Ltd., New York pp. 463-472.

Dong WK, Chudler EH, Sugiyama K, Roberts VJ and Hayashi T (1994) Somatosensory, rnultisensory, and task-related neurons in cortical area 7b(PF) of unanesthetized monkeys, J Neurophysiol 72:542-564.

Dong WK, Hayashi T, Roberts VJ, Fusco BM and Chudler EH (1996) Behavioral outcome of posterior parietal cortex injury in the monkey, Pain 64 579-587.

Dunnett SB, Sirinathsinghi DJS, Heavens R, Rogers DC and Kuehn MR (1989) Monoamine deficiency in a transgenic (Hprt) mouse model of Lesch-Nyhan syndrome, Brain Res 501: 401-406.

Dworkin RH (1994) Pain insensitivity in schizophrenia: a neglected phenomenon and some implications, Schizophr Bull 20:235-248.

Fallon JH and Loughlin SE (1985) Substantia nigra. In: The Rat Nervous System (G Paxinos ed.) Vol. 1, Academic Press Australia, Sydney pp. 353-374.

Fleetwood-Walker SM, Hope PJ and Mitchell R (1988) Antinociceptive actions of descending dopaminergic tracts on cat and rat dorsal horn somatosensory neurones, J Physiol (Lond) 399:335-348.

Gao DM, Jeaugey L, Pollack P and Benabid AL (1990) Intensity-dependent nociceptive responses from presumed dopaminergic neurons of the substantia nigra, pars conpacta in the rat and their modification by lateral hebenula inputs, Brain Res 529:315-319.

Gerfen CR (1992) The neostrial mosaic: multiple levels of compartmental organization in the basal ganglia, Annu Rev Neurosci 15:285-320.

Goldstein M, Kuga S, Kusano N, Meller E, Dancis J and Schwarcz R (1986) Dopamine agonist induced self-mutilative biting behavior in monkeys with unilateral ventromedial tegmental lesions of the brain stem: possible pharmacological model for Lesch-Nyhan syndrome, Brain Res 367:114-120.

Graybiel AM (1990) Neurotransmitters and neuromodulators in the basal ganglia, Trends Neurosci, 13:244-253.

Greenspan JD and Winfield JA (1992) Reversible pain and tactile deficits associated with a cerebral tumor compressing the posterior insula and parietal operculum, Pain 50:29-39.

Guieu R, Pouget J and SerratriceG (1992) Nociceptive threshold and Parkinson's disease, Rev Neurol (Paris) 10:641-644.

Head H and Holmes G (1911) Sensory disturbances from cerebral lesions, Brain 34:102-254.

Hikosaka O (1994) Role of basal ganglia in control of innate movements, learned behavior and cognition-a hypothesis, Adv Behav Biol 41:589-596.

Jones AKP, Brown WD, Friston KJ, Qi LY and Frackowiak RSJ (1991) Cortical and subcortical localization of response to pain in man, using positron emission tomography, Proc R Soc Lond 244:39-44.

Jurna I, Heinz G, Blinn G and Nell T (1978) The effect of substantia nigra stimulation and morphine on (-motoneurones and tail flick response, Eur J Pharmacol 51:239-250.

Kanaan SA, Saadé NE, Haddad JJ, Abdelnoor AM, Atweh SF, Jabbur SJ and Safieh-Garabedian B (1996) Endotoxin-induced local inflammation and hyperalgesia in rats and mice: A new model for inflammatory pain, Pain (In press).

Kemel ML, Desban M, Gauchy C, Glowinski J and Besson MJ (1988) Topographical organization of efferent projections from the cat substantia nigra pars reticulata, Brain Res 455:307-323.

Kenshalo DR Jr, Chudler EH, Anton F and Dubner R (1988) SI nociceptive neurons participate in the encoding process by which monkeys perceive the intensity of noxious thermal stimulation, Brain Res 454:378-382.

Kenshalo DR, Jr and Isensee O (1983) Responses of primate SI cortical neurons to noxious stimuli, J Neurophysiol 50:1479-1496.

Kenshalo DR, Jr and Willis WD Jr (1991) The role of the cerebral cortex in pain sensation. In: Cerebral Cortex, Vol. 9 (A Peters ed) 0New York, Plenum pp. 153-212.

Kilpatrick IC, Starr MS, Fletcher A, James TA and MacLeod NK (1980) Evidence for a GABAergic nigrothalamic pathway in the rat, Exp Brain Res 40:45-54.

Koller WC (1984) Sensory symptoms in Parkinson's disease, Neurology 34:957-959.

Laplane D, Levasseur M, Pillon B, Dubois B, Baulac M, Mazoyer B, TranDinh S, Sette G, Danze F and Baron JC (1989) Obsessive-compulsive and other behavioural changes with bilateral basal ganglia lesions: a neuropsychological, magnetic resonance imaging and positron tomography study, Brain 112:699-725.

Lee JL and Wang AD (1991) Post-traumatic basal hemorrhage: analysis of 52 patients with emphasis on the final outcome, J Trauma 31:376-380.

Li J, Ji Y-P, Qiao J-T and Dafny N (1992) Suppression of nociceptive responses in parafascicular neurons by stimulation of substantia nigra: an analysis of related inhibitory pathways, Brain Res 591:109-115.

Lin MT, Wu JJ, Chandra A and Tsay BL (1981) Activation of striatal dopamine receptors induces pain inhibition in rats, J Neural Transm 51:213-222.

Lombard MC, Nashold BS Jr and Albe-Fessard D (1979) Deafferentation hypersensitivity in the rat after dorsal rhizotomy: a possible animal model for chronic pain, Pain 6:163-174.

Lombard MC, Nashold BS Jr and Pelissier T (1979) Thalamic recordings in rats with hyperalgesia. In: Advances in Pain Research and Therapy, Vol. 3, Proc. II World Congress on Pain. (JJ Bonica, JC Liebeskind and DG Albe-Fessard eds.) Raven Press, New York pp. 767-772.

Mao J, Mayer DJ and Price DD (1993) Patterns of increased brain activity indicative of pain in a rat model of peripheral mononeuropathy, J Neurosci 13:2689-2702.

Melzack R and Casey KL (1968) Sensory, motivational, and central control determinants of pain. A new conceptual model. In: The Skin Senses, CC Thomas (DR Kenshalo ed.) Springfield pp. 423-439.

Melzack R and Wall PD (1965) Pain mechanisms: a new theory, Science 150:971-979.

Morgan MJ and Franklin KBJ (1990) 6-Hydroxydopamine lesions of the ventral tegmentum abolish D-amphetamine and morphine analgesia in the formalin test but not in the tail flick test, Brain Res 519:144-149.

Ovelmen-Levitt J, Young JN, Rossitch E and Nashold B (1991) The expression of a deafferentation syndrome in the Sprague-Dawley rat: effects of frontoparietal cortical lesions, Pain 47:203-208.

Papez JW (1937) A proposed mechanism of emotion, Arch. Neurol Psychiatry 38:725-743.

Parent A and Hazrati L-N (1993) Anatomical aspects of information processing in primate basal ganglia, Trends Neurosci 16:111-116.

Penfield W and Boldrey E (1937) Somatic motor and sensory representation in the cerebral cortex of man as studied by electrical stimulation, Brain 60:389-443.

Quinn NP, Lang AE, Koller WC and Marsden CD (June 14, 1986) Painful Parkinson's disease, Lancet 1 (No. 8494):1366-1369.

Rampin O and Morain P (1987) Cortical involvement in dorsal horn cell hyperactivity and abnormal behavior in rats with dorsal root section, Somatosens Res 4:237-251.

Rodin BE and Kruger KL (1984) Deafferentation in animals as a model for the study of pain: an alternative hypothesis, Brain Res Rev 7:213-228.

Rosland JH, Hunskaar S, Broch OJ and Hole K (1992) Acute and long term effects of 1-methyl-4-phenyl-1,2,3,6-tetrahydropiridine (MPTP) in tests of nociception in mice, Pharmacol Toxicol 70:31-37.

Saadé NE, Atweh SF, Bahuth NB and Jabbur SJ (1996) Augmentation of nociceptive reflex and chronic deafferentation pain by chemical lesions of either dopaminergic terminals or midbrain dopaminergic neurons, Brain Res (In press).

Saadé NE, Atweh SF, Jabbur SJ and Wall PD (1990) Effects of lesions in the anterolateral columns and dorsolateral funiculi on self-mutilation behavior in rats, Pain 42:313-321.

Saadé NE, Ibrahim MZM, Atweh SF and Jabbur SJ (1993) Explosive autotomy induced by simultaneous dorsal column lesion and limb denervation: a possible model for acute deafferentation pain, Exp Neurol 119:272-279.

Saadé NE, Shbeir SA, Atweh SF and Jabbur SJ (1996) Effects of cerebral cortical and striatal lesions on autotomy following peripheral neurectomy in rats, Physiol Behav 60:559-566.

Saadé NE, Shihabuddin LS, Atweh SF and Jabbur SJ (1993) The role of previous nociceptive input in development of autotomy following cordotomy, Exp Neurol 119:280-286.

Sage JI, Kortis HI and Sommer W (1990) Evidence for the role of the spinal cord systems in Parkinson's disease-associated pain, Clin Neuropharmacol 13:171-174..

Schultz W and Romo R (1987) Responses of nigrostriatal dopamine neurons to high-intensity somatosensory stimulation in the anesthetized monkey, J Neurophysiol 57:201-217.

Snider SR, Fahn S, Isgreen WP and Cote LJ (1976) Primary sensory symptoms in parkinsonism, Neurology 26:423-429.

Talbot JD, Marrett S, Evans AC, Meyer E, Bushnell MC and Duncan GH (1991) Multiple representations of pain in human cerebral cortex, Science 25:1355-1358.

Thierry AM, Chevalier G, Ferron A and Glowniski J (1983) Diencephalic and mesencephalic efferents of the medial prefrontal cortex in the rat: electrophysiological evidence for the existence of branched axons, Exp Brain Res 50:275-282.

Tsai C, Nakamura S and Iwoma K (1980) Inhibition of neuronal activity of the substantia nigra by noxious stimuli and its modification by the caudate nucleus, Brain Res 195:299-311.

Urakami K, Takahashi K, Matsushima E, Sano K, Nishikawa S and Takao T (1990) The threshold of pain and neurotransmitter's change on pain in Parkinson's disease, Jpn J Psychiatry Neurol 44:589-593.

Vaccarino AL and Melzack R (1991) The role of the cingulum bundle in self-mutilation following peripheral neurectomy in the rat, Exp Neurol 111:131-134.

Wall PD, Bery J and Saadé NE (1988) Effects of lesions to rat spinal cord lamina I cell projection pathways on reactions to acute and chronic noxious stimuli, Pain 35:327-339.

Wall PD and Devor M (1981) The effect of peripheral nerve injury on dorsal root potentials and on transmission of afferent signals into the spinal cord, Brain Res 209:95-111.

Wall PD, Devor M, Inbal R, Scadding JW, Schonfeld D, Seltzer Z and Tomkiewicz MM (1979) Autotomy following peripheral nerve lesions: experimental anaesthesia dolorosa, Pain 7: 103-113.

Wall PD, Scadding JW and Tomkiewicz MM (1979) The production and prevention of experimental anesthesia dolorosa, Pain 6:175-182.

Winchel RM and Stanley M (1991) Self-injurious behavior: a review of the behavior and biology of self-mutilation, Am J Psychiatry 148:306-317.

Winn P (1994) Schizophrenia research moves to the prefrontal cortex, Trends Neurosci 17:265-268.

Zimmermann M (1983) Ethical guidelines for investigations of experimental pain in conscious animals, Pain 16:109-110.

Neuronal Organization of Limbic Mechanisms of Pain Sensitivity Regulation

O.G. Baklavadjian, A.G. Darbinian, T.Kh. Taturyan, M.O. Baklavadjian, R.M. Stepanyan
L.A. Orbeli Institute of Physiology, Armenian National Academy of Sciences
Yerevan, Armenia

The neuronal organization of the nociceptive afferent system of the hypothalamus is of special interest. The high content of opoid neuropeptides--endorphins and enkephalins-- in hypothalamic neurons (Sar et al., 1978), and the localization of opoid receptors in the hypothalamus (Atweh, Kuhar, 1977) point to the importance of hypothalamic structures in regulation of pain sensitivity. This is confirmed by a number of findings revealing analgesic effects of stimulating medial diencephalic structures, including the paraventricular region of hypothalamus (Valdman, Ignatov, 1976; Golanov, Kaliushni, 1978; Castens, 1982; Hosobushi et al., 1977; Rhades, Liebeskind, 1978; Richardson, Akil, 1977; Balagurn, Ralph, 1973). Evidently, the hypothalamic control of pain sensitivity is triggered by a reflex mechanism, elicited by noxious afferent inputs onto nociceptive neurons in the hypothalamus. However, the literature contains no information on the peculiarities of responses of single units from lateral and medial areas of posterior, tuberal and anterior hypothalamus to noxious and non-noxious afferent signals, converging on hypothalamic nociceptive neurons.

In a series of microelectrophysiological experiments, responses of single units from lateral and medial areas of posterior, tuberal and anterior hypothalamus to electrical stimulation of dental pulp (noxious impulses) and sciatic nerve Aβ afferents (non-noxious impulses) were recorded in anesthetized cats. It was shown that 80.7%, 81.5% and 71.4% of units, respectively responded to stimulation of tooth pulp noxious afferents in posterior, tuberal and anterior hypothalamus. Marked predominance of excitatory responses in posterior hypothalamus and almost an equal proportion of excitatory and inhibitory responses in tuberal and anterior hypothalamus was found. The shortest latency of responses was recorded in postero-lateral hypothalamus. Nociceptive responses in the lateral hypothalamus were of shorter latency than responses of medial hypothalamic units.

Fig. 1 presents oscillograms of the responses from neurons of medial (A) and lateral (B) areas of posterior (1), tuberal (2) and anterior (3) hypothalamus to single tooth pulp stimulation. In A and B, the left column shows recordings of single stimulations, the right column shows the recordings of three stimulations superimposed.

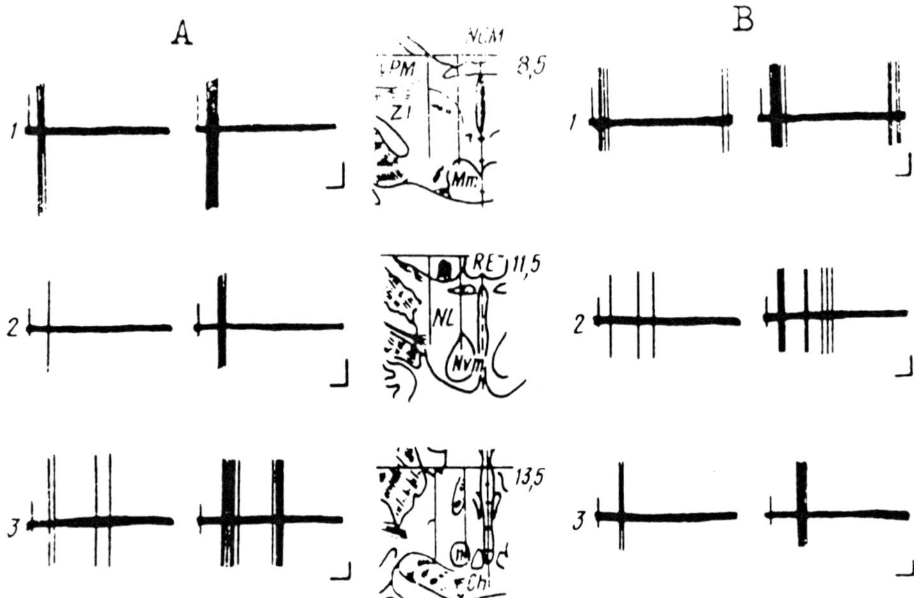

Figure 1. Responses of neurons of medial (A) and lateral (B) areas of posterior (1), tuberal (2) and anterior (3) hypothalamus to single tooth pulp stimulation.
Calibration: 250 μV, 40 ms. In the scheme-localization of microelectrodes in frontal plan 8.5, 11.5 and 13.5 of the atlas of Jasper and Ajmone-Marsan. Mm-nucleus mamillaris; HL-lateral hypothalamus; Nvm-ventromedial nucleus; Ha-anterior hypothalamic nucleus; Ch-chiasm.

A high degree of convergence (85.8%) of noxious and non-noxious (sciatic nerve Aβafferents) impulses was revealed. It is important to note that polysensory convergent type neurons were modally unspecified, i.e. responded with an identical "pattern" of discharge to noxious and non-noxious stimuli, indicating the non-specific character of responses of the majority of polysensory neurons. Only 14.2% of hypothalamic units were monomodal and specific nociceptive neurons.

The reactions of polysensory converging type neurons of posterior (1), tuberal (2) and anterior (3) hypothalamus to single tooth pulp (A) and sciatic nerve Aβafferents (B) stimulation are presented in Fig. 2. It can be seen that in stimulation of tooth pulp noxious and sciatic non-noxious afferents identical "patterns" of responses are recorded, this testifies to the non-specific properties of convergent neurons of posterior, tuberal and anterior hypothalamus.

Increase in latency of responses of hypothalamic neurons to noxious tooth pulp stimulation in caudo-rostral and lateral-medial directions evidently is related to conduction of pain afferent signals along the ascending channels of medial forebrain bundle in the lateral hypothalamus. Recording of short latency responses of some neurons of postero-lateral hypothalamus (3.6-6.5 ms) suggests that ascending nociceptive signals are conducted through olygosynaptic pathways. Low liability and reproducibility of responses to paired stimulation indicate that, in the main, ascending trigemino-reticulo-rubro-hypothalamic polysynaptic pathways are involved in conduction of pain afferent inputs to the hypothalamus.

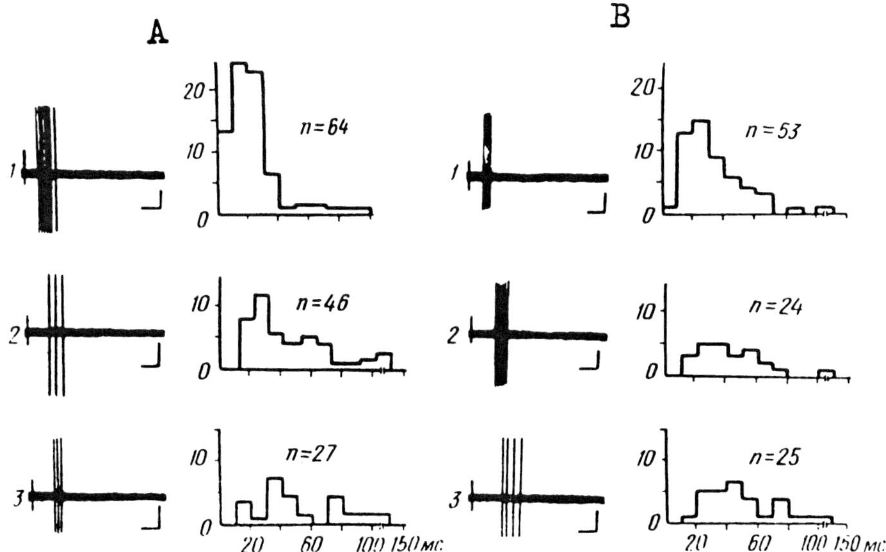

Figure 2. Responses of converging type neurons of posterior (1), tuberal (2) and anterior (3) hypothalamus to single tooth pulp (A) and sciatic nerve Aβ afferent (B) stimulation.
Calibration: 250 μV, 40 ms. On the right of A and B--histograms of latency of neuron reactions.
Abscissa--latency period in ms; ordinate--number of neurons; n--number of reacting neurons with excitatory type of reaction.

The electrophysiological properties of the neurons studied (considerable convergence of nociceptive and pattern of firing discharge) allow most of the neurons of the hypothalamus to be regarded as secondary, unspecified type, reflecting processes of interaction at the hypothalamic level. Such convergence at the thalamo-cortical level is defined as "projected" convergence (Albe-Fessard, and Fessard, 1963). The presence of few neurons with selective reaction to noxious and non-noxious signals indicate the existence of a second type of convergence, reflecting the presence of independent conduction channels of noxious and non-noxious afferent signals in the hypothalamus--heterosynaptic hypothalamic neurons with "local" convergence. Data on presence of purely nociceptive neurons are worth noting. Such neurons reacting only to nociceptive signals are reported in the centrum medianum of the thalamus and in the bulbar nucleus reticularis giganto cellularis (Yokota, 1976; Yong, Gottschaldt, 1976). Our data indicate that in the hypothalamus there are pure nociceptive specific neurons, neurons of integrating type with homosynaptic inputs, and heterosynaptic neurons which take part in interaction and integration of noxious or non-noxious sensory information.

In a series of experiments, we studied the effects of high-frequency stimulation of medial and lateral areas of posterior, tuberal, and anterior hypothalamus as well as of periaqueductal gray (PAG) on digastric muscle EMG responses as a component of the nociceptive jaw-opening reflex elicited with tooth pulp stimulation. It was found that the nociceptive digastric muscle EMG response was suppressed by stimulation of all hypothalamic structures. The threshold of the inhibitory effect was lower in the PAG stimulation. Hypothalamic stimulation-produced antinociception was reversed by specific opiate antagonist naloxone, the effect of PAG stimulation being less sensitive to naloxone.

Effects of tetanic stimulation (100 Hz) of posterior (A), tuberal (B), anterior (C) hypothalamus and PAG (D) on nociceptive diagstric muscle EMG response of are shown on Fig. 3. Fig. 4 shows that after bilateral lesion of PAG, the antinociceptive effect of the hypothalamus was only slightly reduced.

Complete inhibition of EMG nociceptive response, similar to the effect of hypothalamus and PAG stimulation was induced by intravenous administration of opiate agonist-phenaridine, synthesized in the Institute of Fine Organic Chemistry of Armenian Academy of Sciences.

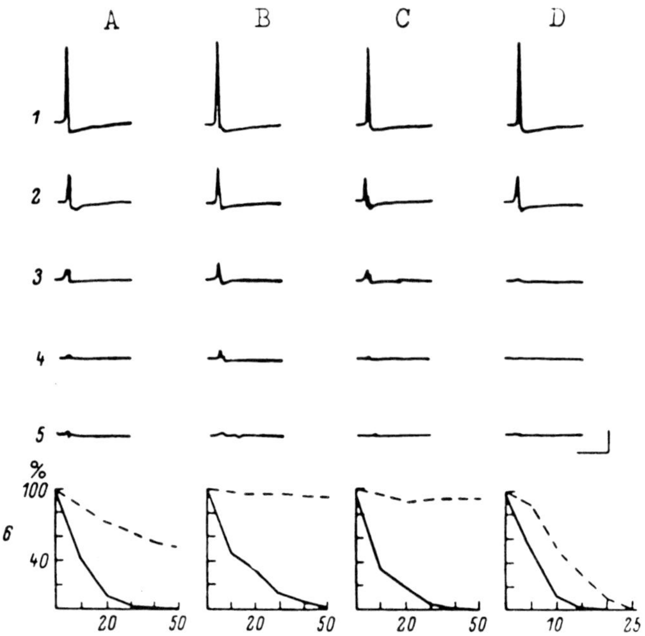

Figure 3. Effects of tetanic stimulation of posterior (A), tuberal (B), anterior (C) hypothalamus and PAG (D) on nociceptive EMG-response of the digastric muscle. 1. background of the EMG-response; 2. –5. electrical stimulation with intensity of 10, 20, 30, 40 V, respectively; 6. averaged curves of decrease of amplitude of EMG-response in % of initial value before (solid lines), and after (broken lines), injection of naloxone. Abscissa--intensity of stimulation; ordinate--amplitude of EMG-response in %. Calibration: 300 μV, 12 ms.

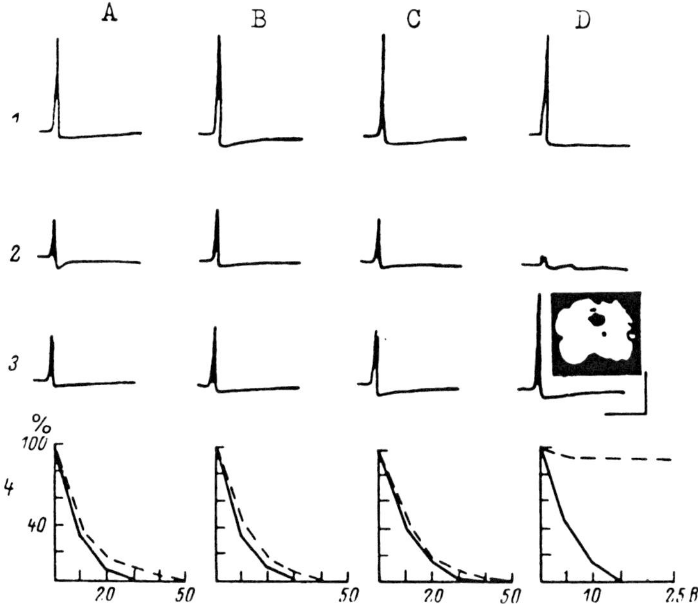

Figure 4. Effects of tetanic stimulation of posterior (A), tuberal (B), anterior (C) hypothalamus and PAG (D) before and after bilateral lesion of PAG.
background of EMG-response; 2. stimulation of hypothalamus and PAG with intensity of 10 V;
3. after lesion of PAG; 4. averaged curves of decrease of amplitude of EMG-response in percentage of initial value before (solid lines), and after (dashed lines), lesion of PAG. On D, 3. histological verification of the lesion of PAG. Calibration: 300 µV, 12 ms.

Fig. 5 illustrates the inhibitory effect of hypothalamus (A-1), PAG (A-2) and phenaridine (A-3) on the amplitude of nociceptive EMG-response, and increase of amplitude of nociceptive EMG-response after lesion of PAG (A-4) and injection of naloxone (A-5). In diagram B are presented the averaged effects of oscillograms A 1-5. Below is presented the hypothetical schema of neuronal organization of hypothalamic antinociceptive efferent system.

Hypothalamic inhibition of nociceptive jaw-opening reflex (inhibition of the digastric muscle EMG nociceptive response) is realized by presynaptic and postsynaptic mechanisms of inhibition. In a series of experiments, we have shown that conditional stimulation of hypothalamus increases the amplitude of the antidromic evoked potential in the tooth pulp evoked by test stimulation of caudal trigeminal nucleus at intervals of 10-50 ms and the increase of the amplitude to primary afferent depolarization of noxious afferents. The two mechanisms of hypothalamic inhibition of pain sensitivity are shown on the scheme of fig. 5--dotted line with black circle, postsynaptic mechanism, dotted line with white circle, presynaptic mechanism.

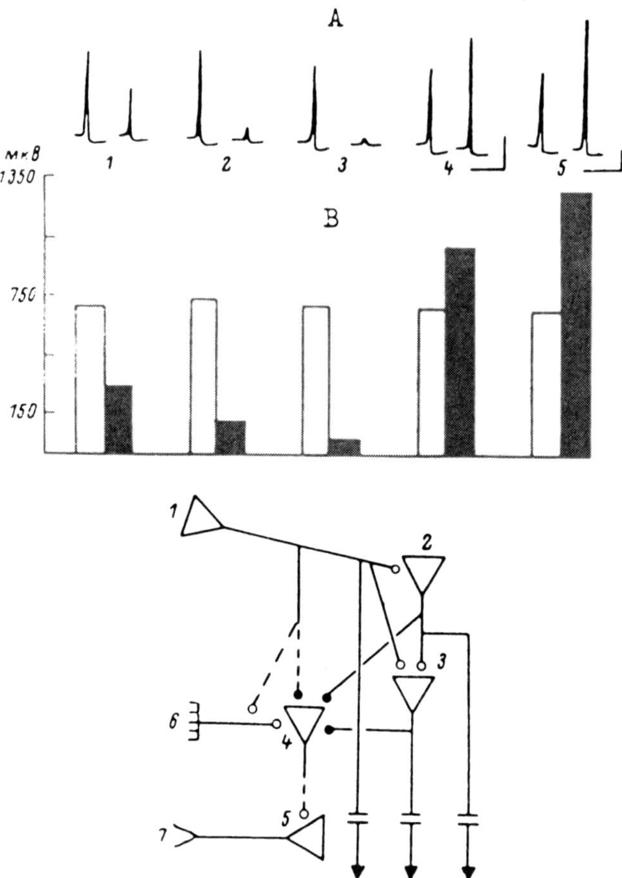

Figure 5.

A: Inhibitory effect of hypothalamus (1), PAG (2) and phenaridine (3) on the amplitude of EMG-response and increase of EMG-response after lesion of PAG (4) and administration of naloxone (5).
B: Diagrams of averaged values of effects as illustrated on corresponding oscillograms under A. Ordinate-amplitude of EMG-responses, μV.
Below: Hypothetical scheme of neuronal organization of hypothalamic antinociceptive efferent system. Neurons: 1. of posterior hypothalamus; 2. of PAG; 3. of n. raphe; 4. caudal sensory trigeminal nuclei; 5. of motor trigeminal nuclei; 6. tooth pulp; 7. Digastric muscle. Arrows show pathways to spinal cord. White circles--excitatory; black--inhibitory synapses.
Calibration: 300 μV, 12 ms.

Increased excitability of tooth pulp afferent terminals in caudal sensory trigeminal nucleus in case of stimulation of PAG and nucleus raphe was established by Dostrovsky et al. (1981). Therefore the presynaptic inhibition is one of the mechanisms of modulation of nociceptive transmission in sensory trigeminal nucleus.

In a series of experiments, we studied the comparative effectiveness of the inhibitory influence of tetanic stimulation of hypothalamus, amygdala and limbic cortex on nociceptive EMG-responses of the digasteric muscle. It was found that inhibition of the EMG-component of the jaw-opening nociceptive reflex is most pronounced in the case of stimulation of the medial and lateral regions of the hypothalamus, the inhibitory effect of central and medial nuclei of amygdala is less pronounced, and the effect of limbic cortex is the weakest. In fig. 6 are shown the effects of tetanic stimulation of the hypothalamus (A) and amygdala (B-G) on the EMG response of the jaw-opening reflex.

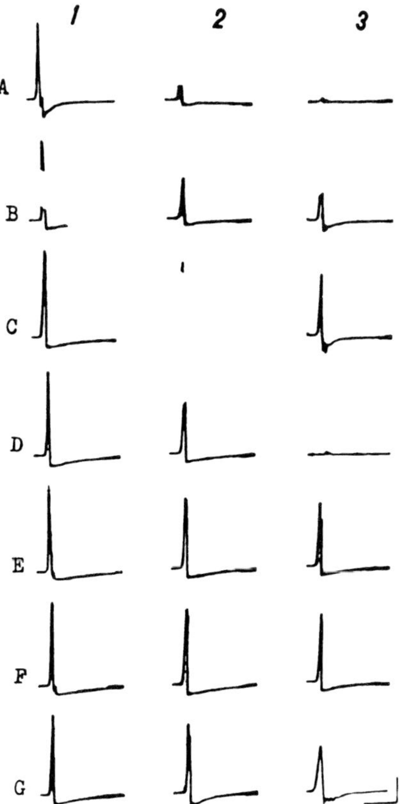

Figure 6. The influence of tetanic stimulation of the hypothalamus (A) and amygdala (B-G) on EMG-response of jaw-opening reflex.
A. stimulation of hypothalamus; B. of medial; C. cortical; D. central; E. basomedial; F. lateral; G. basolateral amygdala. 1. background; 2., 3. stimulation of the hypothalamus with intensity of 10 and 20 V, respectively; B.-G. 2., 3. strength of stimulation of amygdala 30 and 50 V, respectively.
Calibration: 300 μV, 12 ms.

Fig. 7 shows the effect of tetanic stimulation of hypothalamus (A) and limbic cortex (B-D) on EMG-response of jaw-opening pain reflex. It is seen that tetanic stimulation of hypothalamus with the strength of 20V induces complete inhibition of EMG-response while stimulation of limbic cortex with the strength of 50 V decreases the amplitude of the response only to 20%.

In a series of experiments, it was shown that the mechanisms of antinociceptive effect of tetanic stimulation of hypothalamus is not related to the concomitant increase of blood pressure, since the inhibitory effect on the digasteric muscle EMG-component of nociceptive jaw-opening reflex to tooth pulp noxious stimulation also persists after stabilization of systemic arterial pressure, i.e.under the condition of an open baro-reflex loop.

Fig. 8 shows that the effect of tetanic stimulation of hypothalamus on the amplitude of the EMG-responses of pain reflex (3) remains without changes after stabilization of blood pressure by intravenous injection of ganglion blocking agent, which points to a direct, primary, not baro-afferent mechanism for the inhibition of the activity of nociceptive neurons of trigeminal sensory nuclei.

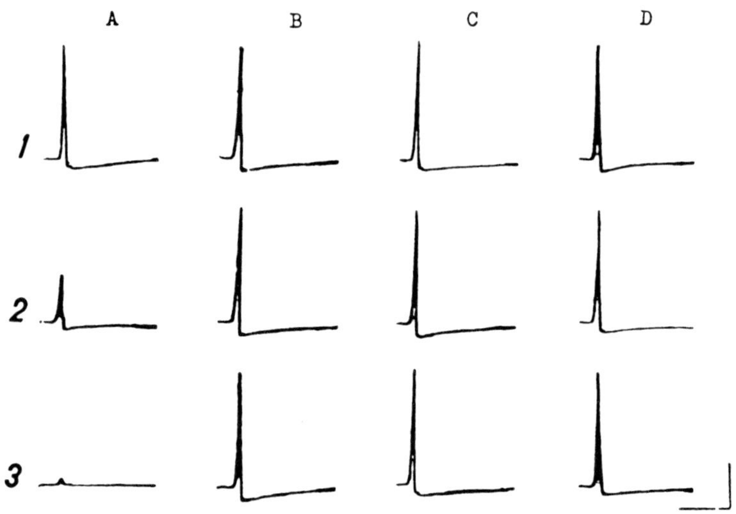

Figure 7. The influence of tetanic stimulation of hypothalamus (A) and limbic cortex (B -D) on EMG-response of the jaw-opening pain reflex. A. stimulation of hypothalamus; B.- D. stimulation of area 23, 24 and 25 of limbic cortex, respectively; 1. background; A. 2.-3. stimulation of hypothalamus with strength of 10 and 20 V, respectively; B.-D. 2., 3. stimulation of limbic cortex with strength of 30 and 50 V, respectively. Calibration: 300 μV, 12 ms.

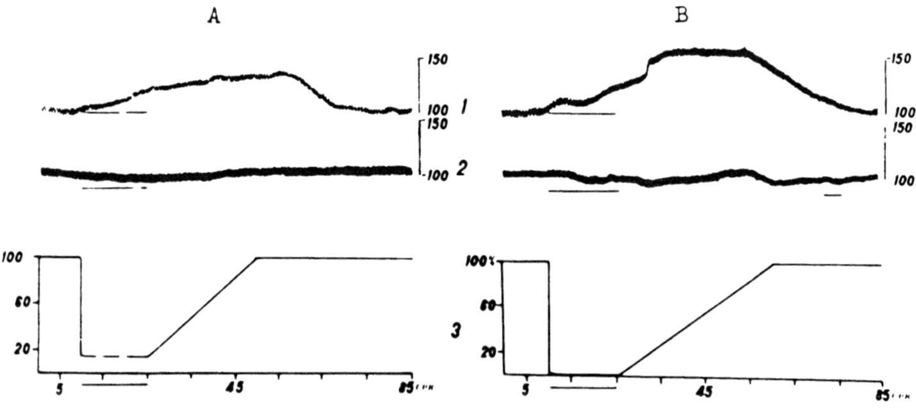

Figure 8. Changes in the amplitude of EMG-response of pain reflex and of blood pressure evoked by tetanic stimulation of postero-lateral hypothalamus before (1) and after (2) stabilization of blood pressure. A., B. intensity of 10 and 20 V, respectively. 1. blood pressure before and 2. after stabilization; 3. diagrams of changes of amplitude of EMG-response of pain reflex after stabilization of blood pressure. On abscissa--time in sec., on ordinate--relative amplitude of EMG-response in percentage (100% is the initial value). On the right--calibration of arterial pressure, mm Hg. Horizontal lines--time of stimulation.

Of special interest are our findings which point out the monoaminergic mechanisms of hypothalamic stimulation-produced analgesia. In a series of experiments, it was shown that noradrenaline, injected intravenously, induced a large increase of blood pressure accompanied by pronounced inhibition of the pain reflex. Angiotensin causes the same degree of blood pressure elevation without changes in the amplitude of EMG-response of the pain reflex. It may be concluded that the antinociceptive effect of noradrenaline is related to the direct action of the drug on the adrenoceptive structures of the hypothalamic antinociceptive system. These findings are in agreement with the findings of the analgesic effect produced by electrical stimulation of catecholaminergic nuclei in the rat brain (Segal, Sanberg, 1977). The role of monoaminergic mechanisms were shown earlier by a study elucidating the effects of noradrenaline, dopamine and serotonin on PAG-stimulation-produced analgesia (Akil, Liebeskind, 1975). Evidently, analgesia from rostral brain stem stimulation is mediated through descending monoaminergic structures of the hypothalamus (Rhodes, Liebeskind, 1978).

Fig. 9 shows the dynamics of changes in the amplitude of EMG-response of pain reflex and of blood pressure evoked by stimulation of postero-lateral hypothalamus (A., B.) and by injection of noradrenaline (C) and angiotensin (D).

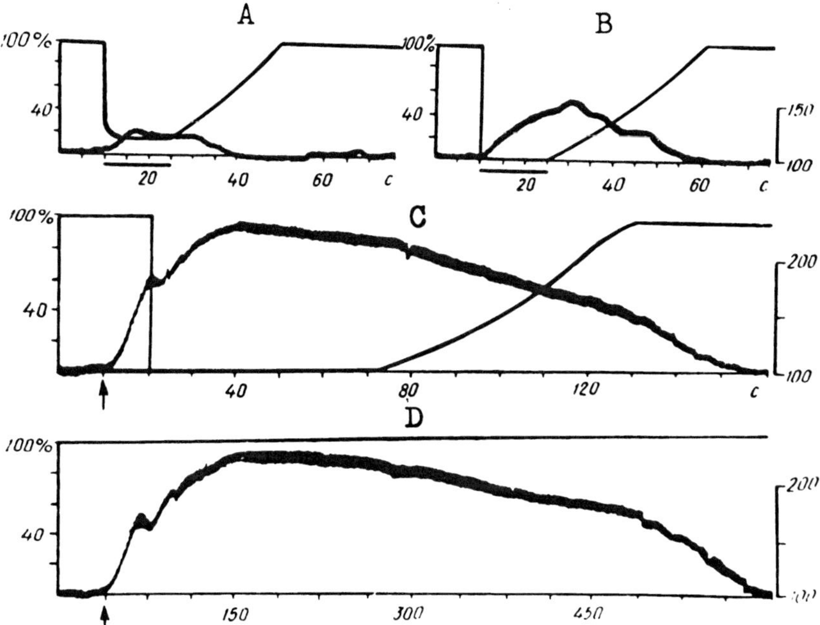

Figure 9. Changes in the amplitude of EMG-response of pain reflex and of blood pressure evoked by stimulation of postero-lateral hypothalamus with intensity of 10 (A) and 20 V (B); and by intravenous injection of noradrenaline (C), and angiotensin (D).
The remaining marks are as in fig. 8.

It can be seen that the increase of blood pressure in the case of intravenous injection of noradrenaline at a dose of 30 mg/kg evokes strong depression of the nociceptive jaw-opening reflex, while the injection of angiotensin at a dose of 0.15 mg/kg induced the same increase of blood pressure like noradrenaline, without changing the amplitude of the nociceptive EMG-response.

Plenary discussion

Wall P.: How is it known that the hypothalamic stimulus does not spread to nearby structures?

Baklavadjian H.: We use for stimulation of hypothalamic structures bipolar electrodes with interelectrode distance of 0.5 mm. The spread of current with such bipolar electrodes is not more than 0.7 mm. The stimulation therefore is local, but we can't exclude stimulation of fibers of passage. But the inhibitory effect of hypothalamic stimulation is much stronger than the effect of amygdala stimulation, implying that the effect is not related to activating amygdala pathways passing through the hypothalamus. Of course, control experiments are necessary with microinjection of L-glutamate, that stimulates only the cell bodies, and not the passing fibers.

References

Akil H, Liebeskind JC (1975) Monominergic mechanisms of stimulation-produced analgesia. Brain Res 94, N2, pp. 279-296.

Albe-Fessard D, Fessard A (1963) Thalamic integrations and their consequences at the telencephalon level. In "Progress in brain research", vol. 1. Brain mechanisms Amsterdam pp. 114-154.

Atweh S, Kuhar M (1977) Autoradiographic localization of opiate receptors in rat brain. II. The brain stem. Brain Res 129 N1, pp. 1-12.

Balagura S, Ralph T (1973) The analgesic effect of electrical stimulation of the diencephalon and mesencephalon. Brain Res 60, N2, pp. 369-379.

Carstens E (1982) Inhibition of spinal dorsal horn neuronal responses to noxious skin heating by medial hypothalamic stimulation in the cat. Brain Res 48, N3, pp. 808-822

Dostrovsky JO, Sessle BJ, Hu JW (1981) Presynaptic excitability changes produced in brain stem endings of tooth pulp afferents by raphe and other central and peripheral influences. Brain Res 218, N1-2, pp. 141-160.

Golanov EV, Kaliushni LB (1978) The analgesic effect of electrical stimulation of dorsomedial hypothalamus in rabbits. Dokl Acad Nauk USSR 242, N2, pp. 469-472.

Hosobuchi Y, Adams E, Linchitz R (1977) Pain relief by electrical stimulation of the central gray matter in humans and reversal by naloxone. Science 197, N2, pp. 183-186.

Rhodes DL, Liebeskind J (1978) Analgesia from rostral brain stem stimulation in the rat. Brain Res 143, N3, pp. 521-533.

Richardson DE, Akil H (1977) Pain reduction by electrical brain stimulation in the periventricular gray matter. J Neurosurg 47, N2, pp. 184-194.

Sar M, Stumpf W, Miller R (1978) Immuno-histochemical localization of enkephalin in rat brain and spinal cord. J Comp Neurol 182, N1, pp. 17-37.

Segal M, Sanberg D (1977) Analgesia produced by electrical stimulation of catecholamine nuclei in the rat brain. Brain Res 123, N2, pp. 369-372.

Valdman AV, Ignatov YD(1976) Central mechanisms of pain. Leningrad Nauka p. 194.

Yokota T (1976) Two types of tooth pulp units in the bulbar lateral reticular formation. Brain Res 104, N2, pp. 325-329.

Young DW, Gottschaldt KM (1976) Neurons in the rostal mesencephalic reticular formation of the cat responding specifically to noxious mechanical stimulation. Sxp Neurol 51, N3, pp. 628-636.

Pain Mechanisms and Management
S.N. Ayrapetyan and A.V. Apkarian (Eds.)
IOS Press, 1998

The Endogenous Pain Control System: Facilitating and Inhibitory Pathways

D. Lima, A. Almeida and I. Tavares
Institute of Histology and Embryology,
Faculty of Medicine, University of Oporto
Porto, Portugal

Abstract. Since the first studies on the antinociceptive role of the periaqueductal gray matter and nucleus raphe magnus, several regions have been included in the endogenous pain control system based on the ability of local stimulation to depress nociceptive reflexes or inhibit nociresponsive dorsal horn neurons. There is increasing evidence, however, on the occurrence of excitatory mechanisms which are likely to act in parallel with the inhibitory ones in order to enhance pain reactions or promote a balanced response adequate to the specific nature of the painful event. Such a bidirectionally organized system may play a role in the genesis of sensitization of central neurons during repetitive or prolonged noxious stimulation by favoring descending facilitating actions in such nociceptive conditions. The present study congregates new data on the functional anatomy of caudal medullary nuclei, which point to both the specific organization of each component of the pain control system, and the common arrangement in recurrent loops capable of counteracting the modulatory effect triggered in each one.

Reciprocal connections were shown to occur between subareas of the dorsal reticular nucleus (DRt), nucleus tractus solitarius (NTS) and caudal ventrolateral reticular formation (caudal VLM), and specific spinal dorsal horn regions, particularly lamina I. Asymmetrical, putative excitatory synaptic contacts were observed between DRt and lamina I neurons at both spinal and medullary levels, suggesting that in this case the reciprocal loop may function as a reverberating circuit aimed at facilitating nociceptive transmission. Accordingly, behavioral studies pointed to the involvement of the DRt in pain facilitation. Electrical or chemical lessening of the nucleus resulted in the increase of pain threshold in the tail-flick and hot plate tests, and decrease of pain behavior during the acute and tonic phases of the Formalin test. Conversely, stimulation of the nucleus by local instillation of glutamate produced a decrease in pain threshold during the tail-flick test. Data based on double retrograde tracing showed, however, that lamina I neurons activating the DRt are also connected with nuclei in the caudal mesencephalon, indicating that the DRt can be simultaneously engaged in promoting a potent antinociceptive effect.

As to the reciprocal connections concerning the NTS and caudal VLM, studies on their anatomy and neurochemistry are still lacking. Nevertheless, the possibility that they mediate descending inhibition upon activation by nociceptive input arriving from the spinal cord is suggested by the fact that inhibitory actions can be induced by stimulating both areas. However, the antinociceptive action elicited from the caudal VLM, which is mediated by spinal α_2 adrenoreceptors and, in a smaller extent, 5-HT receptors, cannot be conveyed by the direct spinopetal descending pathway. Neurons containing 5-HT do not occur in the caudal VLM, whereas noradrenergic neurons of the A1 group could not be labelled retrogradely from the spinal cord. Tracing studies revealed that dysynaptic pathways relayed in the A_5 and the rostral ventromedial medulla are probably conveying, respectively, the noradrenergic and 5-HT antinociceptive effects. Again, negative feedback circuits capable of controlling the ascending triggering effect appear to occur at both the caudal VLM and the spinal cord. Axonal collaterals of spinal-projecting A_5 neurons contact ventrolateral medullary neurons acting upon them. Spinal neurons connected with the caudal ventrolateral medulla receive appositions from descending noradrenergic and serotoninergic fibers.

Introduction

The way in which the central nervous system processes nociceptive signals is one of the best examples of the odd role it plays in the defensive/adaptive relations of the human being with its environment. Both perception and reflex or voluntary behaviours characteristic of painful situations display variable expressions according to a multitude of extrinsic and internal factors. Among the first are the quality, intensity, and duration of the stimulus as well as other sensory events occurring simultaneously. The latter include arousal, affective and volitive conditions, cognitive conditions related to learning and memory, and autonomic conditions such as cardiovascular and respiratory functioning. Conversely, the painful experience determines immediate and long lasting changes in several organic functions.

The endogenous pain control system, first recognized by its ability to depress pain behaviour and inhibit nociresponsive dorsal horn neurons (Basbaum and Fields, 1984), has proved in recent years to present the characteristics expected of a system capable of playing such integrative functions. It is composed of several structures distributed along the brainstem, diencephalon and telencephalon, which receive nociceptive input from the spinal cord (reviewed by Hammond, 1986; Jones, 1992) and give rise to descending mono- or poly-synaptic spinopetal pathways (reviewed by Jones, 1992). Moreover, a complex network of frequently bidirectional projections keeps the different components largely interconnected (reviewed by Gebhart and Randich, 1990; Jones, 1992). Nociceptive signals generated by noxious stimulation of peripheral tissues can in this way be distributed through brain areas involved in very different functions, and thus influence their activity according to the painful event taking place. By feeding back the nociceptive transmission system at the spinal cord dorsal horn, each component can modify the ascending signal in a way probably related to its functional state. Integration of the modulatory processes taking place at each station may be achieved by activation of the pathways interconnecting the different elements of the system, whereas convergence of different descending actions onto spinal dorsal horn neurons probably allows ultimate integration at a cellular level of the multiple modulatory actions triggered supraspinally.

In a few pain control areas, excitatory actions were shown to occur in parallel with the well-documented inhibitory actions. Electrical stimulation of the nucleus raphe magnus (NRM) excited neurons in spinal lamina VIII, whereas stimulation of the latter excited NRM neurons (Cervero and Wolstencroft, 1984). Excitation of spinothalamic and spinomesencephalic cells was observed following stimulation of the midbrain, pontine or medial medullary reticular formation (Giesler et al., 1981; Haber et al., 1980; Yezierski, 1990), as well as of the sensorimotor cortex (Yezierski et al., 1983). The anterior pretectal nucleus exerts an excitatory effect upon nociceptive specific (NS) lamina I cells, and an inhibitory one upon wide-dynamic-range (WDR) deep dorsal horn neurons (Rees et al., 1995). On the other hand, differences in the spinal afferent pathways to the components of the pain control system in what concerns both their laminar origin and the structural neuronal groups involved (reviewed by Jones, 1992; Lima, 1997), are suggestive that each one plays a specific role in nociceptive integration.

Taken together, data suggest that the final effect of the endogenous pain control system upon nociceptive transmission is the result of the balance of multiple negative and positive actions elicited from several brain sites with particular neuronal organization, which is determined by the stimulation conditions and the functional state of each pain control area. The systematic study of each one of its components as to the anatomy, neurochemistry and physiology of the circuits in which they are involved is of major relevance to the understanding of the mechanisms underlying pain control.

This study reports some particular features of the functional anatomy of the caudal medullary pain control centers. Emphasis is given to the structural organization specific of each one, the reciprocal nature of the neuronal circuits involved and the occurrence of facilitating or functionally uncharacterized pathways.

Reciprocal connections between caudal medullary nuclei and the spinal dorsal horn

In the caudal medulla oblongata, the NTS (Lewis et al., 1987; Randich et al., 1988; Morgan et al., 1989; Aicher and Randich, 1990; Du and Zhuo, 1990; Ren et al., 1990), the DRt (Bouhassira et al., 1992; Almeida et al., 1996a,b) and the caudal VLM (Gebhart and Ossipov, 1986; Janss and Gebhart, 1987; 1988) were shown by behavioral (Gebhart and Ossipov, 1986; Janss and Gebhart, 1987; Lewis et al., 1987; Randich et al., 1988; Morgan et al., 1989; Aicher and Randich, 1990; Almeida et al., 1996a,b) or electrophysiological studies (Janss and Gebhart, 1987; Du and Zhuo, 1990; Ren et al., 1990; Bouhassira et al., 1992) to belong to the supraspinal pain control system.

Injections of the tracer cholera toxin subunit B (CTb) in superficial spinal dorsal horn laminae (I-III) or in the entire dorsal horn resulted in retrograde neuronal labelling in the three nuclei (Tavares and Lima, 1994). In the NTS, labelled neurons were located in the subnucleus comissurallis, bilaterally (Fig. 1A). Similar numbers of labelled cells were obtained following superficial or total injections of the dorsal horn, suggesting that the NTS descending pathway is essentially directed to superficial laminae (Fig. 1A) (Tavares and Lima, 1994). As to the spinal-NTS pathway (Menétrey and Basbaum, 1987; Esteves et al., 1993), the spinal path and termination areas were determined by the use of the anterograde tracer biotinylated-dextran (Esteves et al., unpublished observations). Fibers ascending from superficial laminae, which, according to retrograde studies (Menétrey and Basbaum, 1987; Esteves et al., 1993), originate exclusively from lamina I, were shown to travel in the dorsal funiculus (DF), and terminate in the subnucleus commissuralis, bilaterally (Fig. 1A) (Esteves et al., unpublished observations). Those arising from deep laminae (IV-VI; Menétrey and Basbaum, 1987; Esteves et al., 1993) coursed through the dorsolateral fasciculus (DLF) and terminated in the subnucleus lateralis, ipsilaterally (Fig. 1A) (Esteves et al., unpublished observations). Studies based on the induction of the c-*fos* proto-oncogene revealed that spinal neurons projecting to the NTS are activated by several kinds of cutaneous (Lima et al., 1994) and visceral noxious stimulation (Esteves et al., unpublished observations).

In the DRt, neurons labelled by CTb from the superficial dorsal horn were confined to the ipsilateral dorsal most part of the nucleus (DRtd) (Fig. 1B), a small area around the ventral border of the cuneate nucleus (Tavares and Lima, 1994). A few neurons labelled from the deep dorsal horn occurred also in the DRtd, ipsilaterally, but the majority was situated in the ventral part of the DRt (DRtv), bilaterally (Fig. 1B) (Tavares and Lima, 1994). The spinal-DRt pathway (Lima, 1990; Villanueva et al., 1991) was recently shown with biotinylated-dextran to comprise two components: a dorsal one originated in the superficial dorsal horn (mainly lamina I; Lima and Coimbra, 1990; Villanueva et al., 1991) and terminating ipsilaterally in the DRtd, and a ventral one arising from the deep dorsal horn (laminae IV-VI; Villanueva et al., 1991) and projecting to the DRtv, bilaterally, and, in lesser extent, to the DRtd, ipsilaterally (Fig. 1B) (Almeida et al., 1995). Injections in different funiculi demonstrated that fibers directed to the DRtd coursed mainly in the DF (Almeida et al., 1995). This is in agreement with earlier retrograde tracing studies showing that practically no lamina I neurons could be labelled from the DRt caudally to DF lesions (Lima, 1990). Fibers directed to the DRtv, as well as those few connecting the deep dorsal horn with the DRtd, coursed in the DLF (Almeida et al., 1995). A large proportion of DRt-projecting spinal neurons expressed c-*fos* following cutaneous or visceral stimulation (Almeida and Lima, 1997).

The descending projection from the caudal VLM was shown by retrograde tracing to arise exclusively from a small area of the reticular formation (VLMlat) located between the lateral reticular nucleus (LRt) and the ventral pole of the spinal trigeminal nucleus, pars caudalis (SP5C), and to reach both superficial and deep dorsal horn laminae, mainly ipsilaterally (Fig. 1C) (Tavares and Lima, 1994). Anterograde studies demonstrated recently that the descending system targets spinal laminae I and IV-V (Tavares et al., 1996b). Axonal fibers ascending from the spinal cord to the caudal VLM (Menétrey et al., 1983; Lima et al., 1991) were segregated mediolaterally at their termination sites so that those arising from laminae I-II terminated in the VLMlat, those originated in laminae IV-VI in the lateral portion of the LRt (Fig. 1C), and those from the ventral horn in the medial portion of the LRt (Lima et al., 1991). Both electrophysiological (Menétrey et al., 1984) and c-*fos* (Tavares et al., 1993) studies revealed that spinal-caudal VLM neurons can be activated by nociceptive input.

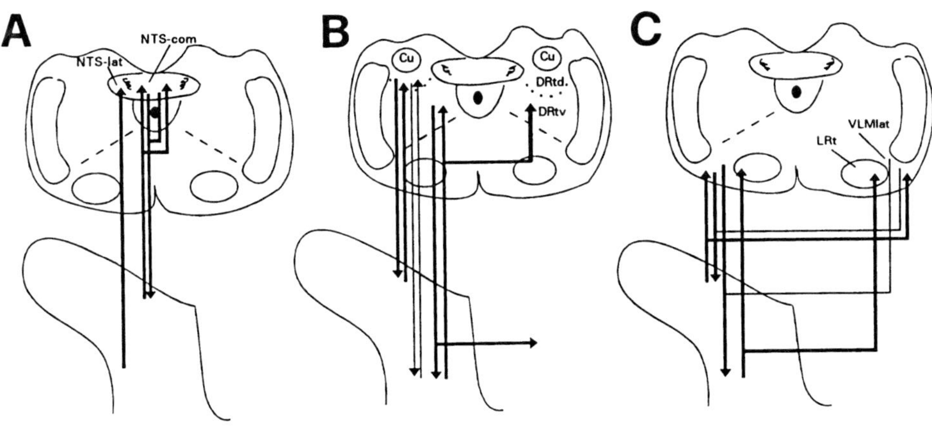

Figure 1. Diagramatic representation of the descending and ascending pathways connecting the spinal dorsal horn with the nucleus tractus solitarius (A), dorsal reticular nucleus (B) and caudal ventrolateral reticular formation (C). Cu - cuneate nucleus; DRtd - dorsal portion of the dorsal reticular nucleus; DRtv - ventral portion of the dorsal reticular nucleus; LRt - lateral reticular nucleus; NTS-com - subnucleus commissuralis of the nucleus tractus solitarius; NTS-lat - sub nucleus lateralis of the nucleus tractus solitarius; VLMlat - lateral portion of the caudal ventrolateral reticular formation.

The above referred findings show that the spinal dorsal horn and the three pain control nuclei of the caudal medulla oblongata are bidirectionally connected in a well organized manner as to the spinal laminae involved (Fig. 1). In all cases, reciprocal connections with specific areas of each medullary target concern lamina I particularly. The deep dorsal horn is either reciprocally linked with more widely distributed regions, as in the case of the DRt, or does not take part in reciprocal pathways. By showing that the neuronal populations of the superficial and deep dorsal horn are differentially connected supraspinally and under distinct supraspinal effects, these data are highly suggestive of the differential involvement of each spinal region in pain processing.

Taken together, the anatomical results presented favor the hypothesis that, contrary to deep dorsal horn neurons (with the exception of those projecting to the DRt), neurons in lamina I are under feedback control from their targets in the caudal medulla. As far as the NTS and the caudal VLM are concerned, it remains to be clarified whether such feedback systems are responsible for the inhibitory actions that can be elicited from each one of them, or if such effects are the responsibility of polysynaptic pathways. Polysynaptic pathways were indeed shown to be involved in the hypoalgesia triggered from the caudal VLM (see below). Nevertheless, studies are needed to determine the precise role of the direct descending tracts, namely their possible facilitating nature. The fact that, in certain nociceptive conditions, stimulation of those nuclei has an antinociceptive effect does not rule out the possibility that they are also involved in excitatory actions. Depending on the intensity of stimulation of the rostral ventromedial medulla (RVM), inhibition or facilitation of either the responsiveness of spinal neurons to noxious stimulation or of the latency of the tail-flick response have been obtained (Zhuo and Gebhart, 1990; 1992).

The dorsal reticular nucleus as a pain facilitating center

Contrary to what has been observed in other brain areas involved in the control of nociceptive transmission (reviewed by Basbaum and Fields, 1984; Jones, 1992), stimulation of the DRt by local instillation of glutamate produced a decrease in pain threshold as measured by the tail-flick test (Fig. 2A) (Almeida et al., 1996b), whereas lesioning the nucleus with quinolinic acid increased the pain threshold during both the tail-flick (Fig. 2 B, C) and the hot plate (Fig. 2 D,E) tests (Almeida et al., 1996b). Decreased pain behaviour was also observed during the acute and tonic phases of the formalin test following chemical or electrical lesions of the DRt (Fig. 3). However, on the earlier acute phase (0-5 min after formalin injection), the effect was exclusively ipsilateral, while during the tonic phase (10-60 min) it occurred bilaterally (Fig. 3) (Almeida et al., 1996a).

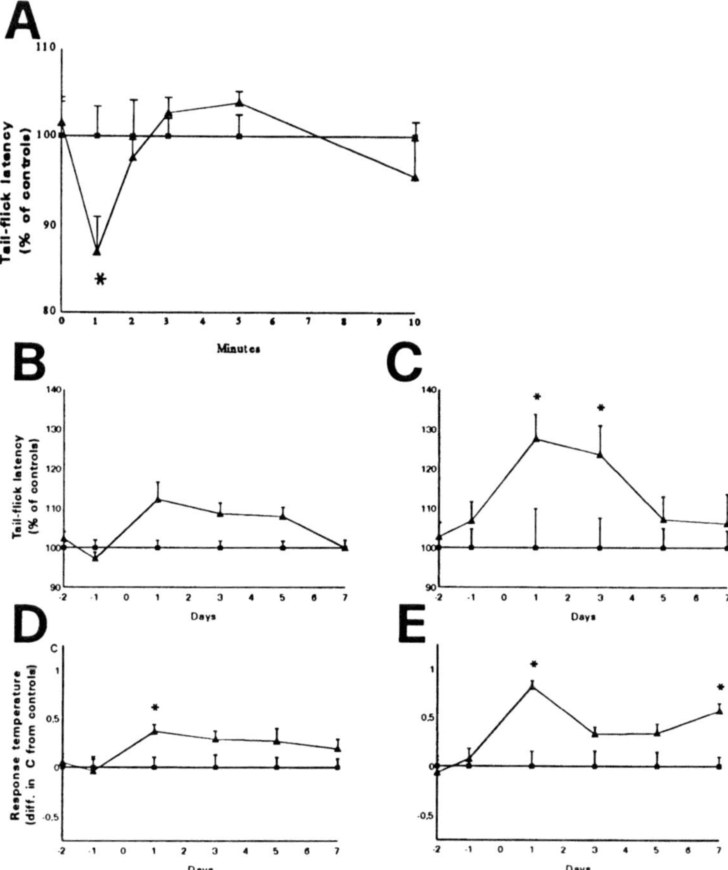

Figure 2. Tail-flick latency (A-C) and hot plate temperature threshold (D, E) following unilateral stimulation by glutamate (A), or unilateral (B, D) or bilateral (C, E) lesioning by quinolinic acid (B-E) of the dorsal reticular nucleus. * = p<0.05

These data suggest that, although the DRt facilitates nociception in both acute and inflammatory conditions, different pathways are probably conveying each effect. As referred above, two descending systems project from the DRt to the spinal cord dorsal horn. One is exclusively ipsilateral and connects the DRtd mainly with the most superficial laminae, while the other is bilateral and links the DRtv with deep laminae (Fig. 1B). It is, therefore, likely that the facilitating effects upon acute and tonic pain are mediated, respectively, by the dorsal and ventral DRt-spinal pathways. With regard to the dorsal pathway, combined LM and EM tracing studies have shown that fibers descending from the DRt establish asymmetrical synaptic contacts upon lamina I neurons projecting back to it (Fig. 4A) (Almeida et al., 1993). Considering the excitatory nature of this structural type of synapses (Todd and Spike, 1993) together with the fact that DRt-projecting lamina I neurons are c-*fos* activated following noxious stimulation of the skin or viscera (Almeida and Lima, 1997), these anatomical data indicate that DRt neurons exert a positive feed-back action upon transmission of nociceptive input to the DRt. Curiously, spinal axons terminating in the DRtd also establish asymmetrical synaptic contacts upon neurons projecting back to the spinal dorsal horn (Fig. 4B) (Almeida et al., unpublished observations). The reciprocal connection between the DRtd and lamina I thus appears to constitute a reverberating circuit aimed at amplifying the ascending nociceptive signal (Fig. 5), and may therefore be the anatomical substrate for the pain facilitating effect elicited from the DRt, particularly in what concerns acute pain. In this respect, it should be noted that the fact that DRt-projecting lamina I neurons must be under a facilitating action is supported by the finding that the percentage of cells retrogradely labelled from the DRt which express c-*fos* following several kinds of cutaneous or visceral noxious stimulation is much higher than the one observed from other spinal targets (Lima, 1997).

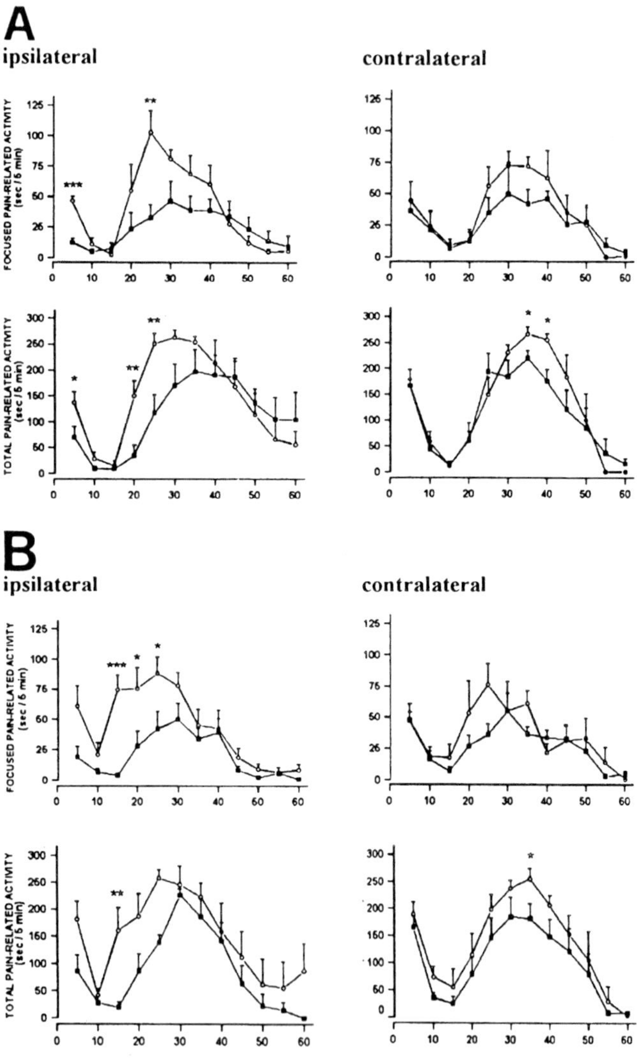

Figure 3. Pain behaviour evaluated by the focused pain-related activity (licking, biting and shaking the injected paw) and total pain-related activity (those parameters plus lifting the injected paw) during the acute (0-5 min) or tonic (10 -60 min) phases of the formalin test, after ipsilateral or contralateral electrical (A) or quinolinic acid (B) lesions of the dorsal reticular nucleus.
* = p<0. 05 - * * = p<0. 0 1; * * * = p< 0. 00 1.

As to the action exerted by the DRtv-deep dorsal horn pathway, no data are available at the moment. The depression of C fiber-evoked inhibition of heterosegmental WDR neurons observed following lesioning of the DRt (Bouhassira et al., 1992) suggested the involvement of the nucleus in diffuse noxious inhibitory controls (DNIC) (LeBars et al., 1979). This phenomenon has been taken as resulting in pain facilitation by promoting contrast enhancement (LeBars et al., 1988; 1992), and is therefore consistent with the proposal of a pain facilitating role for the DRt. Since DNIC is exerted bilaterally (Bouhassira et al., 1992) upon WDR neurons (LeBars et al., 1979; Bouhassira et al., 1992), which prevail in the deep dorsal horn (Menétrey et al., 1977; Laird and Cervero, 1989), it could be conveyed by the ventral DRt descending pathway. It remains, however, to be ascertained whether the inhibitory action mediating DNIC depends on a direct DRt-spinal pathway or involves propiospinal neurons which inhibit WDR neurons heterosegmentally upon activation by DRt descending axons at the homosegmental level. If this is the case, the ventral DRtv-spinal system may also be excitatory and thus be capable of transporting the facilitating effect upon nociceptive transmission during inflammatory pain. Future anatomical and electrophysiological studies are needed to clarify this issue.

Amplification of the nervous signal through the spinal-DRt-spinal loop may result on the transmission of intensified nociceptive input to brain areas targeted by the DRt (Fig. 5). The DRt sends projections to the parafascicular and ventromedial nuclei of the medial thalamus (Fig. 5) (Bernard et al., 1990), which play an important role in affective-aversive reactions to pain (Casey et al., 1974; Mitchell and Kaelber, 1966; 1967). Facial and oral motor nuclei, as well as areas involved in motor control such as the inferior olive and the cerebellum, also receive projections from the DRt (Fig. 5) (Bernard et al., 1990; Newman and Ginsberg, 1992). It is possible that, by amplifying the nociceptive signal, the spinal-DRt-spinal circuit is particularly devoted to the genesis of prompt and intense responses to pain, particularly aversive reactions and vocalizations and facial expressions which normally accompany noxious events.

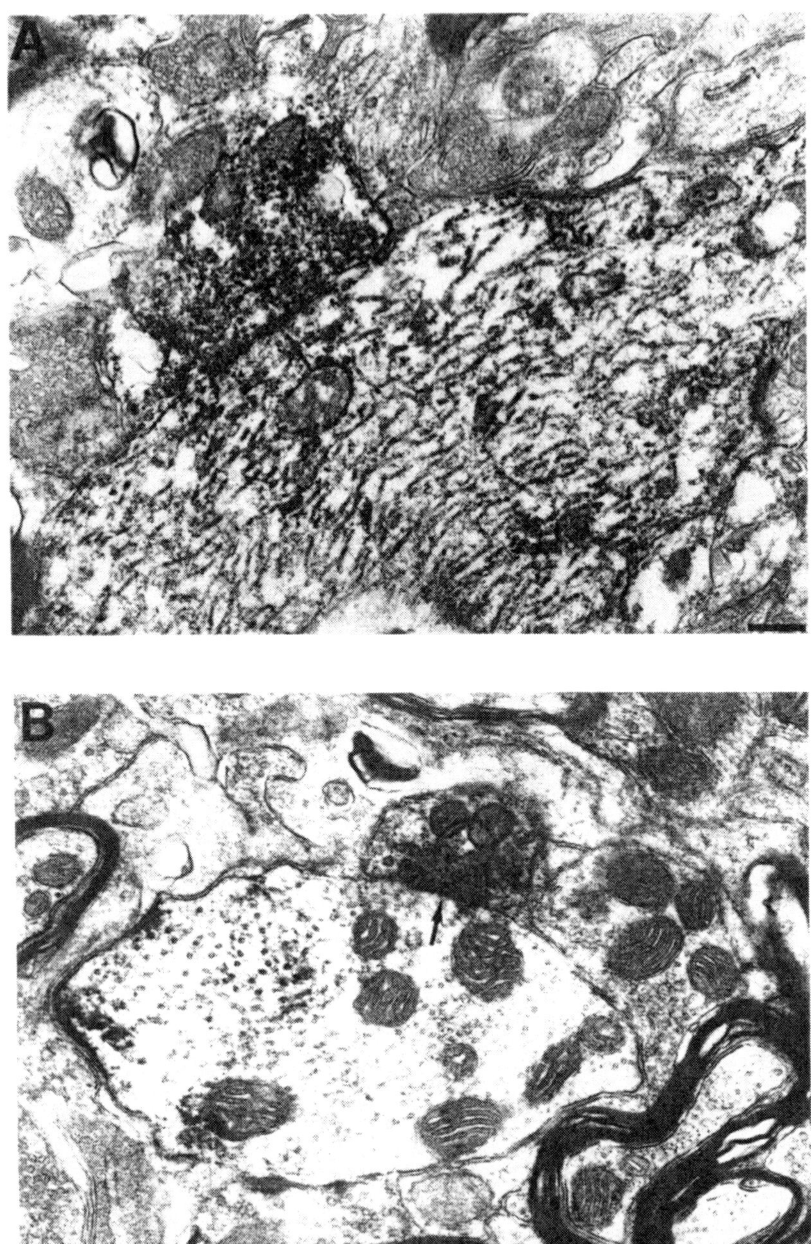

Figure 4. Neuronal profiles in spinal cord lamina I (A) or the dorsal part of the dorsal reticular nucleus (B) labelled by cholera toxin subunit B (CTb) injected in the dorsal reticular nucleus (A) or the spinal dorsal horn (B). Axonal boutons labelled anterogradely present round synaptic vesicles and establish asymmetrical synaptic contacts (arrows) with retrogradely labelled perikaria (A) or dendritic profiles (B). Scale bar equals 0.3 μm.

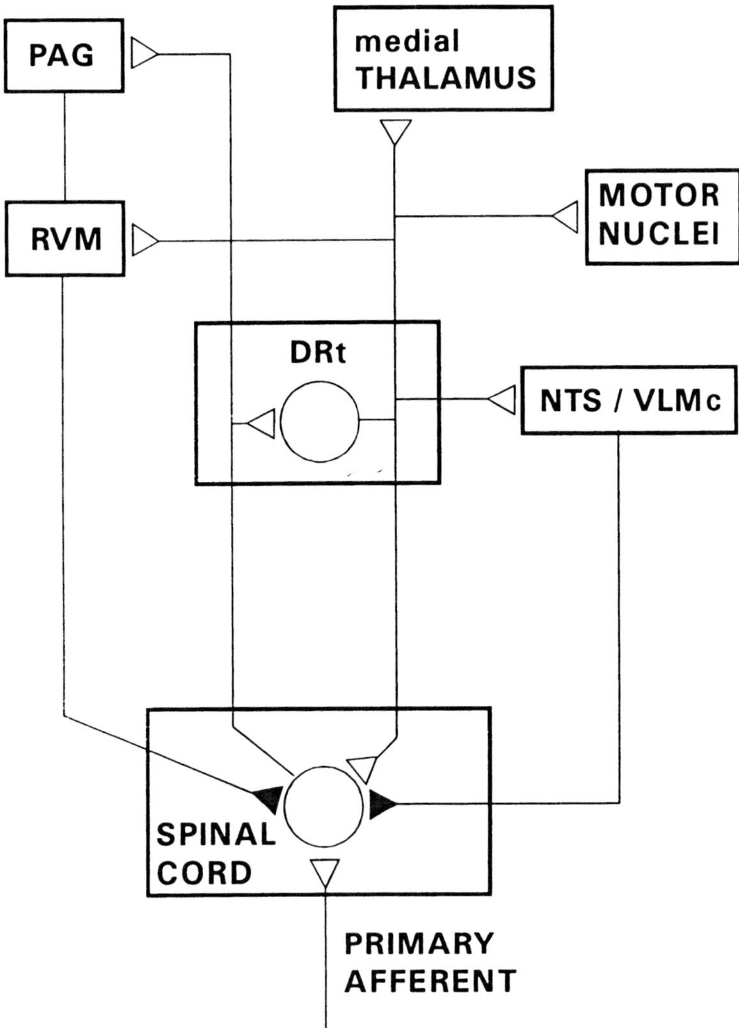

Figure 5. Diagram representing the postulated neuronal circuitry mediating the nociceptive-modulatory effects of the dorsal reticular nucleus (DRt). Primary afferent nociceptive input activates a reverberating spinal -DRt-spinal loop, which results in amplification of the signal transmitted from the DRt to aversive (medial thalamus) or motor areas, and from both the DRt and spinal cord dorsal horn to antinociceptive brain areas which inhibit nociresponsive spinal neurons. NTS - nucleus tractus solitarius; PAG - periaqueductal gray; RVM - rostral ventromedial medulla; VLMc - caudal ventrolateral reticular formation.

The DRt is connected as well with other pain control centers, such as the NTS (Esteves et al., 1993), the caudal VLM (Tavares et al., unpublished observations) and the gigantocellular reticular nucleus (Fig. 5) (Bernard et al., 1990). On the other hand, by the use of double retrograde tracing techniques, some lamina I neurons projecting to the DRt were shown to project also to the caudal mesencephalon (Fig. 5) (Almeida et al., unpublished observations). Through activation of such a circuitry, intensification of the nociceptive signal by the spinal-DRt-spinal loop can also result in the enhancement of descending antinociceptive actions. The possibility that in this case, as in other pain control systems, the final effect depends on the balance between inhibitory and excitatory effects, and that this balance is determined, at least in part, by stimulus conditions, should be investigated in future studies.

Multiple pathways from the caudal ventrolateral reticular formation

The direct pathway descending from the caudal VLM to the spinal dorsal horn (Tavares and Lima, 1994; Tavares et al., 1996b) was thought to originate from the A_1 noradrenergic cell group, and thus to convey the spinal α_2-mediated hypoalgesia triggered by stimulation of the caudal VLM (Dahlström and Fuxe, 1965; Satoh et al., 1977; Fleetwood-Walker et al., 1983). However, studies combining retrograde tracing from the spinal cord with immunocytochemical detection of enzymes of the noradrenergic metabolic pathway not only failed to reveal colocalization of both markers (Westlund et al., 1981; 1983, Kwiat and Basbaum, 1992; Tavares et al., 1996c), but also demonstrated that the A_1 group is topographically distinct from the spinal-projecting neuronal cluster (VLMlat), being located dorsomedially to the latter (Fig. 6A) (Tavares et al., 1996c).

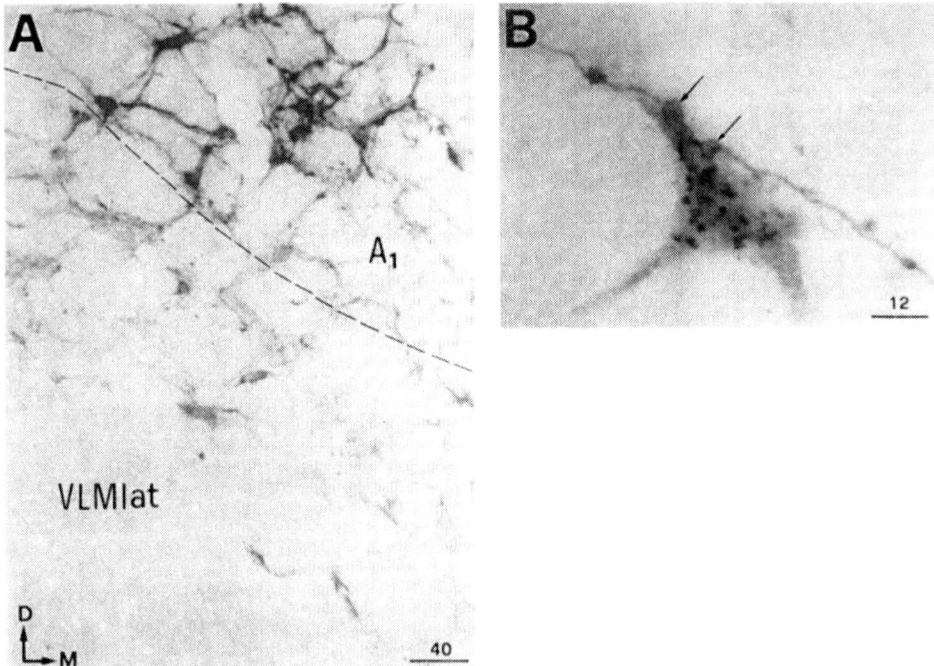

Figure 6. A: Neurons in the caudal ventrolateral reticular formation immunoreactive for dopamine- β-hydroxylase (blue; A₁) or retrogradely labelled with cholera toxin subunit B (CTb) from the spinal dorsal horn (brown; VLMlat). B: Neuron of the A₅ noradrenergic group immunoreactive for dopamine- β-hydroxylase (blue) and retrogradely labelled from the spinal dorsal horn with CTb (black dots), receiving oppositions from varicosities of axonal fibers labelled anterogradely with biotinylated dextran from the VLMlat (brown). Scale bars are expressed in μm.

Fibers labelled anterogradely with biotinylated-dextran from the caudal VLM were shown to establish asymmetrical synaptic contacts with neurons of the A_5 group which were both immunoreactive for dopamine-β-hydroxylase (DBH) and labelled retrogradelly with CTb from the spinal dorsal horn (Figs 6B, 7) (Tavares et al., 1996c). Such synaptic arrangement could not be observed in other DBH-positive areas of the brainstem, suggesting that the antinociceptive noradrenergic effect elicited from the caudal VLM is conveyed by a dysynaptic pathway relayed in the A_5 (Fig. 8) (Tavares et al., 1996c). As to the less intense spinal 5-HT receptor-mediated hypoalgesic effect of the caudal VLM (Gebhart and Ossipov, 1986; Janss and Gebhart, 1987), a dysynaptic pathway relayed in the RVM is probably involved (Fig. 8). Fibers labelled with biotinilated-dextran from the VLMlat apposed also to RVM neurons labelled retrogradely from the spinal cord (Tavares et al., 1996c).

Retrograde labelling from the A_5 revealed that caudal VLM neurons projecting to it are confined to the VLMlat (Tavares et al., 1997). Nociceptive input capable of triggering the descending noradrenergic antinociceptive effect must thus arise from superficial dorsal horn layers (Lima et al., 1991). Neurons in both laminae I and II expressed the c-*fos* proto-oncogene following mechanical or thermal noxious stimulation of the skin (Tavares et al., 1993). However, while lamina I neurons are most certainly engaged in the activation of the system (Willis, 1985) (Fig. 8), the role of lamina II neurons is far beyond being clarified. Lamina II is largely populated by inhibitory neurons (Todd and Spike, 1993) some of which (inverse 1-1) were proposed to modulate locally nociceptive transmission by depressing the tonic inhibitory action exerted by 3 (inverse 3) neurons upon activation by the arriving nociceptive input (Cervero et al., 1979) (Fig. 8). Based on the enhancement of the responses of dorsal horn neurons to noxious stimulation following lesioning of the caudal VLM, but not of other brainstem areas involved in pain control, this medullary region was proposed to be responsible for supraspinal tonic inhibition of nociceptive transmission (Hall et al., 1982). The possibility that lamina II neurons projecting to the VLMlat play a double inhibitory effect upon tonic spinal and supraspinal inhibitory actions (Fig. 8) deserves to be investigated in future studies.

By combining immunodetection of DBH with double labelling by fluorogold injected in the dorsal horn and CTb injected in the VLMlat, A_5 neurons projecting to the spinal cord and receiving appositions from CTb-labelled VLMlat axons were shown to be also labelled retrogradely from the VLMlat (Tavares et al., 1997). According to the results of retrograde plus anterograde tracing with CTb from the A_5, fibers projecting from this noradrenergic nucleus to the VLMlat are apposed to VLMlat neurons projecting back to it (Tavares et al., 1997). A negative noradrenergic feed-back loop made up by collaterals of the A5 descending antinociceptive pathway and impinging upon VLMlat neurons triggering the A5 descending action, thus, appears to occur (Fig. 8). Inhibitory projections from the RVM to the VLMlat were also demonstrated (Qvist et al., 1983; Nicholas and Hancock, 1990; Sim and Joseph, 1992; Murphy and Behbehani, 1993), but it has not been investigated whether they collateralize from the NRM-spinal pathway (Basbaum and Fields, 1984) (Fig. 8). On the other hand, VLMlat-projecting spinal neurons received appositions from descending fibers immunoreactive for DBH or 5-HT (Tavares et al., 1996a), spinal neurons contacted by noradrenergic fibers being more numerous (50%) than those contacted by 5-HT fibers (19%) (Tavares et al., 1996a). The antinociceptive descending inputs thus seem to be feedback inhibiting neurons at the origin of the triggering ascending signal at both the medullary and spinal levels (Fig. 8). Circuits of this kind, probably dedicated to tuning up pain modulatory actions have been observed in several other antinociceptive regions (reviewed by Jones, 1992).

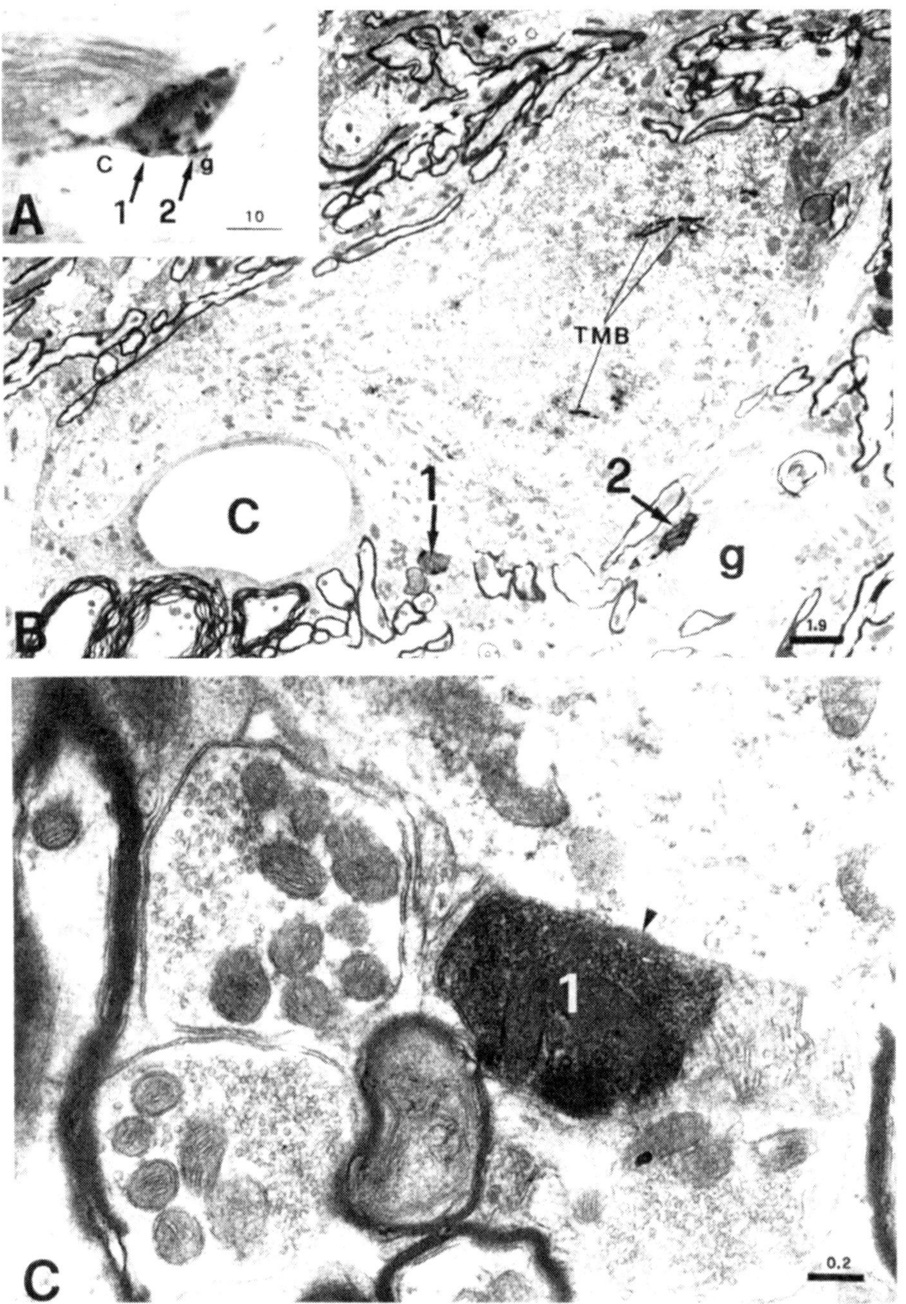

Figure 7. An A_5 neuron immunoreactive for dopamine-β-hydroxylase and retrogradely labelled with cholera toxin subunit B (CTb) from the spinal dorsal horn, is shown in **A** to be apposed by an axonal varicosity (1) labelled anterogradely with biotinylated dextran from the VLMlat. **B** and **C** are higher magnifications of the neuron in A. CTb revealed by tetramethylbenzidine (TMB) appears as black cristals (B). Biotinylated dextran revealed by diaminobenzidine (DAB) darkens the axoplasm and plasma membranes (C). Note the asymmetrical nature of the synaptic contact (arrow head). c - capillary; g - glial cell. Scale bars are expressed in μm.

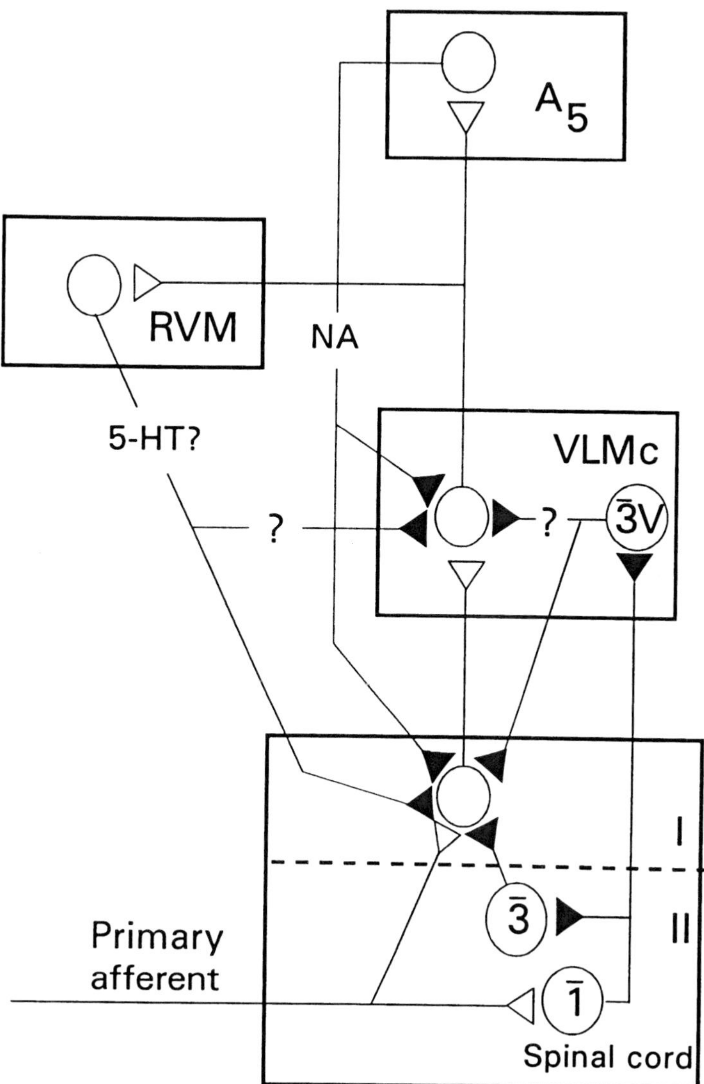

Figure 8. Diagram representing the postulated neuronal circuitry mediating the nociceptive-modulatory effects of the caudal ventrolateral reticular formation (VLMc). On the right side, the spinal-VLMc connections involving lamina II neurons. Neurons of the type $\overline{1}$ (which are activated by nociceptive input and inhibited by innocuous input - Cervero et al., 1979) inhibit neurons exerting tonic inhibition of spinal nociceptive transmission at both the spinal ($\overline{3}$)and VLMc ($\overline{3}$V)levels upon activation by nociceptive primary afferents. On the left side, the A_5 and RVM circuits conveying, respectively, the noradrenergic and 5-HT antinociceptive effects triggered in the VLMlat upon the arrival of nociceptive input transmitted by lamina I neurons. 5-HT - 5-hydroxytriptamine; NA - noradrenalin; RVM - rostral ventromedial medulla.

Integrative functions of the endogenous pain control system

The multiplicity and functional diversity of brain areas taking part in the pain control system strongly suggest that the system is not only, or even primarily involved in controlling nociceptive transmission upon the arrival of nociceptive input, but is rather engaged in integrating nociception with several other brain functions. This implies that, on one hand, those functions can be altered in response to a noxious event, and, on the other hand, changes in the functional state of each brain center can influence nociceptive processing.

To test this latter possibility, the role of the caudal VLM in the genesis of hypertension-dependent hypoalgesia was evaluated. Hypertension produced experimentally in rats by surgical or pharmacological approaches was accompanied by a decrease in the numbers of spinal neurons expressing c-*fos* following noxious stimulation of the skin, as compared to normotensive rats (Fig. 9) (Tavares et al., 1995). This finding was taken as indicating that rises in pain threshold observed in hypertensive subjects, either humans (Zamir and Shuber, 1980; Ditto et al., 1993) or experimental animals (Zamir and Segal, 1979; Zamir et al., 1980; Thurston and Randich, 1990), are due to depression of the response capacity of nociceptive spinal neurons. By lesioning the VLMlat with quinolinic acid, the hypertension-related decrease in c-*fos* expression did not occur (Fig.9), while lesion of the nucleus per itself had no effect (Fig.9). The caudal VLM is known to play a pivot role in the baroreceptor reflex by inhibiting the vasopressor region in the rostral ventrolateral medulla (reviewed by Blessing and Li, 1989; Chalmers and Pilowski, 1991).

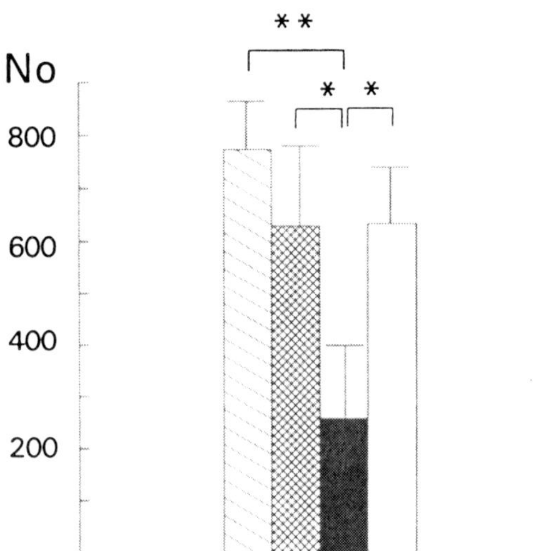

Figure 9. Numbers of Fos-immunoreactive cells occurring in the spinal dorsal horn in rats subjected to sham operation of the renal artery plus injection of saline in the VLMlat (normotensive non-lesioned) - diagonally lined, sham operation of the renal artery plus injection of quinolinic acid in the VLMlat (normotensive lesioned) – cross-hatched, renal artery occlusion plus injection of saline in the VLMlat (hypertensive non-lesioned) - solid black, renal artery occlusion plus injection of quinolinic acid in the VLMlat (hypertensive lesioned) - stippled.

According to the data presented, VLMlat neurons respond to rises in blood pressure by activating not only the baroreceptor reflex but also a descending antinociceptive pathway acting upon nociresponsive spinal neurons.

Conclusion

The data presented on the functional anatomy of the neuronal circuits subserving nociceptive processing in the NTS, DRt and caudal VLM point to the specificity of their structural organization and functional role, while emphasizing common neuronal arrangements such as the occurrence of feedback counteracting circuits and the profusion of interconnections encompassing extramedullary pain control centers. The three medullary regions were shown to differ as to the afferent and efferent spinal systems, although reciprocal connections with the marginal zone, or lamina I, appear to be common to all of them. A pain facilitating role mediated by a reverberating spino-bulbo-spinal circuit was attributed to the dorsal reticular nucleus. The antinociceptive effects elicited from the caudal VLM were revealed to be conveyed by polysynaptic spinopetal pathways, and to be triggered not only by noxious events but also by changes in cardiovascular parameters. Recurrent negative circuits targeting either brain stem relays or the spinal dorsal horn, which are likely to be engaged in tuning up the pain control action, were demonstrated.

Similar studies on the structural organization of the other components of the endogenous pain control system, particularly devised to uncover neuronal arrangements specific of each one or common to the entire system, and to reveal the way in which nociceptive transmission influences or is influenced by the functional state of each component, will be determinant to the better understanding of central processing of nociceptive input.

References

Aicher SA, Randich A (1990) Antinociception and cardiovascular responses produced by electrical stimulation in the nucleus tractus solitarius, nucleus reticularis ventralis, and the caudal medulla. Pain 42:103-119.

Almeida A, Lima D (1997) Activation by cutaneous or visceral noxious stimulation of spinal neurons projecting to the medullary dorsal reticular nucleus in the rat: a c-*fos* study. Europ J Neurosci 9:686-695.

Almeida A, Tavares I, Lima D (1995) Projection sites of superficial or deep dorsal horn in the dorsal reticular nucleus. Neuroreport 6:1245-1248.

Almeida A, Tavares I, Lima D, Coimbra A (1993) Descending projections from the medullary dorsal reticular nucleus make synaptic contacts with spinal cord lamina I cells projecting to that nucleus: an electron microscopic tracer study in the rat. Neuroscience 55:1093-1106.

Almeida A, Størkson R, Lima D, Hole K, Tjølsen A (1996a) The medullary dorsal reticular nucleus facilitates acute and tonic pain induced by formalin. Abstracts of the 8th World Congress on Pain 472. Seattle:IASP Press.

Almeida A, Tjølsen A, Lima D, Coimbra A, Hole K (1996b) The medullary dorsal reticular nucleus facilitates acute nociception in the rat. Brain Res Bull 39:7-15.

Basbaum AI, Fields HL (1984) Endogenous pain control systems: brainstem spinal pathways and endorphin circuitry. Ann Rev Neurosci 7:309-338.

Bernard JF, Villanueva L, Carroué J, Le Bars D (1990) Efferent projections from the subnucleus reticularis dorsalis (SRD): a *Phaseolus vulgaris* leucoagglutinin study in the rat. Neurosci Lett 116:257-262.

Blessing WW, Li Y-W (1989) Inhibitory vasomotor neurons in the caudal ventrolateral region of the medulla oblongata. In: The central neural organization of cardiovascular control (Ciriello J, Caverson MM, Polosa C eds), pp 83-98. Amsterdam:Elsevier.

Bouhassira D, Villanueva L, Bing Z, Le Bars D (1992) Involvement of the subnucleus reticularis dorsalis in diffuse noxious inhibitory controls in the rat. Brain Res 595:353-357.

Casey KL, Keene JJ, Morrow T (1974) Bulboreticular and medial thalamic unit activity in relation to aversive behavior and pain. In: Adv Neurol 4:197-205.

Cervero F, Iggo A, Molony V (1979) An electrophysiological study of neurones in the substantia gelatinosa Rolandi of the cats spinal cord. Q J Exp Physiol 64:297-314.

Cervero F, Wolstencroft JH (1984) A positive feedback loop between spinal cord nociceptive pathways and antinociceptive areas of the cats brain stem. Pain 20:125-138.

Chalmers J, Pilowsky P (1991) Brainstem and bulbospinal neurotransmitter systems in the control of blood pressure. J Hypertens 9:675-694.

Dahlstrom A, Fuxe K (1965) Evidence for the existence of monoamine-containing neurons in the central nervous system. II: Experimentally induced changes in the intraneuronal amine levels of the bulbospinal neuron systems. Acta Physiologica Scandinavica 64:1-36.

Ditto B, Edwards MC, Miller S, D'Antono B, Blum S (1993) The effects of sodium loading on blood pressure and pain responses to the cold pressor test. J Psychom Res 37:771-780.

Du HJ, Zhou SY (1990) Involvement of solitary tract nucleus in control of nociceptive transmission in cat spinal cord neurons. Pain 40:323-331.

Esteves F, Lima D, Coimbra A (1993) Structural types of spinal cord marginal (lamina I) neurons projecting to the nucleus of the tractus solitarius in the rat. Somatosens Motor Res 10:203-216.

Fleetwood-Walker SM, Coote JH, Gilbey MP (1983) Identification of spinally projecting neurones in the A1 catecholamine cell group of the ventrolateral medulla. Brain Res 273:25-33.

Gebhart GF, Ossipov MH (1986) Characterization of inhibition of the spinal nociceptive tail-flick reflex in the rat from the medullary lateral reticular nucleus. Journal Neurosci 6:701-713.

Gebhart GF, Randich A (1990) Brainstem modulation of nociception. In: Brainstem mechanisms of behavior (Klemm WR, Vertes RP eds), pp 315-352. New York: Jonh Wiley & Sons, Inc.

Giesler GJ, Yezierski RP, Gerhart KD, Willis WD (1981) Spinothalamic tract neurons that project to medial and/or lateral thalamuc nuclei: evidence for a physiologically novel population of spinal cord neurons. J Neurophysiol 46:1285-1306.

Haber LH, Martin RF, Chung JM, Willis WD (1980) Inhibition and excitation of primate spinothalamic tract neurons by stimulation in region of nucleus reticularis gigantocellularis. J Neurophysiol 43:1578-1593.

Hall JG, Duggan AW, Morton CR, Johnson SM (1983) The location of brainstem neurones tonically inhibiting dorsal horn neurones of the cat. Brain Res 244:215-222.

Hammond DL (1986) Control systems for nociceptive afferent processing. The descending inhibitory pathawys. In: Spinal afferent processing (Yaksk T ed), pp 363-390. New York: Plenum Press.

Janss AJ, Gebhart GF (1987) Spinal monoaminergic receptors mediate the antinociception produced by glutamate in the medullary lateral reticular nucleus. J Neurosci 7:2862-2873.

Janss AJ, Gebhart GF (1988) Quantitative characterization and spinal pathway mediating inhibition of spinal nociceptive transmission from the lateral reticular nucleusin the rat. J Neurophysiol 59:226-247.

Jones SL (1992) Descending control of nociception. In: The initial processing of pain and its descending control: spinal and trigeminal systems (Gildenberg PL ed), pp 203-295. Basel: Karger.

Kwiat G, Basbaum AI (1992) The origin of brainstem noradrenergic and serotonergic projections to the spinal cord dorsal horn in the rat. Somatosens Motor Res 9:157-173.

Laird JMA, Cervero F (1989) A comparative study of the changes in receptive-field properties of multireceptive and nocireceptive rat dorsal horn neurons following noxious mechanical stimulation. J Neurophysiol 62:854-863.

Le Bars D, Dickenson AH, Besson JM (1979) Diffuse noxious inhibitory controls (DNIC). I. Effects on dorsal horn convergent neurones in the rat. Pain 6:283-304.

Le Bars D, Villanueva L (1988) Electrophysiological evidence for the activation of descending inhibitory controls by nociceptive afferent pathways. Prog Brain Res 77:275-299.

Le Bars D, Villanueva L, Bouhassira D, Willer J-C (1992) Diffuse noxious inhibitory controls (DNIC) in animals and man. Path Physiol Exp Therapy 4:55-65.

Lewis JW, Baldrighi G, Akil H (1987) A possible interface between autonomic function and pain control: opioid analgesia and the nucleus tractus solitarius. Brain Res 424:65-70.

Lima D (1990) A spinomedullary projection terminating in the dorsal reticular nucleus of the rat. Neuroscience 34:577-589.

Lima D, Coimbra A (1990) Structural types of marginal (lamina I) neurons projecting to the dorsal reticular nucleus of the medulla oblongata. Neuroscience 34:591-606.

Lima D (1997) Functional anatomy of spinofugal nociceptive pathways. Pain Reviews 4:1-19.

Lima D, Esteves F, Coimbra A (1994) C-*fos* activation by noxious input of spinal neurons projecting to the nucleus of the tractus solitarius in the rat. In: Proceedings of the 7th World Congress on Pain (Gebhart GF, Hammond D, Jensen TS eds), pp 423-434. Seattle: IASP Press.

Lima D, Mendes-Ribeiro JA, Coimbra A (1991) The spino-latero-reticular system of the rat: projections from the superficial dorsal horn and structural characterization of marginal neurons involved. Neuroscience 45:137-152.

Menétrey D, Basbaum AI (1987) Spinal and trigeminal projections to the nucleus of the solitary tract: a possible substrate for somatovisceral and viscerovisceral reflex activation. J Comp Neurol 255:439-450.

Menétrey D, De Pommery J, Besson JM (1984) Electrophysiological characteristics of lumbar spinal neurons backfired from the lateral reticular nucleus in the rat. J Neurophysiol 52:595-609.

Menétrey D, Giesler J, G.J., Besson J-M (1977) An analysis of response properties of spinal cord dorsal horn neurones to nonnoxious and noxious stimuli in the spinal rat. Exp Brain Res 27:15-33.

Menétrey D, Roudier F, Besson JM (1983) Spinal neurons reaching the lateral reticular nucleus as studied in the rat by retrograde transport of horseradish peroxidase. J Comp Neurol 220:439-452.

Mitchell CL, Kaelber WW (1966) Effect of medial thalamic lesions on responses elicited by tooth pulp stimulation. Am J Physiol 210:263-269.

Mitchell CL, Kaelber WW (1967) Unilateral vs bilateral medial thalamic lesions and reactivity to noxious stimuli. Arch Neurol 17:653-660.

Morgan MM, Sohn JH, Lohof AM, Ben-Eliyahu S, Liebeskind JC (1989) Characterization of stimulation-produced analgesia from the nucleus tractus solitarius in the rat. Brain Res 486:175-180.

Murphy AZ, Behbehani MM (1993) Electrophysiological characterization of the projection from the nucleus raphe magnus to the lateral reticular nucleus: possible role of an excitatory amino acid in synaptic activation. Brain Res 606:68-78.

Newman DB, Ginsberg CY (1992) Brainstem reticular nuclei that project to the cerebellum in rats: a retrograde tracer study. Brain Behav Evol 39:24-68.

Nicholas AP, Hancock MB (1990) Evidence for projections from the rostral medullary raphe onto medullary catecholaminergic neurons in the rat. Neurosci Lett 108:22-28.

Qvist H, Dietrichs E, Roste LS, Walberg F (1983) A projection from the raphe nuclei to the lateral reticular nucleus in the cat. Arch Ital Biol 121:249-257.

Randich A, Roose MG, Gebhart GF (1988) Characterization of antinociception produced by glutamate microinjection in the nucleus tractus solitarius and the nucleus reticularis ventralis. J Neurosci 8:4675-4684.

Rees, H, Terenzi G, Roberts MHT (1995) Anterior pretectal nucleus facilitation of superficial dorsal horn neurones and modulation of deafferentation pain in the rat. J. Physiol 489:159-169.

Ren K, Randich A, Gebhart GF (1990) Modulation of spinal nociceptive transmission from nuclei tractus soilitarii: a relay for effects of vagal afferent stimulation. J Neurophysiol 63:971-986.

Satoh K, Tohyama M, Yamamoto T, Sakumoto T, Shimizi N (1977) Noradrenaline innervation of the spinal cord studied by the horseradish peroxidase method combined with monoamine oxidase staining. Exp Brain Res 30:175-186.

Sim LJ, Joseph SA (1992) Efferent projections of the nucleus raphe magnus. Brain Res Bull 28:679-682.

Tavares I, Albino-Teixeira A, Lima D (1995) Hypertension inhibits noxious-evoked c-*fos* expression in the rat spinal cord. Neuroreport 6:1664-1668.

Tavares I, Lima D (1994) Descending projections from the caudal medulla oblongata to the superficial or deep dorsal of the rat spinal cord. Exp Brain Res 99:455-463.

Tavares I, Lima D, Coimbra A (1993) Neurons in the superficial dorsal horn of the rat spinal cord projecting to the medullary reticular formation express c-*fos* after noxious stimulation of the skin. Brain Res 623:278-286.

Tavares I, Lima D, Coimbra A (1996a) Catecholaminergic and serotonergic input to spinal dorsal horn neurons projecting to the caudal ventrolateral medulla of the rat. Abstracts of the 8th World Congress on Pain 448. Seattle:IASP Press.

Tavares I, Almeida A, Lima D, Coimbra A (1996b) Differential spinal projections from the caudal ventrolateral medulla oblongata. Europ J Neurosci Suppl 9:95.

Tavares I, Lima D, Coimbra A (1996c) The ventrolateral medulla of the rat is connected with the spinal cord dorsal horn by an indirect descending pathway relayed in the A_5 noradrenergic cell group. J Comp Neurol 374:84-95.

Tavares I, Lima D, Coimbra A. (1997) The pontine A_5 noradrenergic cells which project to the spinal cord dorsal horn are reciprocally connected with the caudal ventrolateral medulla. Europ J Neurosci *in press*.

Thurston CL, Randich A (1990) Acute increases in arterial blood pressure produced by occlusion of the abdominal aorta induces antinociception: peripheral and central substrates. Brain Res 519:12-22.

Todd AJ, Spike RC (1993) The localization of classical transmitters and neuropeptides within neurons in laminae I-III of the mammalian spinal dorsal horn. Prog Neurobiol 41:609-645.

Villanueva L, de Pommery J, Menétrey D, Le Bars D (1991) Spinal afferent projections to subnucleus reticularis dorsalis in the rat. Neurosci Lett 134:98-102.

Westlund KN, Bowker RM, Ziegler MG, Coulter JD (1981) Origins of spinal noradrenergic pathawys demonstrated by retrograde transport of antibody to dopamine-b-hydroxylase. Neurosci Lett 25:243-249.

Westlund KN, Bowker RM, Ziegler MG, Coulter JD (1983) Noradrenergic projections to the spinal cord of the rat. Brain Res 263:15-31.

Willis WD (1985) The pain system. The neural basis of nociceptive transmission in the mammalian nervous system. Basel:Karger.

Yezierski RP (1990) Effects of midbrain and medullary stimulation on spinomesencephalic tract cells in the cat. J Neurophysiol 63:240-255.

Yezierski RP, Gerhart KD, Schrock BJ, Willis WD (1983) A further examination of effects of cortical stimulation on primate spinothalamic tract cells. J Neurophysiol 49:424-441.

Zamir N, Segal M (1979) Hypertension-induced analgesia: changes in pain sensitivity in experimental hypertensive rats. Brain Res 160:170-173.

Zamir N, Shuber E (1980) Altered pain perception in hypertensive humans. Brain Res 201:471-474.

Zamir N, Simantov R, Segal M (1980) Pain sensitivity and opioid activity in genetically hypertensive rats Brain Res 184:299-310.

Zhuo M, Gebhart GF (1990) Characterization of descending inhibition and facilitation from the nuclei reticularis gigantocellularis and gigantocellularis pars alpha in the rat. Pain 42:337-350.

Zhuo M, Gebhart GF (1992) Characterization of descending facilitation and inhibition of spinal nociceptive transmission from the nuclei reticularis gigantocellularis and gigantocellularis pars alpha in the rat. J Neurophysiol 67:1599-1614.

Pain Mechanisms and Management
S.N. Ayrapetyan and A.V. Apkarian (Eds.)
IOS Press, 1998

Thalamocortical Connections of the Cingulate and Insula in Relation to Nociceptive Inputs to the Cortex

A. Vania Apkarian and Ting Shi
SUNY Health Science Center
Neurosurgery Research Laboratories
and
Computational Neuroscience Program
Syracuse, NY, USA

The role of the cerebral cortex in pain perception has become an important research topic over the last few years. Early clinical studies of the subject by neurologists, primarily by Head and Holmes in the 1920s, rejected the idea that the cerebral cortex participates in pain perception, and emphasized that the thalamus plays a more important role in conscious pain perception. Although electrophysiological studies in monkeys have indicated the presence of nociceptive neurons in the somatosensory cortex (Kenshalo et al., 1980), their small numbers and relatively flat responses to a stimulus failed to convince scientists that this region is crucial for pain perception. Recent brain imaging studies show the activation of a large number of cortical regions in acute pain conditions and in various pain syndromes. The specific roles of these various areas in pain perception remain to be identified (see essays by Amassian, Apkarian, and by Wall in this book). Here we present the results of some anatomic studies in the squirrel monkey, where thalamic inputs to the insula and the cingulate cortex were examined in relation to the spinothalamic pathway and in relation to the thalamic projections to the primary somatosensory cortex. Such anatomic and electrophysiologic studies are needed to close the gap that exists between our knowledge regarding cortical activations in humans, and the response properties of these regions and their connectivities to nociceptive pathways.

Recent brain imaging studies in humans, including studies utilizing positron emission tomography (PET) and functional magnetic resonance imaging (fMRI), have emphasized the role of both the insular and cingulate cortex in human pain perception (see Apkarian, 1995, Talbot et al., 1991, Vogt et al., 1996, Hsieh et al., 1995). Also, recent anatomic and physiological studies by Craig (1994) have shown that spinal cord lamina I neurons project to cells in a specific subportion of the posterior part of the lateral thalamus (VMpo), which in turn project to the anterior portion of the insula. Neurons in VMpo respond to thermal and noxious stimuli, and this region of the posterior complex has been identified in human thalamic tissue. Craig (1994) demonstrates that the portion of the anterior insula, where VMpo projects to, may be differentially activated in cold pain and in the illusion of pain in the thermal grill paradigm. The studies by Hsieh et al. (1995) and by Vogt et al. (1996) emphasize that the cingulate cortex may be crucial in pain perception. Although both the cingulate and the insular cortex are known to receive afferents from the thalamus, few studies show evidence for nociceptive inputs to these regions. Here, we report the results of retrograde tracer studies in squirrel monkeys which received injections either into the insular or the cingulate cortex. The results indicate that a specific portion of the cingulate cortex receives heavy input from the lateral thalamic somatosensory region, VPI--a region important in pain perception--and that portions of the insular cortex also receive inputs from VPI, but more heavy projections from the posterior complex.

Materials and methods

For this study four squirrel monkeys were used; two of them were female (SG1 and SG2), the other two were male (SG3 and SG4). Their weights ranged from from 0.375 kg to 0.670 kg. All animals were initially anesthetized with a mixture of acepromazine and ketamine and maintained with isofluorane. In animals with primary somatosensory cortex (SI) injections, a retrograde tracer was injected following electrophysiological identification and localization of the hand and foot representation in this cortical area. Cingulate cortex injections were also guided by electrophysiology, however, these injections were placed in regions where any somatosensory responses could be obtained. The insular injections were performed guided by local landmarks only. To limit the injections to the insular gray matter, the lateral sulcus was dissected and the superior temporal sulcus partially removed, thus exposing the insula.

In animal SG1, the retrogradely transported fluorescent tracer Diamidino Yellow (DY) was injected in three locations within the midportion of the cingulate cortex. This injection targeted the lower bank of the cingulate sulcus; recordings performed prior to the injection showed responses to hindlimb and tail stimuli. A second set of fluorescent tracer injections (green beads) was placed in the hand and foot respresentation of the SI cortex ipsilateral to the cingulate injection (see insert in figure 1).

In animal SG2, three different retrograde fluorescent tracers were injected into the posterior ventral insula: two tracts with DY were placed in the anterior portion of this cortical area, two tracts with Rhodamine beads (RB) in the medial portion and two tracts with Fast Blue (FB) in the posterior portion (see insert in figure 2).

Squirrel monkey SG3 received a series of injections of the anterograde tracer biotinylated dextran (BD) into the spinal cervical enlargement from C5 to T1 (10 tracts, 3 injections each). Five weeks later, the retrograde tracer FB was injected at 14 locations in the hand region of SI, contralateral to the spinal injections, and DY was injected in the anterior portion of the insular cortex (see insert in figure 3).

In squirrel monkey SG4, DY was injected in 19 tracts in the hand and foot areas of SI and three other fluorescent tracers were injected into different regions of the cingulate cortex: Green beads in the anterior portion, Fast Blue in the middle portion, Fluorogold in the posterior portion.

All animals except SG4 were perfused with heparinized saline, followed by 4% paraformaldehyde and 0.025% glutaraldehyde in 0.1M phosphate buffer pH 7.2. For animal SG4, the fixative contained 4% paraformaldehyde and 0.5% glutaraldehyde in phosphate buffer. The tissue was removed and stored overnight in buffer or post-fixed in fixative solution. Fifty micrometer thick sections were cut on a freezing microtome (SG1 and 2) or a vibratome (SG3 and 4) and sections were processed in alternate series to visualize the different tracers. The labeled cells and terminals were plotted using a computer interfaced fluorescent microscope. The label was superimposed on anatomic outlines of the thalamus and cortex determined by Nissl staining and cytochrome oxidase staining.

Results

Cingulate cortex connections with the insula

In animal SG1, the cingulate injections covered primarily the ventral bank of the cingulate sulcus, although some of the tracer also spread to the dorsal bank. The injections were made in the mid-portion of the cingulate cortex, antero-posteriorly at the level of hand representation in SI. Anteriorly, the ipsilateral label from the cingulate injections included the dorsal and ventral banks of the cingulate sulcus, as well as the supplementary motor cortex and premotor cortices. This label is attributed primarily to the spread of the injections to the dorsal bank of the cingulate sulcus. In the contralateral midline cortex, label was limited to the ventral bank of the cingulate sulcus (not shown).

Since the hand SI was injected with a different tracer, the relative proximity of the label from the two sources could be compared in the superior operculum of the lateral sulcus (including areas PV and SII), and in the insula (see figure 1A). In the anterior insula (left panel in figure 1A), cells labeled from SI and cingulate were sparse and intermixed. More posteriorly (panels 2-4 in figure 1A), SII cells were almost exclusively labeled from the SI injection; whereas insular label originated only from the cingulate injection. Most posteriorly (right panel in figure 1A), cells labeled from the SI injection were seen both in SII and the insula. At this level, cells labeled from the cingulate injection were intermixed with those labeled from the SI injection in both SII and insula. It should be noted that labeling in more anterior and more posterior cortical regions was not examined.

Thalamic connections with the cingulate cortex

Thalamic labeling following the cingulate injection in animal SG1 was limited to the posterior regions (figure 1B). Only sparse labeling was observed in VLo, in the lateral border of VPL, and the most ventral rim of VPI (top three panels of figure 1B). More posteriorly, (bottom three panels of figure 1B) sparse labeling was seen in LP and in the lateral most portion of VPL, at the same level where the hand portion of VPL was heavily labeled from the SI injection. Most posteriorly, cingulate projecting cells were found in the lateral portion of CL and the ventrolateral region of MD. In PuO, cells labeled from the cingulate injection were limited to the dorsal and lateral portion of this nucleus, whereas cells labeled from SI were distinct and localized in the ventral and medial portions. Cells labeled from the cingulate injection were also seen in the most anterior extent of PuM, mainly in the lateral and ventral portions (not shown). Cingulate projecting neurons were not seen in more posterior areas of the thalamus.

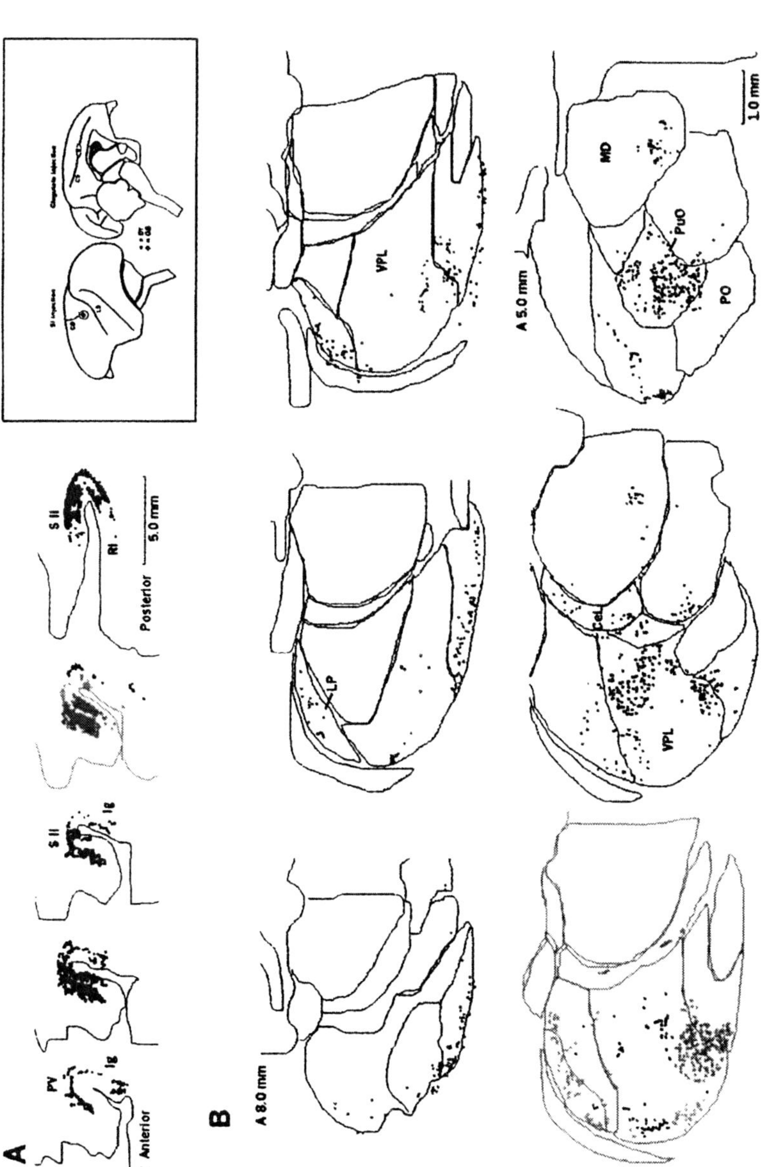

Figure 1. Cortical and thalamic projections to the somatosensory cingulate cortex, in comparison to the SI hand region projecting cells. Insert shows the approximate location of the retrograde fluorescent dye injections: in the cingulate cortex (* = Diamidino Yellow) shown in a midline outline of the brain, and in the hand region of SI (◆ = Green Beads) shown on a lateral view of the squirrel monkey brain. **A:** Labeled cells from both injections in the cortex surrounding the lateral sulcus, illustrating label in the superior operculum and in the insula. Dark or blue dots are cells labeled from the SI hand injection; lighter or red dots are cells labeled from the cingulate injection. **B:** Thalamic label from both injections. The color scheme is the same as in A.

In animal SG4, only the anterior portion of the cingulate sulcus and gyrus was injected with multiple fluorescent dyes. Following this injection, thalamic label was limited to the anterior and medial nuclei, e.g. AV, AM, Cdc, Re, Cif, and MDpc. Since this pattern of labeling was very similar to earlier results reported by other laboratories, the data is not presented. For a detailed description of the labeling, see Vogt and Pandya 1987 (see top panel of figure 2.9 in Vogt and Gabriel, 1993).

Thalamic inputs to the insula

In animal SG2 three retrogradely transported fluorescent dyes were injected in the posterior and ventral portion of the insula. The three dyes were placed along the same dorso-ventral orientation, at three antero-posterior positions within the insula (figure 2 insert). Retrogradely labeled thalamic cells were confined to the most posterior and lateral nuclei. Small numbers of labeled cells were seen in the ventral region of VPI and just outside VPI ventrally. Much higher numbers of cells were seen in the most posterior region of PO, the medial region of PuM, LiM and GM. Labeling from all three insula injections were intermixed, specially in PuM, LiM, PO, and GM (figure 2).

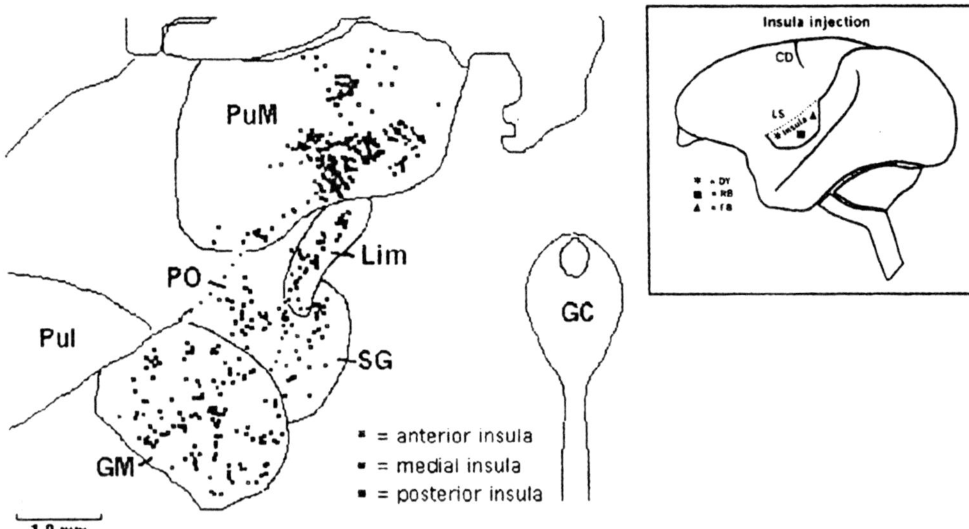

Figure 2. Thalamic topography of insula projecting cells. Insert shows the insula injection sites for three retrograde fluorescent dyes (* = Diamidino Yellow injection, (■ = Rhodamine Beads, ▲ = Fast Blue). Insula projecting cells are shown in one posterior thalamic section. The darkest or the green dots are cells projecting to the most anterior injection, the intermediate dark or red dots are cells projecting to the intermediate injection and the lightest or blue dots are cells projecting to the most posterior injection. Note that at least in PuM. Lim and PO and SG the labeled cells are intermixed.

In animal SG3, the insular injection was placed in its anterior part. Also the hand SI was injected as well as the hand spinothalamic terminations from the spinal cord cervical enlargement. Thus the location of cell projecting to the insula could be compared to those of spinothalamic terminals. Again the insula projecting cells were confined to the most posterior nuclei of the thalamus (figure 3). In this case, however, the labeled cells were mostly concentrated on the medial and ventral rim of VPMpc and VPI.

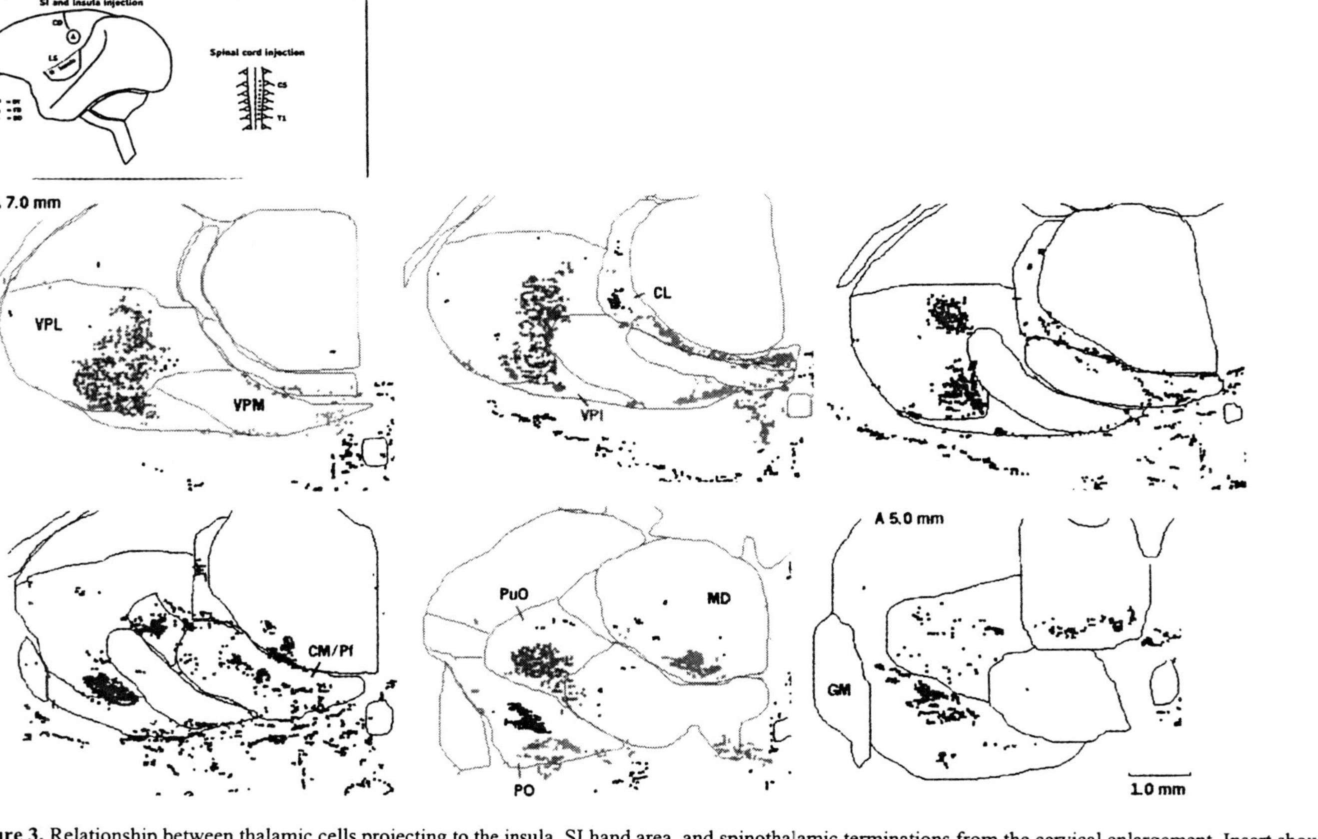

Figure 3. Relationship between thalamic cells projecting to the insula, SI hand area, and spinothalamic terminations from the cervical enlargement. Insert shows injection sites for fluorescent dyes in the insula (* = Diamidino Yellow) and SI hand area (▲ = Fast Blue), and the anterograde tracer injected in the contralateral cervical enlargement (● = Biotin Dextran). The thalamic label is shown in 6 posterior slices. The darkest or green dots are insula projecting cells, the intermediate density or blue dots are SI hand projecting cells, and the lightest or red dots are the spinothalamic terminations.

The labeling in this region created a continuous rim of cells, outlining the most ventral border of VPMpc, VPM, and VPI. Although these labeled cells were in close proximity to spinothalamic terminals, obvious overlap between the insular projecting cells and spinothalamic terminal labeling was rarely observed. Insular projecting cells were also located in PO, in the middle of the nucleus close to its ventral border. Multiple groups of these insular projecting PO cells overlapped with labeled spinothalamic terminals. Insular projecting cells were also found in the ventral midline thalamus, overlapping with spinothalamic terminal label. There was no overlap between SI hand region projecting neurons and the insula projecting neurons.

Discussion

The pattern of labeling presented in these animals may be interpreted as outlining thalamocortical loops that may be crucially involved in processing nociceptive information. The cingulate inputs from VPI are consistent with results in the cat reported earlier by Yasui et al. (1988), but to our knowledge this has not been observed in the monkey. The VPI and VPMpc projections to the insula reported here are consistent with those described by Cechetto and Saper (1987) in the rat. In the rat, these projections were correlated with the response properties of the target neurons in the insula where a topographically organized visceral representation was shown. Cechetto and Saper did not investigate the somatic nociceptive properties of these neurons. At least in the squirrel monkey, our electrophysiological studies (Apkarian and Shi, 1994) show that about 50% of VPI neurons have somatic nociceptive responses, and a large proportion of these cells respond exclusively to noxious stimuli. Similar results have been obtained by Vahle-Hinz and Kniffki (personal communication) in the cat. We have not studied visceral responses of VPI neurons in the monkey, but it is likely that the cells projecting to the cingulate and the insula are a homogeneous population responsive to visceral innocuous inputs and somatic noxious inputs. The portion of the cingulate which receives projections from VPI is a region quite comparable, but perhaps more posterior to the cingulate area in the rabbit, where nociceptive responsive cells have been described by Sikes and Vogt (1992). Thus, the ventral border of VPI may be a region that transmits somatic nociceptive inputs to the cingulate and the insula, and these two cortical areas in turn interconnect at least through insular-cingulate projections. The main doubt that remains regarding this hypothesis is the lack of robust overlap between the VPI and VPMpc cells projecting to the insula and spinothalamic terminations in this region. Our earlier studies have shown strong overlap between SI projecting VPI neurons and spinothalamic terminals (Gingold et al., 1991, Apkarian and Shi, 1994). Thus an alternative possibility is that the insular projections are pure visceral inputs, whereas the cingulate projecting neurons, which are more scattered within VPI, transmit somatic nociceptive inputs.

This thalamocortical network would mediate nociceptive inputs preferentially from the superficial laminae of the spinal cord to the lateral thalamus and then to the cingulate and the insula cortex. Thus, this nociceptive network seems distinct from that described for the more anterior portions of the cingulate cortex, which receives thalamic inputs mainly from midline thalamic nuclei (see Vogt, 1993). In the monkey, the latter should correspond to the anterior portion of Brodmann's area 24c. In the squirrel monkey, the cingulate sulcus connections outlined above are from regions just medial and anterior to the central dimple, which is the middle portion of Brodmann's area 23c. This region is too posterior to be part of the cingulate motor area (Dum and Strick, 1993) and is most likely an associative somatosensory representation region. The correspondence between physiologic responses and the labeling observed in the lateral VPL attests to the region being somatosensory cortex. Whether this cingulate region corresponds to the posterior portion of area 24 in man is not clear.

The insula projecting cells within PO had more robust overlap with spinothalamic inputs. This is consistent with the studies by Craig (1994) and may in fact correspond to the region of PO which they have called VMpo. It seems that at this level, PO does not project to the cingulate but instead, PuO and MDpc. The spinothalamic terminations in PuO are very scant, whereas this portion of MD contains heavy spinothalamic terminal labeling. Whether these separate nociceptive inputs to the cingulate and insula differentiate between their functional involvement in pain perception remains to be investigated.

The anatomic data presented here seems consistent with the notion that the cingulate and insula cortex are involved in the processing of pain. The results are preliminary and suggestive and need to be tested using single unit electrophysiology. The rapid expansion of human brain imaging studies has created the urgent need to examine many cortical areas, their connectivities and response properties, specifically from a pain processing viewpoint. Moreover, the human studies point to a large gap in our knowledge regarding both the thalamus and the cortex in chronic pain states, above and beyond the responses observed for acute 5-10 s duration nociceptive stimuli. The time course of pain is much longer than the stimuli that have been used for its study, especially in animal electrophysiology. As a result, we are in the unfortunate predicament of being unable to apply the results of animal studies to the understanding of the human brain responses to pain.

Abbreviations:

Ig	= granular insular cortex
PV	= cortical parietal ventral area
Ri	= retroinsular cortex
S II	= second somatosensory cortex
CL	= thalamic centrolateral n.
CM/Pf	= thalamic centromedian/parafascicularis n.
GC	= central grey
GM	= thalamic medial geniculate n.
Lim	= thalamic limitans n.
LP	= thalamic lateral posterior n.
MD	= thalamic mediodorsal n.
PO	= thalamic posterior n.
PuI	= thalamic pulvinar inferior n.
PuM	= thalamic pulvinar medialis n.
PuO	= thalamic pulvinar oralis n.
SG	= thalamic suprageniculate n.
VPI	= thalamic ventroposterior inferior n.
VPL	= thalamic ventroposterior lateral n.
VPM	= thalamic ventroposterior medial n.

References

Apkarian AV (1995) Functional imaging of pain: new insights regarding the role of the cerebral cortex in human pain perception. Sem in The Neurosci 7:279-293.

Apkarian AV, Shi T (1994) Squirrel monkey lateral thalamus: I. Somatic nociresponsive neurons and their relation to spinothalamic terminals. J Neurosci 14:6779-6795.

Cechetto DF, Saper CB (1987) Evidence for a viscerotopic sensory representation in the cortex and thalamus in the rat. J Comp Neurol 262:27-45.

Craig AD (1994) A thalamic nucleus specific for pain and temperature sensation. Nature 372:770-773.

Dum RP, Strick PL (1993) Cingulate motor areas. In: Vogt BA, Gabriel M (eds.) (1993) Neurobiology of the cingulate cortex and limbic thalamus. Birkhäuser, Boston, MA.

Gingold SI, Greenspan JD and Apkarian AV (1991) Anatomic evidence of nociceptive inputs to primary somatosensory cortex: Relationship between spinothalamic terminals and thalamocortical cells in squirrel monkeys. J Comp Neurol 308:467-490.

Head H, Holmes G (1911) Sensory disturbances from cerebral lesions. Brain 34:102-254.

Hsieh JC (1995) Central processing of pain, Functional brain imaging studies with PET. Kongl Carolinska Medico Chirurgiska Institutet, Stockholm (Dissertation)

Kenshalo DR Jr., Giesler GJ Jr., Leonard RB, Willis WD (1980) Responses of neurons in primate ventral posterior lateral nucleus to noxious stimuli. J Neurophys 43:1594-1614.

Sikes RW, Vogt BA (1992) Nociceptive neurons in area 24 of rabbit cingulate cortex. J Neurophys 68:1720-1732.

Talbot JD, Marrett S, Evans AC, Meyer E, Bushnell MC, Duncan GH (1991) Multiple representations of pain in human cerebral cortex. Science 251:1355-1358.

Vogt BA (1993) Structural organization of cingulate cortex: areas, neurons, and somatodentritic transmitter receptors. In: Vogt BA, Gabriel M (eds.) (1993) Neurobiology of the cingulate cortex and limbic thalamus. Birkhäuser, Boston, MA.

Vogt BA, Derbyshire S, Jones AKP (1996) Pain processing in four regions of human cingulate cortex localized with co-registered PET and MR imaging. Eur J Neurosci 8:1461-1473.

Vogt BA, Gabriel M (eds.) (1993) Neurobiology of the cingulate cortex and limbic thalamus. Birkhäuser, Boston, MA.

Vogt BA, Pandya DN, Rosene DL (1987) Cingulate cortex in the rhesus monkey: I. Cytoarchitecture and thalamic afferents. J Comp Neurol 262:256-270.

Yasui Y, Kazuo I, Hiroto K, Tadashi I, Noboru M (1988) Cingulate gyrus of the cat receives projection fibers from the thalamic region ventral to the ventral border of the ventrobasal complex. J Comp Neurol 274:91-100.

Pain Mechanisms and Management
S.N. Ayrapetyan and A.V. Apkarian (Eds.)
IOS Press, 1998

Measurement of Tonic Pain in Animals by Evoked Potentials

P. Lebrun, M. Diltoer, F. Colin and J. Manil
Vrije Universiteit Brussel,
Brussels, Belgium

Introduction

The most commonly used tests of pain in animals explore behavioral responses to nociceptive stimuli, either segmental spinal reflexes such as the tail flick (d'Amour and Smith, 1941) or supraspinally mediated typed behavior such as on the hot plate (Woolfe and MacDonald, 1944). Many different variants of these tests have been developed exploiting a variety of similar reflexes, but most suffer from the drawbacks inherent to behavioral assays, among others:

1) Dependency on intact motor function, which can be altered by a side effect of the drug being tested or by non-analgesic effects such as sedation (Carter, 1994, Miaskowski et al., 1991).

2) Endpoints that are not clear-cut and easy to measure.

3) Measurement of nociception rather than the sensation of pain as perceived by the animal.

In human experimentation, scalp-recorded cortical somatosensory evoked potentials (cSEPs) have been shown to provide a good measure of pain (Gehrig et al., 1981, Bromm, 1982) reflecting not only peripheral events but also the higher interpretive processes that influence the overall physiological reaction to noxious stimuli. Late occurring components are of particular interest as they are thought to reflect information processing such as selective attention, classification of stimuli, and memory (Bromm, 1985). Although no component of the cSEP can be said to indicate pain sensation, amplitudes of late components vary reliably with verbal reports of pain sensation, and have been described as correlates of pain (Chapman and Jacobson, 1984). CSEPs are independent of motor function and can be recorded outside the presence of an experimenter.

We have tried to transpose this technique to animals in the hope of providing a better measure of pain, as opposed to nociception. The latter is well approximated by measuring changes in segmental spinal reflexes, but do not include the cognitive or emotional aspects of pain sensation. Behavioral tests measuring supra-spinal responses (eg. hot plate) are more closely related to the sensation of pain as perceived by the animal, but are exquisitely dependent on the observers' interpretation of the animal's behavior and on the motor function of both the animal and the human holding the stop watch.

We have previously shown that components of the cortical somatosensory evoked potential (cSEP) of the rat are related to changes of stimulus intensity above pain threshold and to pain-related behavior. These amplitudes of these components diminish in a dose-related fashion when analgesics were administered in correlation to changes in hot plate latencies (Lebrun et al., 1996).

If these potentials are indeed related to the sensation of pain, it would be expected that they increase in states of hyperalgesia. The aim of this study was to investigate this using an adaptation of the formalin test, a common model of tonic pain in animals (Dubuisson and Denis, 1977). In this test, formalin is injected into the hind-paw of an animal and motor responses counted. There is a biphasic pain response: a transitory early phase lasting 5-10 min. resulting from direct activation of chemonociceptors followed by a quiescent phase, then a tonic phase related to peripheral inflammation and changes in central processing (Haley et al., 1990). This response involves activation of spinal N-methyl-D-aspartate (NMDA) receptors and is reduced by NMDA antagonists (Vaccarino et al., 1993). Peripheral inflammation in the second phase induces progressive tactile hypersensitivity (Ma and Woolf, 1996), a state in which non-nociceptor evoked large fiber afferences are enhanced. This should be measurable by cSEPs, which are responses evoked predominantly by large fiber activity.

Methods

Extradural electrodes were permanently implanted on adult (>250g) male wistar rats through a craniotomy over the parietal cortex. They were allowed one week to recover.

The animals were divided into 3 groups. A vehicle control group of 9 rats were injected with 50ul normal saline s.c. at the base of the tail. 9 rats received 50ul 10% formalin s.c. at the base of the tail, and a third group of 5 rats were pretreated with 5 mg/kg ketamine i.p. 10 min before receiving 50ul 10% formalin s.c. at the base of the tail.

For the recording of cSEPs, the animals were loosely restrained and potentials were evoked by 1 ms square-wave pulses delivered through stainless steel electrodes implanted at the base of the tail at an amplitude twice that necessary to evoke a motor response, and with a frequency of 0.5 Hz. This stimulus intensity activates A-beta and A-delta but not C fibers. The rats had been previously habituated to the proceedure. The signals were amplified though Grass pre-amplifiers (bandwidth 1 - 1 Khz), digitized at 5Khz by an analog-digital acquisition card installed in a PC, and averaged. Each run was the average of 15 stimuli.

Following three control runs, formalin (or saline) was injected in the loose subcutaneous tissue at the base of the tail, and evoked potentials recorded every 5 minutes for 20 min., then once every 10 minutes for an additional 50 min. It should be noted that the stimulation electrodes were at least 2 cm distal to the injection site. The peak to peak amplitude of the pn waves and the baseline to peak amplitudes of the ln wave were calculated and expressed as percent of control amplitude.

Student's t-test was used to evaluate the differences in cSEP amplitude between groups. Differences were considered statistically significant at the P<0.05 level.

Results

The cortical SEP of the rat is composed of 2 major wave complexes (Fig. 1): A positive-negative (pn) wave complex with a latency of 17-22 ms followed by an ample late negative (ln) wave with a latency of 40-50 ms. The impulse conduction velocity of the peripheral nerve fibers mediating these waves was measured by stimulating the tail at two points 50 mm apart. The conduction velocities measured with the first complex were 32.15 ñ 0.76 m/s and 32.68 ñ 0.68 m/s for the positive and negative components respectively. The peripheral conduction velocity calculated from the ln was much slower (17.68 ñ 0.81 ms), and this wave was thought to be the sum of several components resulting from cortical associative processing.

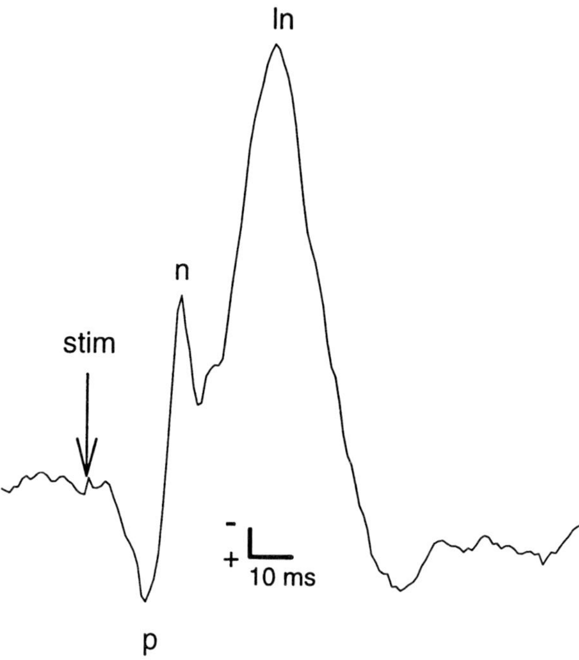

Figure 1. Potential evoked by stimulation of the caudal nerve at A-delta fiber strength. Grand average of 120 stimuli recorded over the contralateral somatosensory cortex referred to the parietal ridge. Inverted electrodes were used.

Formalin produced a biphasic increase in the peak-to-peak amplitude of both pn and ln waves. The first phase started at injection and lasted 15 min, the second was present from 30 to 60 min. The pn wave (Fig. 2) peaked at 145% of control amplitude in the first phase, 140% of control in the second phase. The peak amplitudes of the ln wave (Fig. 3) were 125% and 111% for first and second phases respectively.

When compared to the formalin group, the group pre-treated with ketamine showed a significant reduction of the ln wave in the first phase and the pn wave in the second phase only.

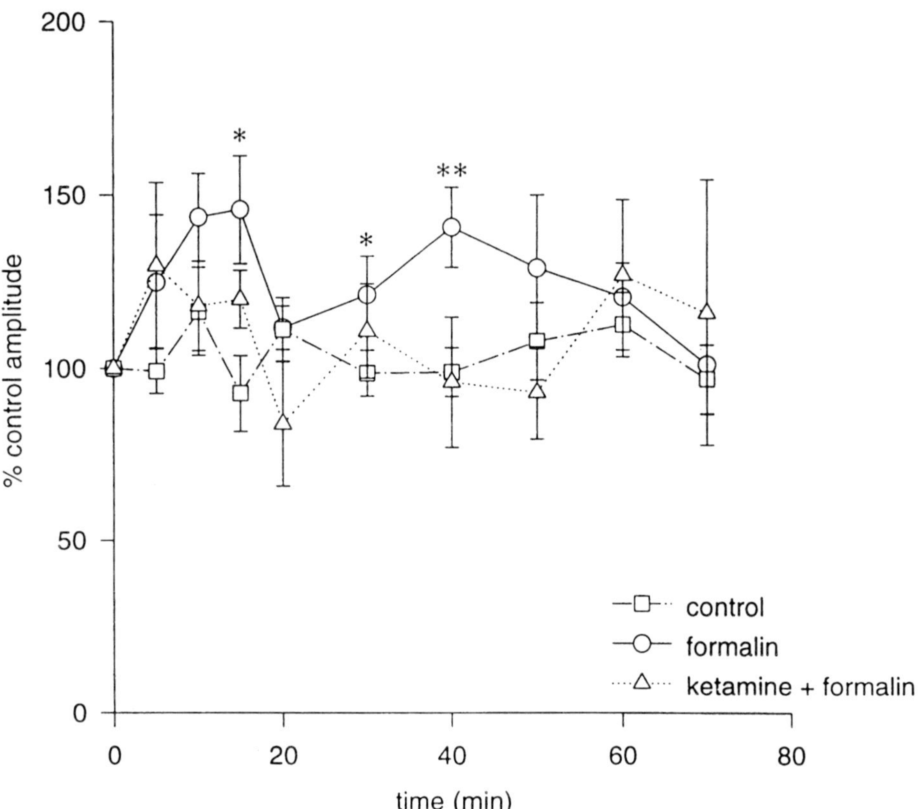

Figure 2. The effects of subcutaneous formalin on pn component of the cSEP. The data are expressed as percentage of the control amplitude (+-SEM) measured during an initial three runs, each rat was his own control. Formalin or saline was injected at time 0. Rats were injected with ketamine 10 minutes prior to formalin. * P<0.05, ** P<0.01 compared to saline.

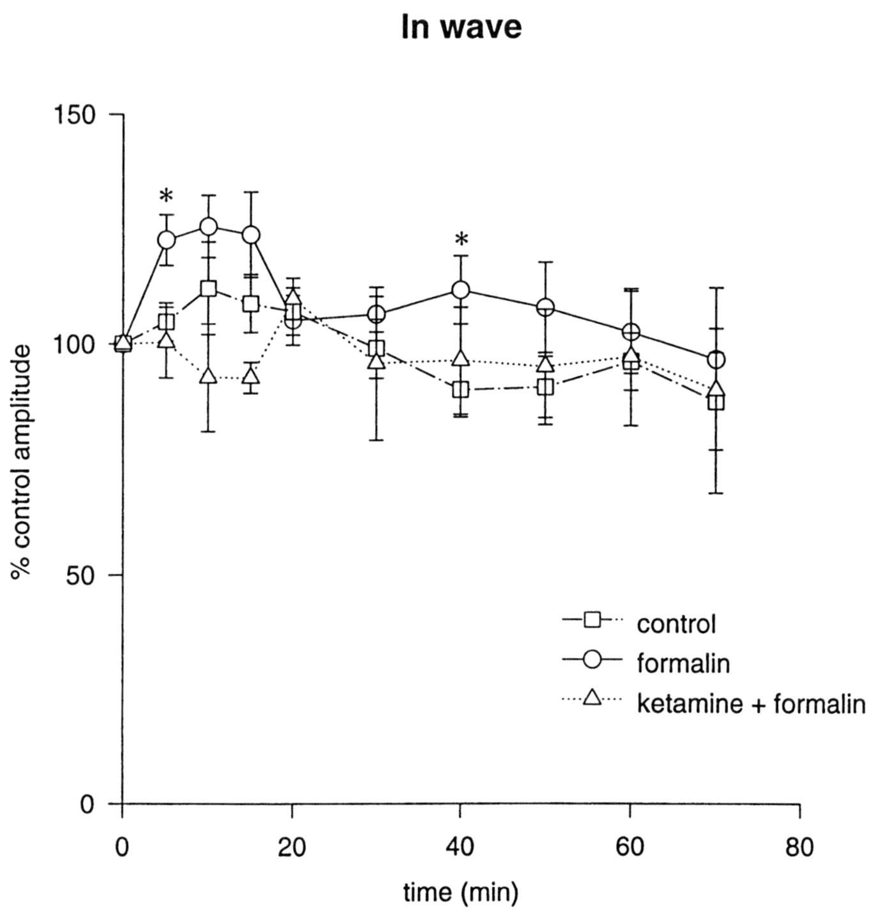

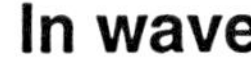

Figure 3. The effects of subcutaneous formalin on ln component of the cSEP. The data are expressed as percentage of the control amplitude (+-SEM) measured during an initial three runs, each rat was his own control. Formalin or saline was injected at time 0. Rats were injected with ketamine 10 minutes prior to formalin. * P<0.05 compared to saline.

Conclusions

This preliminary study demonstrated a typical biphasic increase in the amplitude of the pn wave, an early near field complex evoked by activity in thalamo-cortical fibers and the somatosensory cortex (Dong et al., 1982) after subcutaneous injection of formalin. This effect was blocked by the NMDA antagonist ketamine most efficiently in the second phase, in accordance with reported behavioral (Vaccarino et al., 1993) and electrophysiological (Haley et al., 1990) evidence. NMDA receptors are not involved in the modulation of acute

A-delta fiber afferences in the spinal cord (Dickenson and Sullivan, 1990) and supraspinally, ketamine has been shown to act primarily on the cortex and limbic system rather than on the brainstem or reticular system (Marshall and Wollman, 1991). Ketamine would thus not be expected to influence the first phase of the formalin reaction. Although the pn was not evoked by C fibers, these results confirm that it is a correlate of nociceptive afferences reaching the cortex.

The ln wave also showed a biphasic increase in amplitude having the same time course as the elevation of the pn wave, but of lesser intensity during the second phase. It is not yet clear whether this difference in amplitude is the result of attentional factors or cortical mechanisms of nociceptive suppression. The first phase was blocked by pretreatment with ketamine. This apparently paradoxical effect may be related to the supraspinal (psychoactive) effects of the drug. The dose of 5 mg/kg ketamine i.p. has an analgesic effect when given alone and has been shown to reduce the amplitude of the ln wave by 20%. In human use it has been described as a dissociative agent, from the feeling of dissociation from the environment experienced by the subject. The noxious insult is perceived, but is not interpreted as being painful.

In summary, components of the cortical evoked potential of the rat show promise as an objective and observer-independent measure of hyperalgesia. However, more work towards optimizing this measure is necessary before cSEPs can replace behavioral tests.

References

Bromm B and Scharein E (1982) Principal component analysis of pain-related cerebral potentials to mechanical and electrical stimulation in man. Electroenceph Clin Neurophysiol 53:94-103.

Bromm B (1985) The evoked cerebral potential and pain. In: H.L. Fields, R. Dubner, and F. Cervero (Eds.), Advances in pain research and therapy, Vol. 9, Raven Press (New York) 306-329.

Carter AJ (1994) Many agents that antagonize the NMDA receptor-channel complex in vivo also cause disturbances of motor coordination. J Pharm Exp Ther. 269:573-580.

Chapman CR and Jacobson RC (1984)Assessment of analgesic states: can evoked potentials play a role? In: B. Bromm (Ed), Pain measurement in man. Neurophysiological correlates of pain. Elsevier Science Publishers (Amsterdam).

D'Amour F and Smith DL (1941) A method for determining loss of pain sensation. J. Pharm Exp Ther 72:74-79.

Dickenson AH and Sullivan AF (1990) Differential effects of excitatory amino acid antagonists on dorsal horn nociceptive neurons in the rat. Brain Res 506 (1):31-9.

Dong WK, Harkins SW and Ashleman BT (1982) Origins of cat somatosensory far-field and early near-field evoked potentials. Electroenceph Clin Neurophysiol 53:143-165.

Dubuisson D and Denis SG (1977) The formalin test: A quantitative study of the analgesic effect of morphine, meperidine, and brain stem stimulation in rats and cats. Pain 4:161-174.

Gehrig JD, Colpitts YH and Chapman CR (1981) Effects of local anesthetic infiltration on brain potentials evoked by painful dental stimulation. Anesth Analg 60:779-782.

Haley JE, Sullivan AF and Dickenson AH (1990) Evidence for spinal N-methyl-D-aspartate receptor involvement in prolonged chemical nociception in the rat. Brain Res 518:218-226.

Lebrun Ph, Diltoer M, Colin F and Manil J (1996) Evaluation of the sensitivity of evoked potentials as a method for measuring pain in rats. In: Abstracts - 8th World Congress on Pain. IASP Press (Seattle) p.4

Ma Q-P and Woolf CJ (1996) Progressive tactile hypersensitivity: an inflammation-induced incremental increase in the excitability of the spinal cord. Pain 67:97-106.

Marshall BE and Wollman H (1991) General Anesthetics In: Goodman and Gilman's The pharmacological basis of therapeutics, edited by A. Goodman Gilman, T. W. Rall, A. S. Nies and P. Taylor. N.Y.: MacMillan, p. 276-299.

Miaskowski C, Sutters KA, Taiwo YO and Levine JD (1991) Comparison of the antinociceptive and motor effects of intrathecal opioid agonists in the rat. Brain Res 553:105-109.

Vaccarino AL, Marek P, Kest B, Weber E, Keana JFW and Liebeskind JC (1993) NMDA receptor antagonists, MK-801 and ACEA-1101, prevent the development of tonic pain following subcutaneous formalin. Brain Res 615:331-334.

Woolfe G and MacDonald AD (1944) The evaluation of the analgesic action of pethidine hydrochloride (Demerol). J Pharm Exp Ther 80:300-307.

Pain Mechanisms and Management
S.N. Ayrapetyan and A.V. Apkarian (Eds.)
IOS Press, 1998

Pain Perception and the Role of Thalamocortical Inhibitory Networks across Organizational Scales

A. Vania Apkarian
Department of Neurosurgery
and
Computational Neuroscience Program
SUNY Health Science Center
Syracuse, NY, USA

Over the last three to four years, research in this laboratory regarding the central organization of pain has employed two new techniques. The first technique is functional magnetic resonance imaging (fMRI), which monitors human brain activity at a resolution of $1.5 \times 1.5 \times 6.0$ mm^3 volume of tissue (one voxel). This is the highest spatial resolution with which the human brain physiology can currently be studied, non-invasively. At the level of the cerebral cortex, the resolution of fMRI corresponds to monitoring 6-10 columns or the group activity of 10^6-10^7 neurons at a time. For statistical reasons the activation of a single voxel is not sufficient and only activations of 3-5 connected voxels are accepted as reliable brain activity changes. As a result, the minimum number of responding neurons that can be detected by fMRI must be increased by this factor. Functional MRI primarily monitors changes in blood oxygenation secondary to the metabolic demand of the neuronal activity. Changes in blood oxygenation are achieved by local control of blood flow. Quite likely, the blood flow accompanying neuronal activity covers a tissue area larger than the specific active neurons. The extent of this over-flooding is the amount with which the fMRI neuronal activity scale (about 10^8 neurons) is overestimated. The details of this overestimation remain to be determined.

The second new technique we have recently developed is an electrophysiological one. Thalamic neuronal activity is monitored using four Tungsten electrodes having a fixed relationship to each other. The four electrode tips are fixed at the four diagonal corners of a 115 µm^3 cube. Neuronal activity is collected simultaneously from all four tips as multiunit spikes, and then clustered into individual neurons. Since each action potential is monitored four times from four different locations, the approach increases the confidence with which individual neuronal activity is defined. Moreover, because the spike shape and size are slightly deformed at each of the four tips, these deformations can be used to calculate the location of each identified neuron, in relation to the tips and in relation to the neighboring units. With this approach lateral thalamic groups of neighboring neurons, 4-11 neurons in each group, were studied in the anesthetized squirrel monkey during innocuous and noxious somatic stimuli. The spatial scale of these studies is much better defined than in the fMRI studies. Volumetrically, there is a 10^8 difference in scale between the size of the brain area examined by fMRI as compared to the four-tipped electrophysiological recording. Almost the same scale difference is obtained when one compares the number of neurons monitored with each technique.

Given the enormous scale difference between the two methods, is it possible to explain results obtained by fMRI with electrophysiology? Explaining the larger scale organization from the constituent parts is the basic assumption of reductionist science. Can it be applied at these scales? What about the opposite: can the fMRI results be used to understand the electrophysiological data? Surprisingly, there seems to be a close correspondence between thalamic electrophysiology obtained in the anesthetized squirrel monkey and cortical fMRI results collected in awake humans. The rest of the essay reviews these results. We conclude with an attempt to understand brain organizational principles that must underlie the correspondence across these enormous spatial scales.

Brain imaging studies

Our first brain imaging study of thermal pain was done using single photon tomography (SPECT). Because of the requirements of the technique, the stimulus had to be maintained for three minutes (Apkarian et al., 1992). The results showed decreased activation in the somatosensory cortex of the brain contralateral to the stimulated hand. In the same subjects, an innocuous sensorimotor task was also performed, which resulted in increased activations in approximately the same brain regions. We interpreted these results as indicating that the pyramidal neurons in the somatosensory cortex are inhibited during a sustained painful stimulus or perception. As "pyramidal neurons" we designate all the cortical projecting cells with excitatory connections. The inhibition of these pyramidal neurons would be mediated through a preferential activation of the local inhibitory interneurons. Other investigators have refused to interpret decreased metabolic activity because of the seeming contradiction that activity in interneurons requires energy, which should lead to increased local blood flow. However, the anatomic properties of interneurons imply that their energy requirements may be substantially less than that for pyramidal cells, since the former have small unmyelinated axons, small cell bodies, make up less than 20% of the cortical cells, and individual cells can block activity in multiple pyramidal neurons. As a result, the preferential activation of interneurons must be accompanied by a net decrease in local energy requirements.

Since the majority of the neurons in the somatosensory cortex respond to innocuous rather than noxious stimuli, the results from the SPECT study implied that touch perception may be altered under these sustained pain conditions. We directly tested the latter by examining touch thresholds and supra-threshold touch sensitivity during a mild thermal pain state. These psychophysical studies showed elevated touch thresholds for all vibrotactile channels tested, as well as decreased touch sensitivity. These effects were limited to the hand where the thermal stimulus was applied (Apkarian et al., 1994). In more recent studies (manuscript under preparation) we have also shown that the effects are limited to the proper dermatome, within which its magnitude decreases with distance from the site of the thermal stimulus. These studies confirm the cortical inhibition hypothesis (Apkarian et al. 1992) and indicate that pain and touch dynamically interact with each other. These studies also indicates the existence of a touch gate, similar to the pain gate proposed by Melzack and Wall (1965), the properties of which remain to be systematically studied.

Over the last few years, we had the opportunity to perform fMRI studies. A large effort was dedicated in designing proper innocuous and noxious stimulation paradigms as well as developing fMRI data analyses software. We have now completed a number of fMRI activation studies. The first study, using innocuous vibrotactile stimuli, indicated that fMRI can be used to examine the somatotopy of fingertip representation in the cortex (Gelnar et al., 1997). The study showed that the human primary somatosensory cortex (SI) may be divided into four portions which may be homologues to the multiple body maps observed in the monkey SI (e.g. Kaas et al., 1979). Moreover, the results showed that fingertip representation can be detected in a number of other somatosensory regions, such as the secondary somatosensory cortex, the insula and the posterior parietal cortex.

Studies of cortical activations for pain have been performed by a number of groups using positron emission tomography (PET). These studies indicate the activation of a large number of cortical areas during pain. To test the specificity of these activations, we performed a fMRI study of thermal pain and compared the results to activations following vibrotactile and motor tasks. The results showed cortical activity during pain in many of the same regions of the cortex as reported by the PET studies, such as primary and secondary somatosensory and motor cortices (SI, SII, MI, MII), insula, posterior parietal cortex, supplementary motor area and cingulate cortex. Since fMRI can generate brain activation maps in individual subjects, individual responses can be statistically compared with each other, and the extent of overlap activity across tasks can be compared for different regions within and across subjects (manuscript in preparation, Gelnar et al., 1997, also Gelnar et al., 1996a). In the same study, the extent of cortical decreases in activity was sought, especially in the data obtained using the thermal pain task. Very small decreases were observed, with no consistent patterns. Our current interpretation of the lack of decreased somatosensory activity in this painful stimulation is that the time duration of the thermal stimulus is short, given the size of the stimulus (glabrous skin, digits 2-5). This interpretation is also consistent with results reported in PET studies, where signal decreases were examined when the thermal stimulus was short and intermittent (5s on and 5 s off, Talbot et al. 1991). We have not attempted examining fMRI of thermal pain when the stimulus is maintained for three minutes because of instabilities in fMRI technology.

In another recent study, we compared fMRI pain activations for two thermal stimulators of different sizes (Gelnar et al., 1996b, and manuscript in preparation). Normal subjects were scanned during a thermal pain task where the stimulus was delivered over either a 3 mm^2 or a 1000 mm^2 skin surface area. All subjects were scanned in both conditions. The increased activations in both stimulus conditions were similar and closely matched the results described above. However, there was a large difference in the decreases in fMRI signal. With the large stimulator again there was very little decreased fMRI activity, while with the small surface thermal stimulator large portions of SI and MI were deactivated. These results indicate that the inhibitory effects of thermal painful stimuli have complex temporal and spatial properties, where large scale temporal stimuli and small scale spatial stimuli both inhibit the sensorimotor cortex. This inhibitory mechanism is interpreted as a means of shutting off the discriminatory aspects of pain perception perhaps in an effort to cope with its load. This is consistent with the PET studies by Hsieh et al. (1995), Iadarola et al. (1995) and Di Piero et al. (1991) which show that in chronic pain states the thalamus and sensorimotor cortex are either unchanged or are decreased in activity. Our fMRI studies in chronic sympathetically maintained pain also indicate that the parietal cortical activity seems unaffected, whereas the frontal cortical activity is enhanced in this chronic pain state (Krauss et al., 1997, manuscript in preparation).

Four tipped electrophysiological studies

Single electrode, single unit electrophysiological studies have shown the existence of nociceptive neurons in the lateral thalamus in a number of species. The main outcome of these studies is the demonstration that nociceptive neurons with properties very similar to those found in the spinal cord exist in the thalamus. Thus, although anatomically the thalamus looks like a major integrative region of the brain, the electrophysiology implies that, at least in non-sleep states, the thalamus is simply relaying the nociceptive information further cephalad. The same conclusion is in fact reached for other sensory inflow as well. Even though small differences in post-excitatory rebound are observed for innocuous somatic (Gottschaldt et al., 1983) and for visual inputs (Jones, 1985), by and large the extent of transformation that sensory inputs undergo at the thalamic level seems minimal.

A number of scientists (e.g. Harth, 1993, Grossberg, 1997) have theorized that the thalamus may be the site where conscious perceptions come about because it receives a large cortical feedback as well as inputs from all sensory afferents. This notion is based on the idea that the cortical back-flow would create a differential representation between stored memories regarding a given input and the actual input, and the proper match between the input and stored memories (expectation) would induce conscious perception. Unfortunately, the single unit recordings indicate that such comparisons, at least at the single unit level in the primary sensory nuclei, seem unlikely.

Recent studies in the visual thalamus (lateral geniculate nucleus) indicate that the functional connectivity (correlation) between thalamic neurons is stimulus-dependent and may be controlled by the visual cortex. Sillito et al. (1994) report that when driven by moving, oriented visual stimuli, cortical feedback induces correlated firing in thalamic relay cells and produces coherent firing in those groups of relay cells with receptive field alignments appropriate to signaling the particular orientation of the moving contour to the cortex. Thus, they propose that the cortico-thalamic feedback loop serves to lock or focus the appropriate circuitry onto the stimulus feature. Lesioning the visual cortex abolishes the coherent activity. Consistent with this idea, studies by deCharms and Merzenich (1996) show that auditory cortex neurons show stimulus-dependent connectivity changes, even when the mean firing rate of the neurons does not change with the auditory stimulus.

Our four-tipped electrophysiological recordings enable the examination of the firing and connectivity properties of small groups of neurons within a 100 μm^3 space, as well as mapping of the distance connectivity relationships for different stimuli. This approach was used to study populational properties of lateral thalamic cells (ventral posterior lateral nucleus, VPL) to innocuous and noxious somatic stimuli, in the anesthetized squirrel monkey. The preliminary analyses of the results obtained with the technique show that nociceptive neurons are clustered in groups. If one nociceptive neuron is encountered at a given recording site, then the probability of finding more nociceptive cells is very high (25%). Moreover, the local connectivity rules are very different between sites with no nociceptive neurons (non noci-sites) and those having multiple nociceptive cells (noci-sites). The vast majority of the functional connectivity at non noci-sites is excitatory. At non noci-sites, during spontaneous activity, most excitatory connections occur between neuron pairs located less than 20 μm apart, while during innocuous stimuli the connectivity spreads uniformly across neuron pairs at all distances from less than 10 μm to over 100 μm. In contrast, at noci-sites around 30% of the connectivity is inhibitory. At noci-sites, the incidence of excitatory and inhibitory connections were similar during spontaneous activity and during noxious stimulation (majority of excitatory connections limited to distances less than 35 μm and the inhibitory connections occurring at distances more than 40 μm) and very different from that seen during innocuous stimuli (excitatory connections spread to distances more than 65 μm and the incidence of inhibitory connections much reduced).

Thus, in the VPL, near-neighbor connectivities are dramatically different at non-noci versus noci-sites, and in both regions these connectivities change during somatosensory stimuli. Therefore, we conclude that, at the local populational level, thalamic connectivities differentiate between somatosensory stimuli, and that nociceptive stimuli almost exclusively activate inhibitory connections. Thalamic microcircuitry is comprised of cortex projecting excitatory cells, local inhibitory interneurons, cortical feedback direct excitatory connections, and indirect inhibitory connections through the thalamic reticular nucleus (RTN). As a result the preferential activation of inhibitory connections must be mediated either through preferential connections to the local interneurons or via the preferential activation of the cortical RTN loop. It must be emphasized that the inhibitory connectivity observed in the thalamus seems unique for regions with nociceptive inputs because such inhibitory connectivity has not been observed in the cortex (see e.g. Gerstein et al., 1985), and in the thalamus the majority of correlations described have been excitatory (e.g. Sillito et al., 1994, and Johnson and Alloway, 1996).

Conclusions

The correspondence between the human fMRI studies of cortical representation of pain and the squirrel monkey thalamic connectivity patterns is evident from the above two sections. In both cases painful stimulation seems intimately involved in activating inhibitory connections either in the thalamus or in the cortex.. The spatio-temporal dynamics of this inhibitory connectivity for painful inputs remains to be studied more carefully with both approaches. Still, the close correspondence between the two sets of results is surprising given the enormous difference in spatial scales between the techniques. This correspondence in mechanisms across scales has two important implications: first, it is consistent with the idea that the brain is a network of networks spanning large spatial scales, and second, it implies that the rules of connectivity at small scales apply to larger scales as well, and vice versa. Recent analysis of fMRI data from the viewpoint of embedded networks indicates that multiple scale networks can be extracted across similar tasks (Caplan et al., 1997). Such organization places a strong burden on the current models that we have for performing large scale computations using realistic single neuron models (see e.g. Anderson and Sutton, 1997). A theoretical concept advanced by Bak (1996) which has attracted enormous popularity in physics, is the concept of self-organized criticality. The general idea behind the theory is that complex behavior is the natural consequence of simple natural laws which are scale invariant. If we follow Per Bak's idea and apply it to the data described above the interpretation would translate as follows: A noxious stimulus creates a local thalamic avalanche, where the network connectivity reorganizes to its optimum representation. "Optimum" is used in the sense that it is at its most sensitive organizational state (critical) to respond to the stimulus maximally without becoming totally unstable and unpredictable. The stimulus-caused avalanche of connectivity reorganization propagates across a 10^8 fold spatial scale via thalamo-cortico-thalamic loops and initiates a specific spatio-temporal dynamics associated with pain perception. If the theory is true then understanding neural dynamics in small scales would translate into understanding whole brain dynamics. The above evidence seems consistent with such a notion.

The self-organized criticality model brings a new perspective to pain representation and perception. One corollary is the idea that chronic pain states would be a manifestation of moving away from the critical balance between inhibitory and excitatory connectivity, resulting in exaggerated pain perception. The latter state in fact threatens the survival of the organism. There remains a very large set of questions that need serious consideration and perhaps, the criticality viewpoint can provide insights into their study. For example, why does pain seem to be the only sensory modality for which both thalamic and cortical level inhibitory connections are necessary? How does the balance between inhibitory and excitatory connectivity shift under different acute and chronic pain states? And, what is the underlying physiology or pathophysiology of these changes? Such questions will keep our laboratory busy for a long time.

Plenary discussion

Jabbur S.: Did you observe any changes in the orbital frontal lobe with nociceptive stimuli in your subjects?

Apkarian V.: The interface between the orbital frontal cortex and the underlying sinuses and bone creates magnetic field artifacts. As a result, we have not studied the activity of the region, and we have systematically excluded this region from the human brain imaging data analyses.

Wall P.: What is the role of lamina I projections to the inhibitory responses you observe both in the thalamus in animals, and in humans with fMRI? What is the correspondence between the inhibitory effects observed and the descending modulatory mechanism of diffuse noxious inhibitory control (DNIC)?

Apkarian V.: The human brain imaging data indicate a complicated spatio-temporal organization for the cortical inhibitions, and the role of spinal cord lamina I neurons, in this regard, remains unknown. In the monkey thalamus, the inhibitory connections that we observe are only in ventral posterior lateral thalamic areas where wide dynamic range type neurons are found. These neurons most likely receive their primary inputs from dorsal horn lamina V wide dynamic range type cells, through the ventral spinothalamic tract. Therefore, this inhibitory connectivity seems independent of lamina I inputs.
We have examined the psychophysical correspondence for the inhibitory responses seen by fMRI in the cortex. The results show that the touch threshold and sensitivity increase during pain. This change, however, is limited to the ipsilateral dermatome and decreases with distance. Thus, this inhibition is much more localized. Undoubtedly, however, it is part of a larger spectrum of inhibitory systems of which DNIC is perhaps the most unspecific as far as body position differences are concerned.

Saade N.: What is the somatotopic organization of the neuron groups you describe? Can you distinguish between dorsal column (DC) inputs and dorsal column postsynaptic (DCPS) inputs?

Apkarian V.: The population recording technique limits us to the accuracy with which the receptive fields of individual neurons can be described. However, let me add that the receptive field organization for either wide dynamic range type neurons or neurons with pure innocuous responses, all of which have small well-localized receptive fields, is very similar. At some recording sites, we observe some cells that have receptive fields on one body part, while others have receptive fields located in a distinct other body region. The local inter-connectivity properties of such recording sites remain to be seen if they differ from other sites. The extent of the nociceptive responses being channeled through the spinothalamic tract, the DC or the DCPS are not readily testable in population recordings.

Saade N.: Is there a possible interference between anesthesia used and the two different groups of WDR and nociceptive specific neurons?

Apkarian V.: I do not think so. We have observed very similar incidence counts when single unit recordings are done on squirrel monkeys using a variety of anesthetic cocktails such as gas (Halothane & NO_2 & O_2) or chloralose. Moreover, the incidence of these neurons is very similar to results obtained by Casey et al. in the awake squirrel monkey lateral thalamus.

Saade N.: Can we make a direct correlation between thalamic activation and cortical activation during different types of pain (i.e. acute versus chronic pains).

Apkarian V.: Generally, we see very little activity in the thalamus using fMRI. Although we have not looked for differences in the thalamus between patients with chronic pain and normal subjects, I would speculate that in the chronic situation thalamic activity should be either decreased or unchanged, while in the acute case it should be increased. Interestingly, thalamic connectivity during acute stimulation reveals inhibitory connectivity in the anesthetized monkey.

Amassian V.: The first question is whether the short range firing correlation relate to branching of the incoming axon.

Apkarian V.: In a strict sense, the answer is "Yes!": For a given population of cells, we can tell the difference between coactivation versus unidirectional activation, but we have not carried such analysis any farther. In general, the thalamic connectivity seems much more unidirectional in comparison to cortical connectivities.

Amassian V.: The second is whether the nociceptive cells you have recorded from can perform fine localization of say pinprick, although you used pinch in your experiments.

Apkarian V.: We do not know the pinprick responses for these neurons. However, their receptive fields are small and well localized.

Berkley K.: Where is the pain in the brain?

Apkarian V.: I refuse to answer this question. My data clearly showed that pain is not a unitary event in the brain. Various regions of the cortex are activated in a complicated manner during different pain tasks. The more interesting question is what the specializations of these regions are in the infinite types of pain perceptions that a person can experience. This question will keep us busy for a longtime to come.

References

Anderson JA, Sutton JP (1997) If we compute faster, do we understand better? Behav Res Meth, Instr & Comp 29 (1):67-77.

Apkarian AV, Stea RA, Bolanowski S (1994) Heat-induced pain diminishes vibrotactile perception: A touch gate. Somatosens Motor Res 11 (3):259-267.

Apkarian AV, Stea RA, Manglos SH, Szeverenyi NM, King RB, Thomas FD (1992) Persistent pain inhibits contralateral somatosensory cortical activity in humans. Neurosci Lett 140:141-147.

Bak P (1996) How nature works. The science of self-organized criticality. Copernicus, New York, NY.

Caplan JB, Bandettini PA, Sutton JP (1997) Weight-space mapping of fMRI motor tasks: evidence for nested neural networks. In: Computational Neuroscience '96, James Bower (ed.), Plenum Press.

de Charms RC, Merzenich MM (1996) Primary cortical representation of sounds by the coordination of action-potential timing. Nature 381:610-613.

Di Piero, V., Jones, A.K.P., Iannotti, F., Powell, M., Perani, D., Lenzi, G.L. and Frackowiak, R.S.J., Chronic pain: A PET study of the central effects of percutaneous high cervical cordotomy, Pain 46 (1991) 9-12.

Gelnar PA, Krauss BR, Szeverenyi NM, Apkarian AV (1997) Finger tip representation in the human somatosensory cortex: an fMRI study. J Neurosci (submitted)

Gelnar PA, Krauss BR, Szeverenyi NM, Apkarian AV (1996a) Overlap of medial wall fMRI activity between pain, motor, and vibrotactile tasks in humans. 26th annual meeting of Soc for Neurosci (abstract)

Gelnar PA, Szeverenyi NM, Apkarian AV (1996b) Cortical responses to noxious thermal stimuli depend upon the skin surface area stimulated. 2nd Internat. Conf. on Functional Mapping of the Human Brain (abstract)

Gerstein GL, Perkel DH, Dayhoff JE (1985) Cooperative firing activity in simultaneously recorded populations of neurons: Detection and measurement. J Neurosci 5:881-889.

Gottschaldt K-M, Vahle-Hinz C, Young DW (1983) The extraction of specific stimulus information out of complex afferent signals in subcortical relay stations of the cat's sinus hair system. Forschr Zool 28:113-128.

Grossberg S, Mingolla E, Ross WD (1997) Visual brain and visual perception: how does the cortex do perceptual grouping? Trends Neurosci 20:106-111.

Harth E (1993) The creative loop. How the brain makes a mind. Addison-Wesley, Reading, MA.

Hsieh JC (1995) Central processing of pain, Functional brain imaging studies with PET. Kongl Carolinska Medico Chirurgiska Institutet, Stockholm (Dissertation)

Iadarola MJ, Max MB, Berman KF, Byas-Smith MG, Coghill RC, Gracely RH and Bennett GJ (1995) Unilateral decrease in thalamic activity observed with positron emission tomography in patients with chronic neuropathic pain. Pain 63 (1):55-64.

Johnson MJ, Alloway KD (1996) Cross-correlation analysis reveals laminar differences in thalamocortical interactions in the somatosensory system. J Neurophysiol 75 (4):1444-57.

Jones EG (1985) The thalamus. Plenum Press, New York, NY.

Kaas JH, Nelson RJ, Sur M, Lin C-S, Merzenich MM (1979) Multiple representations of the body within the primary somatosensory cortex of primates. Science 204:521-523.

Krauss BR, Apkarian AV, Thomas PS, Szeverenyi NM (1997) Sympathetically maintained chronic pain (RSD) is a hyperfrontal condition. 27th Annual Meeting Soc for Neurosci (abstract)

Melzack R, Wall PD (1965) Pain mechanisms: a new theory. Science 150:971-979.

Sillito AM, Jones HE, Gerstein GL, West DC (1994) Feature-linked synchronization of thalamic relay cells firing induced by feedback from the visual cortex. Nature 369 (6480):444-5.

Talbot JD, Marrett S, Evans AC, Meyer E, Bushnell MC, Duncan GH (1991) Multiple representations of pain in human cerebral cortex. Science 251:1355-1358.

Neurotransmitter Receptor Mechanisms Involved in Nociceptive Processing in the Thalamus

S.A. Eaton[1] and T.E. Salt[2]
[1]*MRC Anatomical Neuropharmacology Unit*
Oxford, United Kingdom
[2]*Department of Visual Science, Institute of Ophthalmology*
London, United Kingdom

The processing of nociceptive information in the thalamus depends on several key features including a) the types and properties of the neurotransmitter receptors which mediate nociceptive synaptic responses, b) the intrinsic membrane properties of thalamic neurones and c) the functional relationship of the nociceptive neurones with the thalamic reticular nucleus (TRN).

Glutamate receptor pharmacology of nociceptive thalamic neurones

Extracellular recording studies have shown that the majority of neurones in the rat ventrobasal thalamus (VB) are excited by non-noxious, low threshold somatosensory stimulation (e.g. Waite, 1973). Other VB neurones respond exclusively to noxious sensory stimuli or to both noxious and non-noxious stimulation (Peschanski, Guilbaud, Gautron and Besson, 1980; Guilbaud, Peschanski, Gautron and Binder, 1980). Because of their ability to encode some of the features of the noxious stimulus, it has been proposed that VB neurones play an important role in the sensory-discriminative aspect of nociception (Peschanski, Guilbaud, Gautron and Besson, 1980). There are also nociceptive neurons in the thalamus dorsal to the VB (Hill and Pepper, 1978; Guilbaud et al., 1980). Synaptic responses of VB neurones evoked by low threshold, non-noxious, somatosensory stimulation are mediated by specific glutamate receptor subtypes (Salt, 1986; Salt and Eaton, 1991; 1989). Glutamate receptors can be broadly subdivided into three classes i) N-Methyl-D-Aspartate (NMDA) receptors, ii) non-NMDA (AMPA/kainate) ionotropic receptors, and iii) the metabotropic glutamate receptors (Mayer and Westbrook, 1987; Pin and Duvoisin, 1995). Metabotropic receptors can be further subdivided into three groups on the basis of sequence similarity, second messenger coupling, as well as agonist and antagonist preference (Watkins and Collingridge, 1994). In the VB, non-noxious somatosensory synaptic responses are mediated by AMPA/kainate and NMDA glutamate receptor subtypes (Salt, 1986; Salt and Eaton, 1991; 1989). Similarly, in the visual homologue of the VB, the lateral geniculate nucleus (LGN), sensory responses are also mediated by NMDA and AMPA/kainate receptors (Sillito, Murphy, Salt, 1990).

To establish which glutamate receptor subtypes mediate nociceptive synaptic responses of thalamic neurones located within and dorsal to the VB, we have used extracellular recording techniques combined with iontophoretic application of selective glutamate receptor agonists and antagonists. Synaptic responses evoked by noxious thermal stimulation were challenged by iontophoretic application of an antagonist for either NMDA receptors, AMPA/kainate receptors or metabotropic receptors, specifically, group I metabotropic receptors. On each neurone, the antagonist was also tested against responses evoked by iontophoretically applied agonists to establish that a) the antagonist was ejected at a concentration sufficient to antagonise the appropriate neurotransmitter receptor subtype and b) the antagonist was acting *selectively* at the appropriate receptor subtype. Iontophoretically applied agonists for different glutamate receptor subtypes were applied in regular cycles until responses were reproducible. They were then challenged with continuous concurrent iontophoretic application of the antagonist. Ejection parameters were chosen to produce a selective antagonism of the agonist acting at the appropriate receptor type, but not responses evoked by the agonist(s) acting at other types of glutamate receptors. The synaptic response of the same neurone evoked by noxious sensory stimulation was then challenged with the antagonist, using the same ejection parameters. Any reduction in the synaptic response by the antagonist indicated that the receptor types under investigation were involved in the mediation of the synaptic response.

NMDA receptors - the effects of CPP on responses to excitatory amino acids and noxious sensory stimulation

The NMDA receptor antagonist, of 3-((±)2-carboxypiperazin-4-yl)-propyl-1-phosphonic acid (CPP), was tested on 24 neurones against the responses to the NMDA receptor agonist, N-Methyl-DL-Aspartate (NMA) and one or more of the following agonists which act at different receptor types: quisqualate (13 neurones), kainate (eight neurones), acetylcholine (five neurones). CPP abolished or greatly reduced the responses to NMA with little or no effect against responses to kainate, quisqualate or acetylcholine (Table 1 and Figure 1). These controls indicate that the ejection parameters of CPP selectively antagonised NMDA receptors on the neurones under investigation. Using the same NMDA receptor selective ejection parameters, CPP markedly reduced the action potential responses to noxious sensory stimulation of the same neurones (Table 1; Figure 1). These results indicate that NMDA receptors mediate a substantial component of the synaptic response evoked by noxious stimulation.

Table 1. The effects of CPP, (S)-4C3HPG and CNQX on responses to excitatory amino acids and noxious sensory stimulation. Values are mean percentage responses relative to control values, ± standard deviation of *n* trials. Values in parentheses represent the number of neurones.

	Kainate	Quisqualate	AMPA	NMA or NMDA	Noxious Stimulation
CPP	97.7 ± 21.0 (8) *n*=8	91.5 ± 24.5 (13) *n*=18		19.0 ± 20.0 (24) *n*=29	24.1 ± 18.2 (24) *n*=29
(S)-4C3HPG		159.5 ± 33.2 (2) *n*=2	103.7 ± 28.3 (10) *n*=10	118.5 ± 47.7 (12) *n*=12	38.5 ± 26.3 (12) *n*=12
CNQX	26.6 ± 14.9 (16) *n*=18	119.7 ± 69.0 (3) *n*=3	57.2 ± 38.0 (12) *n*=14	87.5 ± 24.4 (17) *n*=19	97.7 ± 13.6 (17) *n*=19

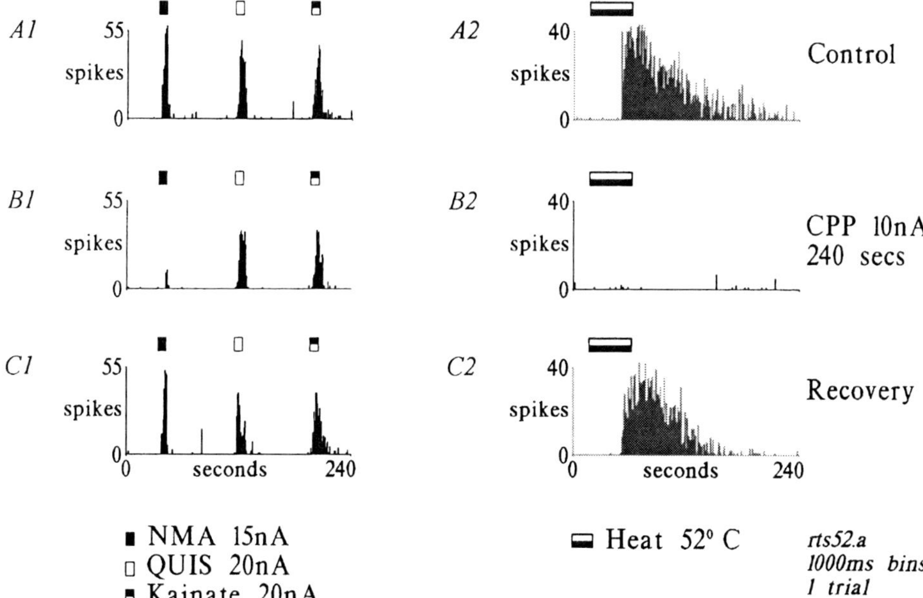

Figure 1. Selective antagonism of the response to iontophoretic application of the NMDA receptor agonist, N-Methyl-D,L-Aspartate (NMA) and the synaptic response to noxious thermal stimulation by CPP. Records are PSTHs of action potential spikes counted into one-second epochs. The bars above the records correspond to the timing and duration of agonist applications or thermal stimulation (see key). *Upper Panels:* A1) Control responses to iontophoretic application of the NMDA receptor agonist NMA and the non-NMDA receptor agonists, quisqualate (QUIS) and kainate. B1) The control synaptic response to noxious thermal stimulation. *Middle panels:* Responses to the same stimuli but during the concurrent iontophoresis of CPP at 10nA for 240 seconds. Note that CPP antagonised responses mediated by the NMDA receptor agonist, NMA, (B1) as well as the synaptic response to noxious stimulation (B2), but did not affect responses to agonists acting at non-NMDA glutamate receptors (B1). *Bottom panels:* Recovery of the response to NMA and the synaptic response to noxious stimulation following termination of CPP ejection.

AMPA/kainate receptors - the effects of CNQX on responses to excitatory amino acids and noxious sensory stimulation

Using the same approach described above for CPP, the AMPA/kainate receptor antagonist, 6-cyano-7-nitroquin oxaline-2,3-dione (CNQX), was used to investigate the potential involvement of AMPA/kainate receptors in synaptic responses evoked by noxious stimulation. On all of the 17 neurones tested, CNQX had little or no effect against the synaptic response at ejection currents which selectively antagonised the responses mediated at AMPA/kainate receptors by iontophoretically applied agonists on the same neurones (figure 2; table 1).

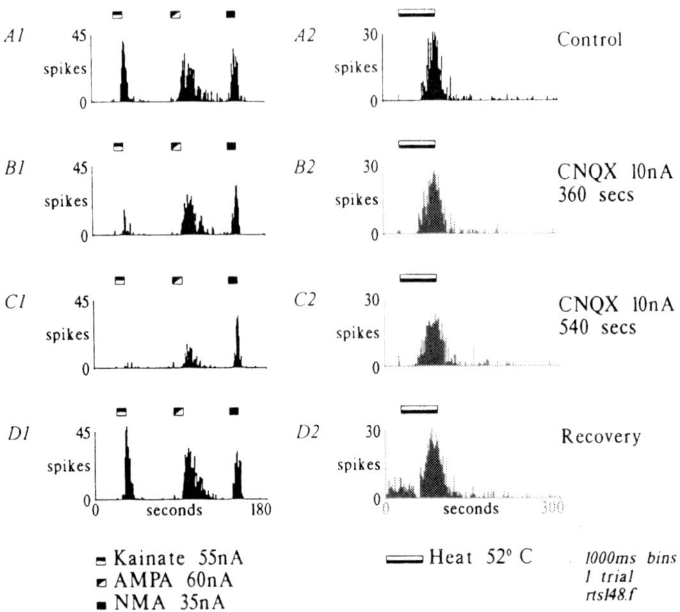

Figure 2. The AMPA/kainate receptor antagonist, CNQX had little effect against the synaptic response to noxious stimulation. For figure details see Figure 1. *Upper Panels:* A1) Control responses to the AMPA/kainate receptor agonists, kainate and AMPA and to the NMDA receptor agonist, NMA. A1) Control synaptic response evoked by noxious sensory stimulation. *Middle panels:* B1) CNQX initially reduced the response to kainate with good selectivity against the response mediated at NMDA receptors by NMA. B2) Using the same ejection parameters, CNQX had little effect against the sensory synaptic response. C1) More prolonged duration ejection of CNQX antagonised responses to both kainate and AMPA, albeit associated with a small reduction in the response to NMA. C2) A small reduction in the synaptic response was comparable to the reduction in the response to the NMDA receptor agonist, NMA. *Bottom panels:* Recovery following termination of CNQX application.

These results suggest that CNQX-sensitive AMPA/kainate receptors have little or no involvement in the mediation of the synaptic response evoked by noxious stimulation.

Group I metabotropic receptors - the effects of (S)-4C3HPG on responses to excitatory amino acids and noxious sensory stimulation

The group I metabotropic receptor antagonist, (S)-4-Carboxy-3-Hydroxyphenylglycine ((S)-4C3HPG), attenuated the responses to the iontophoretically applied group I metabotropic agonist, (1S,3R)-ACPD ((1S,3R)-1-aminocyclopentane-1,3-dicarboxylic acid) on all of the 12 neurones tested and concurrently enhanced or had little effect against the responses to agonists acting at other receptors, NMDA, AMPA or quisqualate (figure 3; table 1). Using the same ejection parameters of (S)-4C3HPG, this group I metabotropic receptor antagonist reduced the synaptic responses to noxious stimulation on all but one of the 12 neurones tested.

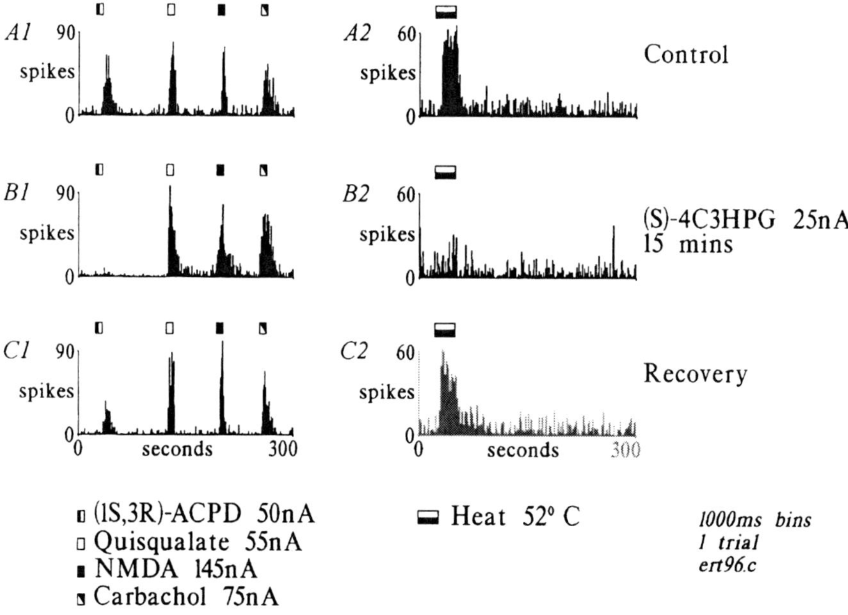

Figure 3. Antagonism of the synaptic response to noxious stimulation by the group I metabotropic receptor antagonist, (S)-4C3HPG. For figure details see Figure 1. *Upper Panels:* Control responses to the group I metabotropic agonist (1S,3R)-ACPD and to quisqualate, NMDA and carbachol (A1) and noxious sensory stimulation (A2). *Middle panels:* The same series of stimuli during the ejection of 4C3HPG; this group I metabotropic antagonist selectively antagonised the responses to (1S,3R)-ACPD (panel B1) and the synaptic response to noxious stimulation (panel B2). *Bottom panels:* Recovery from the effects of the antagonist.

To summarise, these data suggest that a substantial component of the sensory synaptic response evoked by noxious stimulation is mediated by NMDA receptors and group I metabotropic receptors, with little contribution made by AMPA/kainate receptors.

Intracellular recordings from nociceptive thalamic neurones

It is evident that the interaction of synaptic ligand-gated conductances with the intrinsic membrane potential-dependent conductances will be one of the principal determinants of the firing pattern of thalamic neurones evoked by sensory stimuli.

Thalamic neurones exist in two state-dependent firing modes, the so-called oscillatory (burst) and tonically-activated (relay) modes, which are determined by the interplay of the predominant intrinsic membrane conductances associated with each state, which is in turn determined by the membrane potential: oscillatory and relay modes are evident at relatively hyperpolarised and depolarised membrane potentials, respectively. The intrinsic membrane properties of thalamic neurones, the ionic conductances underlying them and the mechanisms responsible for oscillatory behaviour of thalamic neurones have been extensively characterised both *in vivo* and *in vitro* (Steriade and Llinas, 1988; McCormick, 1992; Steriade, McCormick and Sejnowski, 1993; Steriade and Deschênes, 1984). Briefly, burst firing patterns arise following membrane hyperpolarisation sufficient to de-inactivate a low threshold Ca^{2+} current, I_H. This results in a depolarising Ca^{2+} spike (low-threshold spike (LTS)) which can depolarise the membrane potential to the threshold to elicit one or a burst of conventional action potentials: this is often called a burst of rebound spikes. Spontaneous or sensory-evoked inhibitory input to thalamic relay neurones *in vivo* can evoke inhibitory postsynaptic potentials (IPSPs) capable of generating low threshold burst spiking activity (Steriade and Deschenes, 1984). There is substantial evidence to suggest that these IPSP sequences are derived from the TRN, which acts as a pacemaker, sending a rhythmic sequence of bursts of action potentials into the thalamus. IPSP-elicited low threshold Ca^{2+} spikes can also be evoked by sensory stimuli. Thus, in the VB, short duration stimulation of the peripheral receptive field elicits a short latency excitatory postsynaptic potential (EPSP) plus one or two spikes and is followed by a sequence of one or more TRN-derived IPSPs, which can give rise to one or more LTS and associated action potentials (Salt and Eaton, 1990). Similar rebound spikes are evident following visual stimulation in the LGN (Lo, Lu and Sherman 1991).

In relay mode, the interplay of intrinsic membrane conductances prevalent in this state results in a characteristic tonic, non-inactivating firing pattern of action potential spikes. Such firing patterns can be experimentally produced by simple injection of sufficient depolarising current (Steriade and Llinas, 1988). One of the membrane conductances involved in the generation and maintenance of tonic firing patterns is the persistent, non-inactivating Na^+ conductance, NaP which is activated in a regenerative fashion by depolarisation (Jahnsen and Llinas, 1984). In addition, and as suggested by McCormick (1992), the lack of spike train accommodation, presumed to be due in part to the relative lack of potassium currents, I_M and I_{AHP}, may serve to maintain the precision of sensory information transmission during long duration sensory responses. Excitatory glutamate receptor-mediated synaptic input to the thalamic relays can elicit such tonic firing patterns, typically evoked by long duration stimulation (Salt, 1986; Sillito et al., 1990, Turner et al., 1994), and thus it is feasible that synaptic glutamate receptor-mediated depolarisation activates Na_P during sensory responses and that NaP contributes to sensory-evoked responses in the relay thalamic nuclei (Salt and Eaton, 1996).

To examine how the intrinsic membrane properties and synaptic events contribute to the spontaneous and noxious sensory-evoked firing pattern of nociceptive thalamic neurones, standard intracellular recordings were made from 11 nociceptive thalamic relay neurones.

For six of the 11 neurones, spontaneous activity prior to noxious sensory stimulation characteristically consisted of high amplitude, frequent and relatively regular sequences of IPSPs. Individual IPSPs within a sequence could give rise to a rebound slow depolarisation which could itself elicit one or more action potentials in a burst firing pattern (figure 4). Judging by the waveform characteristics and the preceding IPSP, the slow depolarisation probably represents the well-known threshold Ca^{2+} spike (LTS). A tonic firing of action potentials could also be seen in the epochs between the IPSP sequences (figure 4). For the remaining five neurones, the spontaneous inhibitory input was much less marked and resting membrane potential oscillated less extensively.

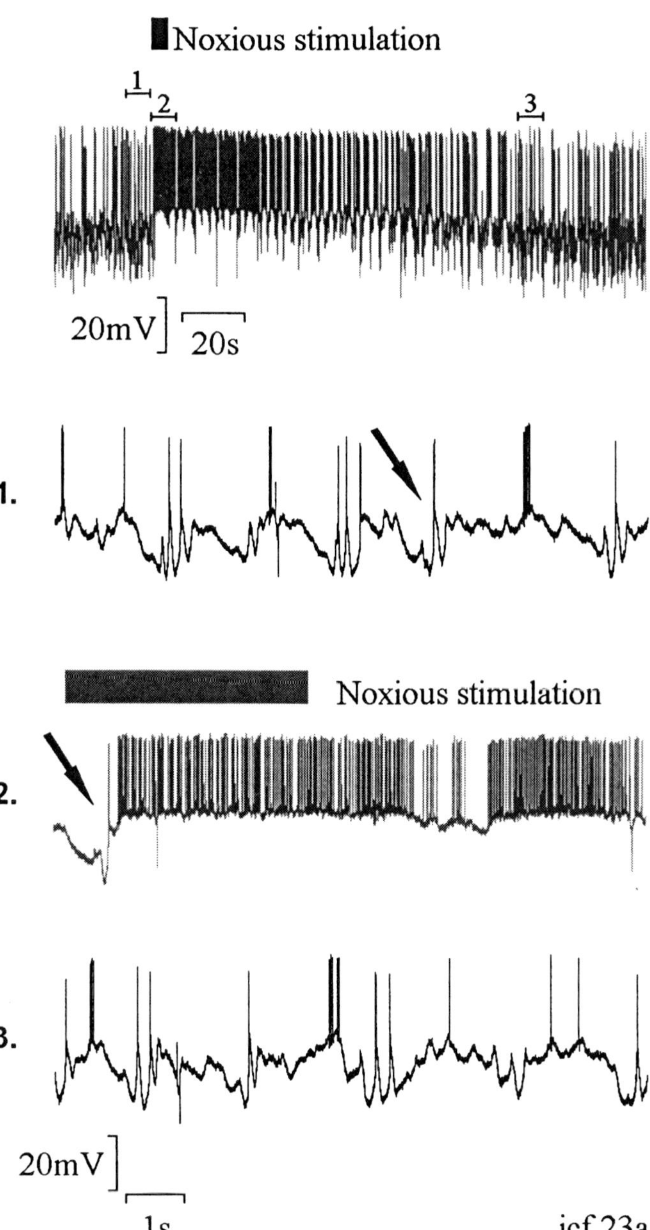

Figure 4. An intracellular recording from a nociceptive thalamic relay neurone. *Upper panel:* The membrane potential changes evoked by noxious sensory stimulation applied at the time shown by the filled bar above the record. Panels 1 - 3 show parts of this same record in more detail, at a different time base before, during and after noxious stimulation, at the times shown by the numbered horizontal bars above the record. Panel 1. Prior to noxious stimulation, spontaneous activity is typified by sequences of inhibitory postsynaptic potentials (IPSPs). IPSPs could generated low threshold calcium spikes which could give rise to regular action potentials (example shown at arrow). Panel 2. Noxious stimulation evoked a depolarising plateau and a tonic firing of action potentials. Immediately before the depolarising plateau an IPSP sequence gives rise to a LTS and associated action potential (at arrow). Note the marked reduction in peristimulus inhibition. Panel 3. Spontaneous activity following the synaptic response to noxious stimulation.

For all neurones, noxious mechanical stimulation evoked a maintained depolarising plateau which evoked a tonic firing of action potentials. It is likely that intrinsic Na and K conductances maintain the tonic pattern of firing, as discussed above. The plateau depolarisation was typically ramp shaped, and typically declined in magnitude with poststimulus time (figure 4). As seen in extracellular studies, the synaptic response typically outlasted the stimulus.

During the initial stage of the response, two features were notable. First, on the majority of neurones, an IPSP preceded the depolarising plateau and was associated with a rebound, depolarising LTS (note that the first spike of the nociceptive response in figure 4 was evoked by a LTS). Second, subsequent IPSPs were greatly reduced during the ensuing *peristimulus* stage of the depolarising plateau on all but two of these neurones. Both facets of this initial inhibition-disinhibition of nociceptive neurones during the peristimulus epoch may be important mechanisms in the initiation of the synaptic response (see discussion). Later stages of the maintained depolarisation and tonic firing were interrupted by IPSPs which progressively increased in magnitude back to prestimulus levels with poststimulus time (figure 4).

These intracellular records illustrate the underlying excitatory and inhibitory synaptic potentials during spontaneous activity and during the noxious sensory-evoked synaptic response and indicate the roles played by the intrinsic membrane properties of thalamic neurones in the integration and transfer of nociceptive information through the thalamus.

Effects of noxious stimulation on somatosensory thalamic reticular neurones

It is clear from the results presented above that inhibitory innervation of these nociceptive neurones plays a central role in both the spontaneous and sensory-evoked activity. In the rat VB, inhibitory interneurones are lacking and inhibitory innervation is derived primarily from the GABAergic thalamic reticular nucleus (TRN) (Barbaresi, Spreafico, Frassoni and Rustioni, 1982; Houser, Vaughan, Barber and Roberts, 1980; Harris and Hendrickson, 1987). Like the dorsal thalamus, the TRN can be anatomically and physiologically subdivided (Shosaku, Kayama, Sumitomo, Sugitani and Iwama, 1989), so that the VB is reciprocally connected with a specific section of the TRN, which shall be referred to here as the somatosensory TRN (sTRN). Considering the key role played by inhibitory innervation of nociceptive thalamic neurones by the TRN, in particular, the loss of peristimulus inhibition, it is interesting that TRN neurones have previously been shown to be inhibited by noxious stimulation (Peschanski, Guilbaud and Gautron, 1980). However, in this study it was not possible to physiologically identify the TRN neurones under investigation and, specifically, they did not respond to low threshold non-noxious somatosensory stimulation.

In order to establish whether neurones in the sTRN can be inhibited by noxious stimulation and to examine whether somatosensory submodalities exhibit functional interactions in the sTRN, the effects of noxious stimulation on both a) the spontaneous activity of sTRN neurones and b) synaptic responses evoked by non-noxious somatosensory stimulation in sTRN have been examined.

Extracellular single neurone recordings were made from sTRN neurones in tonic firing mode. Synaptic responses to low threshold somatosensory stimulation were evoked every at 0.5Hz or 0.25Hz before, during and after concomitant noxious stimulation of 12 or 16 seconds duration. Low threshold sensory stimulation consisted of a 10ms or 20ms jet of air directed at the peripheral receptive field, typically a vibrissa or a small region of body hair. Noxious stimulation consisted of a noxious mechanical stimulus applied to the ipsi- or contralateral hindpaw or ear.

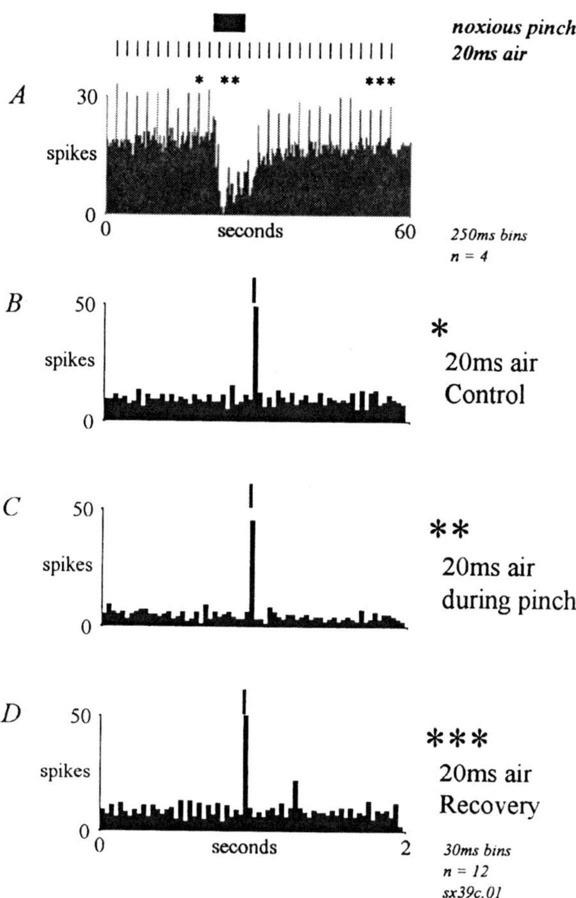

Figure 5. Extracellular recording from a somatosensory thalamic reticular (sTRN) neurone. *Panel A.:* A cumulative PSTH (four trials) showing the synaptic responses to 20ms air jet stimulation of the peripheral low threshold receptive field delivered at 0.5Hz at the times shown by the vertical bars above the record and the effects evoked by noxious sensory stimulation, delivered at the time shown by the filled bar above the record. Noxious stimulation produced a marked peristimulus inhibition of the spontaneous tonic firing of this sTRN neurone. Panels B - D show cumulative PSTH's of the synaptic response evoked by air jet stimulation of the low threshold peripheral receptive field. Each cumulative PSTH is constructed from three air jet responses in four trials (12 air jet responses in total) and are taken immediately before (panel B), during (panel C) and after (panel D) noxious stimulation (at the times shown by the asterisks in panel A. *Panel B.:* Low threshold sensory stimulation evokes a relatively short and constant latency action potential response. *Panel C:* During concurrent noxious stimulation, the synaptic response to air jet stimulation is little affected, despite the marked reduction in the tonic spontaneous activity. *Panel D:* Tonic spontaneous activity returns to control levels after noxious stimulation.

Like thalamic relay neurones, TRN neurones display two state-dependent firing modes, tonic and burst firing modes. In tonic firing mode, the characteristic spontaneous activity of TRN neurones consists of a relatively constant frequency regular firing of action potentials (figure 5, upper panel). In this mode, low threshold non-noxious sensory stimulation evokes 2 - 5 action potentials at relatively short and constant latency from sTRN neurones (figure 5, lower panels). Noxious stimulation produced a marked inhibition of the tonic spontaneous activity (figure 5). For the majority of neurones, an initial excitatory response was evoked at stimulus onset. In contrast to the inhibition of spontaneous tonic firing, noxious stimulation had little effect against the synaptic response evoked by non-noxious sensory stimulation.

The results show that the tonic spontaneous activity of sTRN neurones can be inhibited by noxious stimulation, and that this mechanism might contribute to the peristimulus reduction in inhibitory input during nociceptive responses in the relay thalamus. In addition, the selective attenuation of the spontaneous activity, rather than the non-noxious sensory-evoked activity may represent one mechanism by which the signal to noise ratio of inhibitory input to the relay thalamus may be enhanced during concurrent noxious stimulation. This may represent one mechanism by which attention can be focused during arousal.

Discussion

The results presented here illustrate some of the synaptic receptor mechanisms involved in the processing of nociceptive information in the thalamus.

The pharmacological approach indicates that group I metabotropic receptors and NMDA receptors mediate substantial components of the synaptic response evoked by noxious stimulation. The utilisation of this combination of glutamate receptor subtypes in nociceptive responses contrasts with the combination of receptor subtypes which mediates low threshold somatosensory responses of VB neurones and visual responses in the LGN, the visual homologue of the VB, which are mediated by NMDA receptors and AMPA/kainate receptors subtypes (Salt, 1986; Salt and Eaton, 1991; 1989; Sillito et al., 1990). The finding that somatosensory submodalities can be separated according to their synaptic pharmacology, specifically the utilisation of group I metabotropic receptors in nociceptive responses, might be of potential importance in the development of novel centrally-acting analgesic agents.

Intracellular recording of nociceptive thalamic neurones demonstrates how the synaptic events and intrinsic membrane properties interact to generate the firing patterns of nociceptive neurones during spontaneous and sensory-evoked activity. The spontaneous activity of many of these neurones consisted of a burst firing of one or more action potentials, evoked by the interaction of inhibitory postsynaptic potentials (IPSPs) with membrane conductances inherent to thalamic neurones. The underlying mechanism most likely results from the well known de-inactivation (activation) of a low threshold calcium conductance by hyperpolarising IPSPs. The ensuing low threshold calcium spike (LTS) depolarised the membrane potential sufficiently to generate one or more action potential. Some neurones additionally showed episodes of tonic spontaneous firing, or a mixed tonic and burst firing pattern of action potentials. Tonic firing is characteristic of thalamic neurones when depolarised, for example by excitatory synaptic input. It is interesting to speculate that other intrinsic membrane properties of thalamic neurones might also contribute to the depolarising plateau response evoked by noxious stimulation. In the pharmacological experiments described above, during selective antagonisms of either NMDA receptors or group I metabotropic receptors, on average, the sensory synaptic response to noxious stimulation was reduced on average by more than 50%. This might suggest some form of mutual functional interaction by these receptor subtypes. Membrane depolarisation of thalamic neurones activates a persistent sodium conductance, Na_p. It is possible that the excitatory synaptic drive recruits a depolarising contribution from Na_p. Any reduction in the excitatory synaptic drive by antagonism of the NMDA receptors or group I metabotropic receptors would correspondingly diminish any contribution made by Na_p and this mechanism may account for the disproportionately large antagonism of the synaptic response by both antagonists.

During the synaptic response to noxious sensory stimulation, an initial IPSP sequence (which could give rise to a LTS and associated action potential(s)) often preceded the depolarising plateau. During the ensuing peristimulus period of the depolarising plateau, it was notable that inhibitory input was markedly diminished. The initial inhibition-driven LTS in combination with the subsequent reduction in peristimulus inhibition may play an important role in the initiation of this synaptic response. The results presented above indicate that NMDA receptors are substantially involved in the mediation of this synaptic response. NMDA receptors have a well known, unusual, voltage dependency. This results from a channel block by magnesium ions at relatively hyperpolarised membrane potentials. Membrane depolarisation relieves the voltage-dependent block by Mg^{2+}. Membrane depolarisation by an IPSP-driven LTS might therefore potentially facilitate the utilisation of NMDA receptors during the initiation of the synaptic response. Similarly, a loss of inhibition during the early stages of the synaptic response could promote the contribution made by NMDA receptors. The sequence of inhibitory input might therefore have important implications for the initiation of the synaptic response to noxious stimuli. In the rat, inhibitory interneurones are lacking in the majority of nuclei and inhibitory innervation is derived primarily from the TRN. The initial excitation-inhibition response pattern of TRN neurones, described above, is compatible with the resulting sequence of inhibitory input to nociceptive thalamic relay neurones during noxious stimulation. Accordingly, the response pattern of sTRN neurones to noxious stimulation may play a key role in the initiation of the synaptic responses of nociceptive thalamic relay neurones. In addition, the response pattern of sTRN neurones may be important in the processing of non-nociceptive information during noxious stimulation. The effects of noxious stimulation on sTRN neurones is more complicated than a simple excitation-inhibition sequence. The data presented here show that synaptic responses of sTRN neurones to non-noxious sensory stimulation are largely unaffected during the period when noxious stimulation produced a marked reduction in the spontaneous tonic activity. Consequently, during noxious stimulation, neurones receiving feedback inhibition from this population of sTRN neurones (presumably VB neurones) will be relieved of tonic inhibitory innervation as noxious stimulation reduces the tonic spontaneous activity of sTRN neurones. However, feedback inhibition of VB neurones evoked by non-noxious stimulation would remain unaffected. Such feedback inhibition has been shown to play a pivotal role in the control of response magnitude of non-noxious sensory synaptic responses and in the maintenance of receptive field structure (Salt, 1989; Lee, Friedberg and Ebner, 1994; 1994a). During noxious stimulation, the effects in the sTRN would serve to increase the signal to noise ratio of feedback inhibitory innervation of VB neurones evoked by non-noxious sensory stimulation and this may serve to focus attention during arousal.

In summary, these data describe some of the neurotransmitter receptor mechanisms and systems level mechanisms which operate in the thalamus to process nociceptive information. In the absence of noxious stimulation, the thalamic neurones recorded here can display a mixed pattern of spontaneous firing, consisting of IPSP-driven low threshold calcium spikes and associated action potentials and/or a tonic firing of action potentials, presumably evoked by an underlying depolarisation. The response of thalamic relay neurones to noxious stimulation consists of a long lasting depolarising plateau, mediated by NMDA receptors and group I metabotropic glutamate receptors. It is possible that one of the intrinsic membrane conductances, Na_P, contributes to the depolarising plateau. The peristimulus reduction in inhibitory innervation might be important in the initiation of the depolarising plateau, considering the properties of the receptor subtypes mediating the synaptic response. An initial IPSP-driven LTS seen at the beginning of the synaptic response for many of the neurones in this study might also facilitate initiation of the depolarising response to noxious stimulation. This pattern of inhibitory input to thalamic relay neurones is in accord with the response profile of TRN neurones during noxious stimulation: the initial excitatory response, followed by an inhibition of tonic firing might be expected to mediate such a pattern of inhibitory input to the relay neurones. The effects of noxious stimulation on TRN neurones appears to be more complicated than a simple inhibition of TRN neurones, since responses of the same neurones to non-noxious stimulation are little affected, despite a marked concomitant reduction in the spontaneous tonic activity. The receptor mechanisms which mediate the excitation-inhibition sequence in the TRN and the complex interaction between somatosensory submodalities are currently under investigation.

In conclusion, the functional interactions between i) the neurotransmitter receptor subtypes which mediate the synaptic response of thalamic neurones to noxious stimulation, ii) the intrinsic membrane properties of thalamic neurones and iii) the pattern of inhibitory input from the TRN are primary determinants in the processing of nociceptive information at the level of the thalamus.

Plenary discussion

Besson J.-M.: You described clear pharmacological differences between thalamic responses to noxious and innocuous responses. Have you considered differences between classical non-noxious neurons, wide dynamic range neurons, and nociceptive specific neurons?

Eaton S.: Nociceptive responses are mediated by NMDA receptors and group I metabotropic receptors. Non-nociceptive responses are mediated by AMPA/kainate receptors and NMDA receptors. This seems to be the case for nociceptive specific neurons, non-nociceptive neurons and wide dynamic range type neurons.

Besson J.-M.: Do you think that the involvement of other ascending pathways in nociception is mediated through the same neurotransmitters and receptors?

Eaton S.: It is interesting to speculate that this may be the case, but this would need to be tested directly.

Amassian V.: How much of the difference between nociceptive and non-nociceptive thalamic neurons is a reflection of the very high quantal release per impulse in the dorsal column projection system? In the cuneate nucleus, certain receptor type inputs are driven by one impulse in one afferent fiber, and afferent periodicities are preserved in the output discharges (Amassian et al.) and in ventroposterior unit discharges (Waller). Possibly, one could get some useful data comparing stimulus intensity thalamic response functions by comparing electrical stimulation with spinothalamic projection, the question being how much spatial convergence is needed in the nociceptive input to activate the nociceptive thalamic neurons?

Eaton S.: It is difficult to speculate whether the specific utilization of different receptor types in different sensory sub-modalities is a result of the quantal properties of release. This question appears to make an assumption that the nociceptive responses are mediated by the spinothalamic pathway. We have previously published results suggesting that the context plays a very substantial role in these thalamic nociceptive responses.

Berkley K.: In view of steroidal modulation of GABA-ergic influences, the sex of the rat under study (if female, her estrous stage) is important. What was the sex of the rats you used for the studies?

Eaton S.: Male rats are always used to prevent the introduction of additional variables associated with female hormonal fluctuations.

Carpenter D.: It is surprising that the nociceptive response of the thalamic neurons was blocked by both metabotropic and NMDA receptor antagonists. Where do you believe these receptors to be? Are they on the same cell, pre-or/and post-synaptic?

Eaton S.: There does seem to be some form of functional interaction between these receptors. This could result from one or more of several mechanisms. Firstly, these are extracellular studies. Whilst a very large reduction of the synaptic action potential response is seen, an underlying depolarization mediated by other receptors may still occur but not reach the threshold for action potential generation. Secondly, the contribution made by the different receptor subtypes may generate additional contributions from intrinsic membrane conductances (see discussion in this book). Thirdly, the synaptic response was not abolished on all neurons (see results in this book). It seems likely that these antagonists are acting postsynaptically. However, it is not possible to rule out a contributory action at presynaptic sites.

References

Barbaresi P, Spreafico R, Frassoni C and Rustioni A (1982) GABAergic neurones are present in the dorsal column nuclei but not in the ventroposterior complex of rats. Brain Research 382, 305-326.

Guilbaud G, Peschanski M, Gautron M and Binder D (1980). Neurones responding to noxious stimulation in VB complex and caudal adjacent regions in the thalamus of the rat. Pain 8, 303-318.

Harris RM and Hendrickson AE (1987) Local circuit neurons in the rat ventrobasal thalamus-A GABA immunocytochemical study. Neuroscience 21, 229-236.

Hill RG and Pepper CM (1978) Selective effects of morphine on the nociceptive responses of thalamic neurones in the rat. British Journal of Pharmacology 64, 137-143.

Houser CR, Vaughan JE, Barber RP and Roberts E (1980) GABA neurons are the major cell type of the nucleus reticlaris thalami. Brain Research 200, 341-354.

Jahnsen H and Llinas R (1984) Ionic basis for the electroresponsiveness and oscillatory properties of guinea-pig thalamic neurones in vitro. Journal of Physiology 349, 227-247.

Lee SM, Friedberg MH and Ebner FF (1994) The role of GABA-mediated inhibition in the rat ventral posterior medial thalamus. I. Assessment of receptive field changes following thalamic reticular nucleus lesions. Journal of Neurophysiology 71, 1702-1750.

Lee S M, Friedberg MH and Ebner FF (1994a). The role of GABA-mediated inhibition in the rat ventral posterior medial thalamus. II. Differential effects of $GABA_A$ and $GABA_B$ receptor antagonists on responses of VPM neurons. Journal of Neurophysiology 71, 1716-1726.

Lo F-S, Lu S-M and Sherman SM (1991) Intracellular and extracellular in vivo recording of different response modes for relay cells of the cat's lateral geniculate nucleus. Experimental Brain Research 83, 317-328.

Mayer ML and Westbrook GL (1987) The physiology of excitatory amino acids in the vertebrate central nervous system. Progress in Neurobiology 28, 197-276.

Mayer ML, Westbrook GL and Guthrie PB (1984) Voltage-dependent block by Mg^{2+} of NMDA responses in spinal cord neurones. Nature 309, 261-263.

McCormick DA (1992) Neurotransmitter actions in the thalamus and cerebral cortex and their role in neuromodulation of thalamocortical activity. Progress in Neurobiology 39, 337-388.

Nowak L, Bregestovski P, Ascher P, Herbet A and Prochiantz A (1984) Magnesium gates glutamate-activated channels in mouse central neurones. Nature 307, 462-465.

Peschanski M, Guilbaud G, Gautron M and Besson J-M (1980) Encoding of noxious heat messages in neurons of the ventrobasal thalamic complex of the rat. Brain Research 197, 401-413.

Peschanski M, Guilbaud G and Gautron M (1980) Neuronal responses to cutaneous electrical and noxious mechanical stimuli in the nucleus reticularis thalami of the rat. Neuroscience Letters 165-70

Pin J-P and Duvoisin R (1995) The metabotropic glutamate receptors: Structure and functions. Neuropharmacology 34, 1-26.

Salt TE (1986) Mediation of thalamic sensory input by both NMDA and non-NMDA receptors. Nature 322, 263-265.

Salt TE (1989) Gamma-aminobutyric acid and afferent inhibition in the cat and rat ventrobasal thalamus. Neuroscience 28, 17-26.

Salt TE and Eaton SA (1989) Function of non-NMDA receptors and NMDA receptors in synaptic responses to natural somatosensory stimulation in the ventrobasal thalamus. Experimental Brain Research 77, 646-652.

Salt TE and Eaton SA (1990) Postsynaptic potentials evoked in ventrobasal thalamus neurones by natural sensory stimuli. Neuroscience Letters 114, 295-299.

Salt TE and Eaton SA (1991). Sensory excitatory postsynaptic potentials mediated by NMDA and non-NMDA receptors in the thalamus in vivo. European Journal of Neuroscience 3, 296-300.

Salt TE and Eaton (1996) Functions of iontotropic and metabotropic glutamate receptor in sensory transmission in the mammalian thalamus. Progress in Neurobiology 48, 55-72

Shosaku A, Kayama Y, Sumitomo I, Sugitani M and Iwama K (1989) Analysis of recurrent inhibitory circuit in rat thalamus: neurophysiology of the thalamic reticular nucleus. Progress in Neurobiology 32, 77-102.

Sillito AM, Murphy PC and Salt TE (1990) The contribution of the non-N-methyl-D-aspartate group of excitatory amino acid receptors to retinogeniculate transmission in the cat. Neuroscience 34, 273-280.

Steriade M and Deschênes M (1984) The Thalamus as a Neuronal Oscillator. Brain Research Reviews 8, 1-63.

Steriade M and Llinas RR (1988) The functional states of the thalamus and the associated neuronal interplay. Physiological Reviews 68, 649-742.

Steriade M, McCormick DA and Sejnowski TJ (1993) Thalamocortical oscillations in the sleeping and aroused brain. Science 262, 679-685.

Turner JP, Leresche N, Guyon A, Soltesz I and Crunelli V (1994) Sensory input and burst firing output of rat and cat thalamocortical cells: the role of NMDA and non-NMDA receptors. Journal of Physiology 480, 281-295.

Waite PME (1973) Somatotopic organization of vibrissal responses in the ventro-basal complex of the rat thalamus. Journal of Physiology 228, 527-540.

Watkins JC and Collingridge G (1994) Phenylglycine derivatives as antagonists of metabotropic glutamate receptors. Trends In Pharmacological Sciences 15, 333-342.

Pain Mechanisms and Management
S.N. Ayrapetyan and A.V. Apkarian (Eds.)
IOS Press, 1998

The Mechanisms by which Tissue Damage and Pain are Related

Patrick D. Wall
University College London, St Thomas's Hospital
London, United Kingdom

There are two complementary ways of looking at the origin of pain. The first traditional way is to start with damage to tissue, and to examine the course of the nerve impulses which are generated by the tissue damage and to follow them through the nervous system. The second is to ask what is going on in the brain of someone who says that they are in pain. We will follow both courses.

Approach A: the origin and path of nerve impulses generated by injury

Peripheral tissue
Dramatis personae: smashed cells, myelinated nerve fibers, unmyelinated nerve fibers, sympathetic fibers, motor fibers, mast cells, white cells, serum, fibroblasts, immune system.

Action: Nerve impulses are produced by heat, pressure and chemicals.

Reaction: Smashed cells break down and the arachnidonic acid in their membranes produces prostaglandins and leukotrienes. Excited C fibers emit peptides. Mast cells break down. Blood vessels dilate and leak serum. White cells and fibroblasts invade.

The consequence is that the chemical environment of the sensory nerve terminals changes, aided by the action of the sympathetic system and motor movement. The chemicals include algogens such as histamine and bradykinin, peptides such as Substance P, cytokines, neurotrophins, and immune products. These combine to produce very prolonged firing and sensitization of the nerve ends.

Peripheral nerves
Single cells running from terminals in tissue over peripheral axons, their dorsal root ganglion cells, dorsal root fibers and central terminals in spinal cord.

Action: To carry nerve impulses rapidly and to transport chemicals slowly.

Reaction: In addition to the nerve impulses, the terminals pick up the changed chemicals in the inflamed tissue and transport them to the dorsal root ganglion cells, where they change the metabolism. This in turn noticeably changes the cytoplasmic content of peptides and of substances delivered to the spinal cord. If nearby tissue is denervated, peripheral nerve fibers sprout to invade the abandoned territory. If the axons are damaged, synthesis of cytoplasmic and membrane proteins in the cell body change, and sprouting begins at the damaged end. The new membrane has novel physiological properties, including mechanical sensitivity, adrenaline sensitivity and spontaneous firing. At the same time, similar changes take place in the dorsal root ganglion cell. The consequence is that abnormal impulses are generated at the surviving ends of the axon and in the outgrowing sprouts and in the dorsal root ganglion cell.

The spinal cord

All types of cells in the upper five laminae of the dorsal horn are involved in receiving, processing and transmitting arriving impulses over the dorsal root axons.

Action: To transmit impulses and substances to motor neurones, to other spinal cord segments, and to the brainstem and beyond.

Reaction:

Fast: Immediately after the arrival of an afferent volley, an inhibition is installed which limits the subsequent effect of arriving impulses, both over the axons which have carried the impulses and over their neighbors. This inhibitory mechanism operates both presynaptically on the terminals of the arriving afferents and postsynaptically on the dorsal horn cells, and is produced by the action of the small cells in the substantia gelatinosa.

Slow: A slower-onset inhibitory process is provoked by the arriving volley which involves a loop running from the spinal cord at least as far as the reticular formation and midbrain periaqueductal gray and then descending from these structures back to the spinal cord.

After the arrival of impulses in C fibers, there is a prolonged increase of the excitability in the receiving dorsal horn cells. Cells which previously responded only to intense stimuli now also respond to innocuous stimuli, and they become spontaneously active. This hyperexcitability involves changes in the cell's nucleus, cytoplasm and membrane.

Later, after these impulse-induced changes of excitability, there are the slow consequences of the changed chemical transport along afferent fibers which result in further diminutions of inhibitory mechanisms and increases in excitability, and in some anatomical change.

It will therefore be seen that the dorsal horn is by no means a simple relay. The responses of cells to a noxious stimulus depend on:

a.   the existence of other simultaneous inputs
b.   the setting of the local and descending control circuits
c.   the previous existence of C fiber inputs
d.   the effect of transported substances from the periphery

Target structures beyond the spinal cord

Cells responding to noxious stimuli have been recorded in a bewildering number of structures. These include:

-     pons and medulla: dorsal column nuclei, olive, cerebellum, reticular formation
-     midbrain: parabrachial nuclei, periaqueductal gray, tectum, pretectal nuclei
forebrain: thalamus, hypothalamus, pulvinar, putamen, globus pallidus, amygdala, cortex

I find that this approach ceases to be productive when presented with so many important structures. The traditional explanation has been to assign to each structure some isolated aspect of the phenomenon of pain. These fantasies dressed up as hypotheses or even as statements of fact have claimed to be able to identify the source of the following fractions of pain: alerting, arousal, orientation, descending inhibitory control, autonomic responses, the sensation of pain as distinct from the affective components such as suffering.

At this stage I would prefer to explore the other approach, which starts from the top down, to see whether we can do any better than the conclusion of the bottom-up approach.

Approach B: What brain state is associated with pain?

This approach might seem to be the simple obverse of the first approach. That is to say it is based on the notion that pain is the sensation associated with injury, and injury produces pain. We could then adopt the common-sense approach that there is an injury-detection mechanism, which we have already described, which feeds a number of separate mechanisms

1.   flexion reflexes
2.   autonomic, respiratory, endocrine and immune responses
3.   the sensation of pain followed by perception
4.   the affective responses of misery and suffering
5   behavior, learning, and memory

The majority of scientists take this approach—and, good luck to them! I do not, because I am not convinced that the five categories of response to injury are independent variables, each generated by a separate mechanism which is fed by a common injury detector. I think that the facts suggest that the five responses appear as an integrated package, after a brain process has determined that the whole organism is in a situation where the combined responses are appropriate. One of the reasons for this approach is that there is a very poor correlation between injury and pain in important clinical situations. When patients with acute overt injury arrive at a civil emergency clinic, 20% report no pain at the time of the accident, 40% complain more than might be thought appropriate, and 40% give the expected answer. When patients in pain are given a placebo which they expect will relieve their pain, their pain disappears along with the other four responses. In chronic conditions such as osteoarthritis and cancer, where there is pain and overt tissue damage, there is a very poor relation between the amount of pain and the amount of tissue damage. Finally, there are a number of serious intractable pain states such as migraine, trigeminal neuralgia, deafferentation disorders, and central pains where no origin of a nociceptive input has been identified. For these reasons, it is at least of interest to take the top-down approach to see where it leads.

The results of image studies of people in pain

There have now been a very large number of studies of normal subjects and of patients using positron-emission tomography (PET) and, just beginning, functional nuclear magnetic-resonance images (fNMR). They localize regions of change activity. They show even more widespread activation than had been seen with electrophysiological technique. For example, the following areas are involved:

Cortex:

sensory and motor cortex areas	1-4
premotor cortex	6
parietal cortex	7 and 37-40
frontal cortex	8-10 and 43-47
cingulate cortex	24 and 32
insula	14
occipital cortex	19

Subcortical structures:

thalamus, putamen, caudate nucleus, hypothalamus, amygdala, periaqueductal gray, hippocampus, red nucleus, pulvinar, cerebellar vermis.

All of these areas have been reported as changed in their activity during pain states by a number of research groups. The results could be said to only add to the multiple targets revealed by the neurophysiological approach, and therefore to add to the mystery. Somehow, we have to incorporate this new body of data into any satisfactory theory. The facts include remarkable detail: For example, the expected increase of activity which is observed in the thalamus in normal subjects receiving painful stimuli is observed as a decrease of activity in patients in chronic clinical pain. A surprise target area, the anterior cingulate gyrus, reported as active by many groups, is active only on the right side, irrespective of the side of pain in recent studies, and the same area is less active when the pain is angina but more active in other pain states.

Clearly, this remarkable new tool has provided no simple answers, but has given a wonderfully sophisticated picture which must be incorporated into any adequate model of pain mechanisms.

Do lesions produce analgesia?

If there were specialized parts of the brain entirely devoted to pain, it should follow that local lesions should produce analgesia in isolation. There is no part of the brain which has not been destroyed by vascular accidents or by tumors or by metal fragments. Furthermore, there have been a very large number of neurosurgical deliberate lesions of the expected parts of the brain known to respond to a nociceptive input. There have been many such lesions aimed at spinal cord, brain stem, thalamus, and cortex. These are best reviewed in J.M. Gybels and W.H. Sweet, "Neurosurgical treatment of persistent pain" (Karger 1989). The long-term results are very disappointing in their failure to produce a selective analgesia. The short-term results are always encouraging in their apparent success, which later fades. This story of failure has let to the nearly complete disappearance of neurosurgery by lesion of the CNS for chronic pain. These lesions also failed to dissect out one or more of the components of pain, such as suffering. This result could have been predicted, if the nociceptive input feeds separate targets for the various components associated with reaction to injury. The resulting failure of isolated lesions to dissect off certain components strongly suggests that we must expect a spatially distributed system. The nearest approach to a lesion producing an apparently specific sensory deficit is seen in patients with large strokes involving the right inferior parietal cortex. This area is one of the surprise areas whose activity is markedly changed in PET scans of patients in pain. Neurophysiologists thought the area to be related to orientation, and they may well be right. These patients show a complete neglect of all inputs from the left side of their visual and auditory field and of their body. However, this neglect disappears on vestibular stimulation, which strongly suggests that it is not the sensory system which is disabled but the ability to orient into the source of the sensory stimulus.

What influences pain other than tissue damage?

There are certain manipulations of pain and its associated feelings which tell us little about mechanisms. For example, a patient with pain fears that it is a sign of lethal cancer. The doctor informs the patient that he does not have cancer. The pain remains but is less frightening. This simply means that pain is felt in context, and that the doctor has changed the context. In another example, an arthritic patient fears that the pain associated with movement signals that he is injuring himself and so does not move. A skilled therapist shows the patient that he can move and have pain, but that he does not deteriorate. The pain remains, but the patient's mood improves because he is more mobile. These situations are not independently manipulating different parts of the pain syndrome, but they are changing the context in which the pain is felt.

However, there are other types of change of pain which have been intensively studied by therapists. They all relate to attention, or to a special form of attention which is expectation. A basic rule of all sensory mechanisms is that some process selects from all possible sensory inputs one to which attention is paid. Pain is the preeminent attention-getter. But supposing the patient is distracted; that is to say, some event is biologically more important than the pain. That, I believe, is precisely what is happening to those who suffer accidental, sports-related, or wounding in battle, and yet do not feel pain. They may be fully aware of their injury, but at the time, there is some more important sensory input, such as the possibility of escape. Not only do they feel no pain or suffering, but their skilled movement shows that the injured part is not dominated by the flexion reflex. In other words, these people miss not only pain but also other responses normally associated with injury. Expectation is a prediction of some future relevant sensation. The placebo response is tightly locked to the subject's expectation. If a subject has learned that some manipulation is followed by a loss of pain, then a mock manipulation, which the patient believes to be the true one, produces pain relief. Interestingly, this pain relief is accompanied by autonomic, endocrine, respiratory, and motor relief. Many therapies attempt to provide socially acceptable forms of distraction. Anxiety and depression both increase the expectation that the next event is likely to be painful. In all these states where pain is manipulated top-down, there is a simultaneous coordinated movement of the other correlates of pain in response to injury.

What, then, do we expect to learn from a top-down or bottom-up analysis of pain mechanism? The classical expectation from the time of Aristotle is that we will discover a generator of the pure sensation of pain, another generator of the misery and suffering, and again separate generators of the motor and vegetative reflexes. We have learned from the top-down approach that the separate independent generator expectation may be in error, and that a coordinated package of responses may be what is actually observed. Next, we have learned that the entire package is subject as a whole to the permission of expectation and attention. Third, we have learned that the mechanism must be distributed in space, since no local lesions have been found to abolish pain permanently or any of the other injury-response components. Finally, we have learned from the active brain images that the engaged parts of the brain are even more widespread than was suspected by the physiologists. Perhaps the greatest surprise from the brain images is the clear demonstration of the involvement of areas previously assigned a role in the planning of motor movements. These areas include the motor cortex, premotor cortex, frontal lobe areas, putamen, and cerebellum.

This raises a final question for future exploration: Everyone so far has assumed that the input first encounters a sensory brain, which analyzes the nature of the stimulus. Once this task is completed, the answer to this analysis is handed on to a quite different part of the brain, the motor brain. What is the evidence for this two-stage brain: first sensory, and only then motor planning? Could it not be that the sensory input is analyzed, classified and defined in terms of what the organism might do about the stimulus? That would mean that the separation of motor planning from sensory analysis would be an intellectual error. The hypothesis that sensory analysis is incorporated in the motor-planning system requires thought and experiment. Certainly, the separate target locations for pain and its associated responses have not been located and perhaps do not exist.

Plenary discussion

Amassian V.E.: First, a comment on what these uptake or blood flow strokes mean in terms of neuronal activity. Speaking generally an input to cerebral cortex leads often to one or more short latency regions of increased activity followed by a period of reduced activity (associated with IPSPs), and then sometimes a period of rebound increased activity. Surrounding these initially activated areas are zones of reduced activity. Out of this complex in space and time comes an effect which exceeds, or not, statistical criteria of no demonstrable change. A good example of the problem is provided by the finding (Bernd Meyer's group) that blood flow increases in contralateral cortex following magnetic stimulation of motor cortex even though contralateral cortex has its excitability reduced to separate magnetic stimulation. Therefore 'anomalies' may not be too surprising in the uptake of blood flow studies.

Secondly, the capsaicin experiments may avoid the problems that arise when non painful thermal stimulation is compared with painful thermal stimulation. Simple subtraction of flow will not do. One should study the intensity functions of thermal stimulation that is non-painful, extrapolate to the temperature level used to elicit pain and then do the subtraction.

Wall P.D.: You have asked two crucial questions: Your first relates to the validity of the measure which is certainly in question, and to the spatial and temporal resolution of the technique. PET studies are particularly poor in temporal resolution and therefore, as you say, could give false answers, if the measured phenomenon oscillates. Your second question correctly mocks those who think of pain as an isolated or even isolatable event. Clearly, a pain provoking event will necessarily involve attention, orientation, effectuation and a background state. Furthermore, it will be accompanied by a series of somatic, autonomic and endocrine responses, which may or may not be necessary components of the sensory state. Fortunately experiments now begin to move away from the initial simplistic form to ones designed to dissect out those components which are necessary and sufficient for the sensory state.

Knapp: Since chronic pain is mediated by small C-fiber nerves, are MR & PET imaging studies valid, since they depend on stimulation of large, myelinated nerve fibers?

Wall P.D.: MR and PET measure local blood flow changes secondary to overall changes of activity.

Basbaum A.I.: What might you predict would be the pattern of activity (distributed, to be sure) in a patient with pain asymbolia, i.e. in a condition without pain, but with presumably normal transmission of nociceptive messages. Patients with persistence of autonomic signs would be even better, since you have an independent measure of the integrity of the neural basis of nociception.

Wall P.D.: The answer to your question has not been found, but would be fascinating. A similar study, however, has been done on patients with parietal lesions who neglect all sensory stimuli on one side. It is possible to restore sensation by vestibular stimulation. The change on PET scanning relates only to activity in the frontal lobe.

Basbaum A.I.: If one looks at the imaging studies as a way to do studies in patients comparable to those done for years in the spinal cord , perhaps a more positive outlook is in order. We are probably never going to find a "pain" area, but it is informative to identify sites of distributed processing in normal patients and in patients with different pain conditions.

Wall P.D.: I agree with you. As I have said, I think it is likely that we are dealing with a distributed system, but that is just hand waving speculation until one can specify its nature. A distributed system would require a mechanism to bind together the distributed parts, and a mechanism which could read out and identify the pattern. We have no facts, theory or model relevant to the nervous system. This is a widespread problem in the central nervous system which has been most clearly recognized by those working on hippocampus and cerebellum.

Basbaum A.I.: Regardless of whether the mechanism of action of sumatriptan for migraine is known, the fact is that it is an example of an effective therapy using a drug that targets a subtype of receptor. It is not at all unreasonable to predict that development of other drugs that target receptor subtypes will be developed for pain control. The value of agonist selectivity is well established in the adrenergic receptor domain for cardiovascular problems, why not for nociceptive processing?

Wall P.D.: I agree with you that a search should continue for subtypes of receptors, because they represent a fascinating biological fact whose meaning we do not understand. My point was that the reason for this search should not be that they might provide a specific drug without side-effects. The example you give of sumatriptan, which has been a wonderful help to some patients with migraine, is a poor example because it is not clear that this target of action relates to the tissue for which it was developed. The saddest example is the failure of the massive search on opiate receptors to develop a single superior compound. The example you quote of alpha and beta adrenaline blockers was fully developed by classical pharmacology long before anyone had heard of a receptor.

Seltzer Z.: The scheme you suggest portrays the nervous system as related to an intelligent response automaton pain as a "nocifensor", whereby the task of the brain is merely to seek the proper response to the input. Doesn't this scheme skip the subjective aspect of pain?

Wall P.D.:Let me emphasize again that I am not a behaviorist who thinks that all aspects of pain perception can be detected in overt behaviour. However, I do suggest that the subjective aspect of pain might be expressed in terms of possible future action, rather than in terms of an isolated analysis of preceding events in sensory terms.

Basmadjian G.P.: You were talking about "increased activity" in areas supposedly stimulated by pain. The uptake of activity in these areas is mainly due to superfusion of the tracer. Does this mean that pain stimulation increases perfusion to the area or, is there increased metabolism at the area that demands higher uptake of tracer?

Wall P.D.: I have reported here the results of PET scanning for the oxygen uptake of 0^{15} which measures cerebral blood flow.

References

Wall PD and Melzack R (Eds.) (1994) Textbook of Pain, 3rd ed., Churchill Livingstone, Edinburgh.

Melzack R and Wall PD (1994) The Challenge of Pain, revised ed., Penguin, London.

Pain Mechanisms and Management
S.N. Ayrapetyan and A.V. Apkarian (Eds.)
IOS Press, 1998

Magnetic Transcranial Stimulation Studies in Humans on the Roles of Frontal and Occipital Lobes in Perception, on Estimating Perceptual Delay, and on Temporary Pain Relief with Parietal Stimulation

V.E. Amassian, R.Q. Cracco, M. Vergara, P.J. Maccabee,
M. Somasundaram and J.B. Cracco
Departments of Physiology and Neurology
SUNY Health Science Center at Brooklyn
Brooklyn, NY, USA

Abstract. Magnetic transcranial stimulation of human frontal, occipital and parietal lobes alters perception of nonpainful and painful stimuli, respectively. Single pulse stimulation of the frontal lobe elicits a sense of projected movement, and paresthesias in a minority of subjects, under conditions where afferent feedback was excluded. Because single pulses to the parietal lobe do not elicit a projected sensation, we conclude that the frontal lobes readily access the perceptual system, probably through the strong connections with the intralaminar and other higher level thalamic nuclei. Other influences of the magnetically stimulated frontal lobes on perception are exemplified by the facilitation of phosphenes elicited by small coil stimulation of occipital cortex and the improvement in detection of faintly illuminated letters.

Analysis of the time flow of the representations of flashed linguistic symbols from visual to frontal cortex and their accurate vocalization implies a time delay of less than 1/10 sec for conscious perception of the symbol. Motor programming the sequence of phonemes that characterize the numeral occupies less than 1/20 sec.

Repetitive magnetic stimulation with 10 pulses at 20 Hz of the non-dominant posterior parietal lobe results in reduced ischemic muscle and nail bed pain after, for example, a delay of 3-6 sec which lasts for 30-35 sec. The temporary relief may be accompanied by a pleasurable sensation of warmth, Implying that a full Neglect Syndrome has not been temporarily produced. The basis of pain relief clearly differs from that in visual suppression and requires further study.

Introduction

The introduction of transcranial magnetic stimulation by Barker et al., (1985) provided a relatively painless technique for stimulating the human cerebral cortex non-invasively. Thus, *normal* brains could be stimulated without the complication of plasticity from disease occurring in the patient brain stimulated after surgical exposure. Significantly, Penfield and Roberts (1959) observed only a brief aphasia in two patients after extirpation of Broca's Area. However, trancranial magnetic stimulation is at a disadvantage in that the actual gyri stimulated are not directly visualized, as when the Neurosurgeon places electrodes on the exposed cerebral cortex, nor is the locus of stimulation by the magnetic coil (MC) known with the same precision. (Exceptionally, focal magnetic stimulation was combined with surface MRI cuts to reduce these disadvantages of transcranial stimulation, cf, Levy et al., 1991).

Although, phosphenes from occipital stimulation by the MC were included in the earliest report (Barker et al., 1985), most studies after the introduction of transcranial stimulation dealt with movements elicited by single MC pulse stimulation (for example, reviewed by Rothwell et al., 1991). However, sensory responses to stimulation of the cerebral cortex have long been known. Traditionally, neurosurgeons, for example Penfield and Boldrey (1937), used repetitive electrical stimulation to elicit projected sensations from the human postcentral gyrus. In a careful parametric study, Libet et al, (1964) established minimum *repetitive* train lengths of 0.3-0.5 sec for reported sensations by the patient; a single electrical pulse did not lead to any sensation despite the large electrical cortical response it produced. Similarly, single magnetic pulses applied to the parietal lobe do not elicit a projected sensation. However, single magnetic pulses applied to certain portions of the frontal lobe elicited distally projected sensations (Amassian et al., 1989, 1991). This finding pointed to a significant role of the frontal lobe in readily accessing the perceptual system. In the following report, we describe: (1) The role of the frontal lobes in: (A) Somatosensory sensations, specifically, the projected sense of movement and paresthesias; (B) Facilitating phosphenes from MC stimulation of occipital cortex; (C) Facilitating perception of faintly illuminated linguistic symbols. (2) An estimate of the minimum delay for visual perception based on tracking the time flow of the representation of linguistic symbols from the visual cortex to their vocalization. (3) A *delayed*, temporary relief of acutely induced pain by repetitive parietal lobe stimulation.

Methods

The human subjects stimulated by the MC in all these studies were members of the SUNY Neurology Faculty; the Institutional Review Board approved transcranial magnetic stimulation. Technical details are described more fully in the cited references. Briefly, MC stimulation was usually done by a Cadwell Laboratories (Kennewick, WA, USA) single pulse (MES-10) stimulator, or by a rapid rate (repetitive) prototype model. The MCs used were either round, ovoid, or figure 8 in design; where relevant, they and their dimensions are identified in each experiment. Focal stimulation was secured either by edge stimulation of a round MC, or by stimulation at the junction region of a figure 8 MC. Focal stimulation permits movements of predominantly a single digit to be elicited with near-threshold stimulation (Amassian et al., 1989). By contrast, laying a round or ovoid MC *tangentially* on the scalp permits in principle stimulation of neurons anywhere under the windings, which is potentially an advantage if the functions studied are distributed over a wide cortical area.

Recordings were either EMGs conventionally recorded with surface disc electrodes and RC amplified, or voice recorded with a microphone, amplified and electronically timed, with monitoring of the accuracy of the timing on a digital storage oscilloscope.

The structures stimulated by the magnetic pulse

Summarizing, an electric current pulse passing through a coil of wire generates a magnetic pulse, which then induces an electric field in a volume conductor, such as the brain, with the field direction the reverse of that in the wire. The induced electric field is associated with flow of current directly proportional to the conductance of the volume conductor. Two lines of evidence imply that the structures usually stimulated are the nodes of Ranvier of myelinated axons: The first was obtained by Barker et al. (1991), measurements of the chronaxie of elements excited by motor cortical stimulation being similar to that of peripheral A-alpha motor axons. Subsequently, Rothwell et al. (1992) showed more directly that facilitation of a near threshold magnetic pulse by a subsequent anodic electrical pulse had a decay time constant of 80-100 µs, that is, similar to that of peripheral A-alpha motor axons, thereby approximating the nodal membrane time constant (Tasaki, 1953). In the macaque, the similarity in synaptic modulation of focal *cathodal* and *some* MC elicited direct corticospinal discharge implies that MC excitation can occur near synaptic regions, e.g., at the initial segment (Amassian et al., 1990). However, direct MC excitation can also occur in the macaque white matter and there is evidence against, and none for initial segment excitation in humans as proposed (Eyre et al., 1990).

The mechanism of axonal excitation is presumed to come about through depolarization by outward membrane current at one or more nodes. Membrane current is absent in an axon lying in the axis of a uniform induced electric field, but can occur when: 1) A linear axon is excited near the negative spatial derivative of the induced electric field (Roth and Basser, 1990): This occurs (a) when the induced electric field curves away from the axon, or (b) when the axon lies in an inhomogeneous volume conductor (Maccabee et al., 1993). 2) When the axon bends in a uniform induced electric field, 3) When the axon terminates, eg, in presynaptic arborizations or dendrites, in a uniform electric field directed towards the terminations. (Reilly, 1989, Amassian et al., 1992a, Maccabee et al., 1993). Of these possibilities, axonal bending appears to be a most important low threshold site for excitation in the brain.

The MC could theoretically excite excitatory and, or inhibitory axons with opposite effects on perception, for example, projected sensations, or their suppression. A possible membrane explanation for these effects is suggested by an intracellular analysis of the effects of a brief electrical pulse applied to cat motor cortex. Rosenthal el al., (1967) showed the initial response was a relatively brief EPSP with, or without, action potentials followed by a prolonged IPSP. (Unfortunately, the large stimulus artifact with nearby MC stimulation has so far precluded such direct evidence of the effects of an MC pulse). In the following account, we tentatively attribute the positive sensations to EPSPs and action potentials and the suppressive phenomena to IPSPs

1. The role of the frontal lobes in accessing perceptual systems

Results

(A)   Somatosensory sensations

A focal MC stimulus to the motor or premotor cortex can elicit a projected sense of movement in the contralateral hand. Clearly, the perception of movement might result from afferent feedback from overt movement or from movements too small to be detected visually. A critical control was to stimulate the frontal lobe after inflating a cuff on the upper arm above arterial pressure and waiting 25-35 min for ischemic paralysis (with EMG monitoring) and insentience of the hand to tactile and proprioceptive stimulation. Under such conditions where afferent feedback was excluded, clearly localized projected sensations of flexion or extension were experienced, the magnitude of the perceived movement being related to the intensity of the MC stimulus (Amassian et al., 1989). These findings were confirmed in a subject additionally paralyzed with a muscle relaxant and artificially ventilated (Gandevia et al., 1993).

The projected sense of movement has been mapped under such ischemic block and remapped after relief of the block by readmission of the circulation (Fig. 1). In the hope of extending the time for mapping beyond that tolerable for ischemic block, we attempted to map the central sense of movement in two quadriplegic adults, who had sustained the spinal cord injury two years previously. Surprisingly, reports of digit movement were scarce, perhaps not unrelated to the wide expansion of the motor representation of proximal, spared muscles (Levy et al., 1990). This negative finding is consistent with the lack of a projected sense of movement in a patient with a long history of large afferent fiber loss (Cole and Sedgwick, 1992). Apparently, in the chronic absence of a normal 'validating' afferent feedback, the projected sense of movement map in the body scheme becomes attenuated.

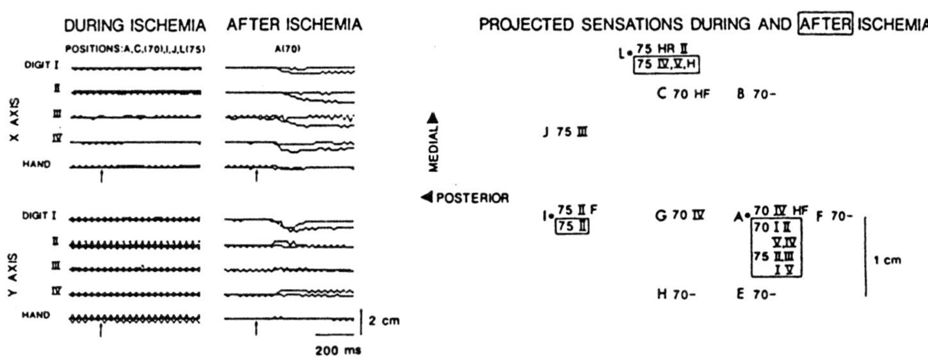

Figure 1. Mapping the projected sense of movement elicited by MC stimulation of motor cortex during ischemic block of distal arm. Left; superimposed traces showing absence and recovery of digit movements, respectively, during and after ischemic block. Right; each position of the tip of an ovoid MC (5.5 x 6 cm, o.d.) is indicated by a black dot with an alphabetical letter (A to L). I is approximately in the interaural axis and 3 cm from the midline. In two other subjects, the digit area was more lateral. (Fig. 1 reproduced from Amassian et al., 1995).

Another type of projected sensation elicited by frontal lobe stimulation is paresthesia, likened by subjects variously to tingling, or to an electrical stimulus to a digital nerve (Amassian et al., 1991). The projected paresthesias differ from the sense of movement in that paresthesias 1) can only be elicited from a minority, probably less than 30% of the population; 2) readily fatigue with repeated stimulation; 3) may only occur in a restricted part of the hand (for example subject 1 in Amassian et al., 1991).

As indicated in the Introduction, *single* MC pulses to parietal lobe fail to elicit a projected sensation. The difference between frontal and parietal lobe MC stimulation is illustrated in Fig. 2. However, *repetitive* MC stimulation of the parietal lobe can elicit projected sensations as was previously known from using repetitive electrical stimulation (for example, Penfield and Boldrey, 1937; Libet et al., 1964).

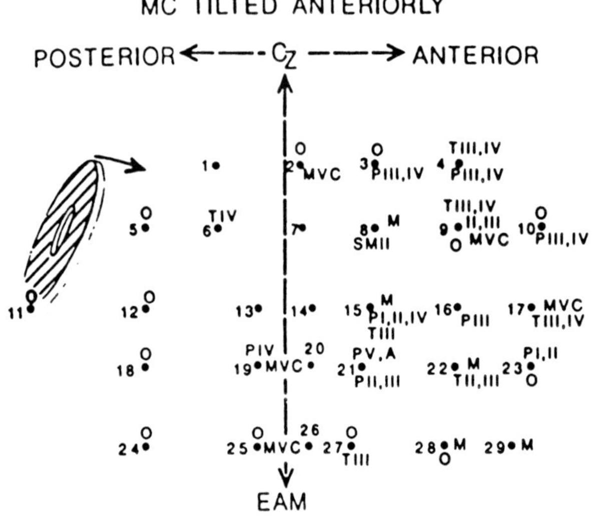

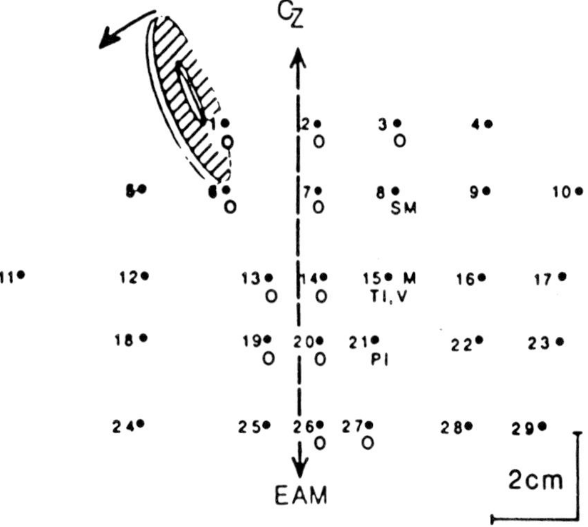

Figure 2. Mapping the cerebral cortex in a subject reporting paresthesias. The edge of a large (14 cm, o.d.), or a smaller (6.5 cm, o.d) round MC was used for focal stimulation. The coils were tilted anteriorly (top), or posteriorly (below) to direct the stimulation towards frontal and parietal lobes, respectively. A numbered black dot indicates the position of the midpoint of the contacting edge; the reported responses to the small and large MCs are indicated above and below, respectively. Any motor responses are indicated to the right of the dot. Abbreviations are: EAM, external auditory meatus; A, arm; P, paresthesias in digit I to IV; T, touch; SM, sense of movement or sensation in a tendon; M and MVC, motor responses in relaxed and voluntarily contracted muscle, respectively. (Fig. 2 reproduced from Amassian et al, 1995).

(B)   Facilitating Phosphenes

A puzzling feature of our early experience with MC stimulation of the occipital lobe was the difficulty in confirming that single pulses elicited phosphenes (cf Barker et al. 1985). The major difference in the diameter of the MCs used most likely explained the difference in findings. With the Magstim Corporation (14 cm, o.d.) MC used by Barker et al., (1985) and Meyer et al., (1991), a 'light' line phosphene is readily elicited, but with the Cadwell Laboratories (9.8 cm, o.d.) MC, such phosphenes are rarely elicited. Two factors may contribute to the difference in findings; with the larger diameter MC: (a) The induced electric field intensity is larger at greater subcortical depth (Barker et al., 1987) and (b) The *superior* MC windings are close to the frontal lobe and its projections; limb movement may accompany the effects on the visual system (Fig. 3).

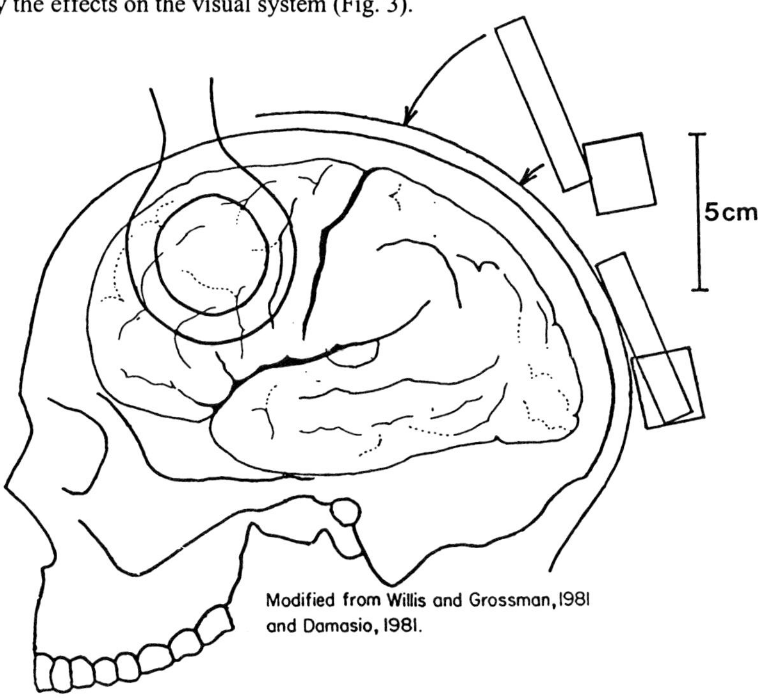

Figure 3. Diagram showing typical frontal and occipital locations of MCs in relations to scalp and brain. Note *lateral* views of brain (modified from Damasio, 1981) and its relation to the skull (modified from Willis and Grossman, 1981) are combined with the *midline* aspects of 14 cm and 9.4 cm round MCs. The arrows indicate the effect of conforming the superior windings of the larger coil to the scalp.

The effect of frontal lobe stimulation on perception of phosphenes elicited by occipital stimulation is of special interest because, unlike projected somatosensory sensations, the MC stimulation of frontal lobe is at a great physical distance from the corresponding primary cortical receiving area. The Cadwell round MC (9.8 cm, o.d.) was oriented with inferior windings symmetrically across the midline over calcarine cortex. The frontal lobe stimulus was given through an ovoid (5.5 x 6 cm, o.d.), or figure 8 MC (5 x 10 cm), with coil windings mainly anterior to motor cortex. The subject was masked and usually had eyes closed. The occipital stimulus alone elicited little or no light phosphenes; when followed by a frontal lobe pulse that alone elicited no visual sensation, the combination resulted in clear white, or colored phosphenes (Amassian et al., 1994). The optimal interstimulus intervals lay between 0-75 ms. The phosphenes were usually complex, for example bundles of light lines, curved or zig zag lines and infrequently were simple spots (Fig. 4).

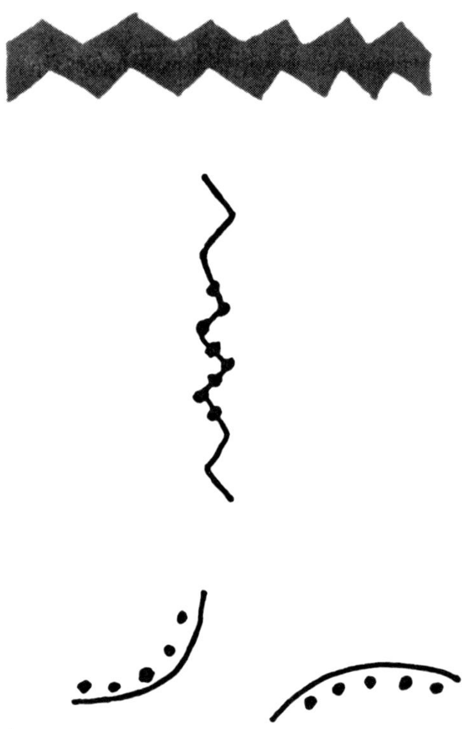

Figure 4. Examples of phosphenes elicited with occipital followed by frontal lobe stimulation after different delays. The phosphenes were light against a dark background.

The question arises as to whether the sites of facilitated phosphenes reflect the sites of the frontal or the occipital MC stimuli. By using a double square MC (7x 14 cm) to deliver the occipital stimulus to one side, it could clearly be shown that the location of the phosphene facilitated by frontal lobe stimulation depended on the site of occipital stimulation. For example, when the junction of the double square MC was horizontally oriented on the *right* occiput just above the inion and with the coil bifurcation close to the midline, the facilitated phosphene was a series of bright lines in the *left* visual field.

(C)   Facilitating visual perception of faint linguistic symbols

A difficulty with frontal lobe facilitation of phosphenes is the dependence on subjective reports, which cannot readily be statistically tested. We therefore adapted the visual suppression paradigm (described below), reducing the luminance of 4 alphabetic letters to a level permitting an average detection of only 1-2 letters per trial. The horizontal array subtended a visual angle of 2.5°. Although flashed on a single 1/60 sec sweep, phototransistor recordings disclosed a rapid decay of luminance of the letters by 2 ms. Anterior frontal cortical stimulation with the ovoid MC (5.5 x 6 cm, o.d.), eg, 20 ms after the visual stimulus, increased the number of letters correctly reported (proportionality test, P values ranged from 0.05 to 0.01). Some subjects reported an apparent brightening of the letters, but such effect was not a necessary condition for the enhanced accuracy of the report.

Unexpectedly, at sites near those improving accuracy, the frontal lobe stimulus was followed by a swift, confident, but erroneous report. The subjects misperceived the letters, but the reponse appeared too swift to exemplify the confabulations seen with certain brain lesions. Possibly enhanced perception of only *portions* of the letters with incorrect synthesis thereof led to the false report (Mari et al, 1996).

Discussion of role of frontal lobes in perception

The remarkable efficacy of single MC pulses delivered to the frontal lobe in accessing or enhancing sensory perception raises a number of questions. The subjects in the above experiments were alert and focused on the required task. Therefore, it is unclear how these findings relate to the attention mechanisms studied by Fuster (1980). Initially, we attributed the projected sense of movement to subcortical connections with specific thalamic or dorsal column nuclei and related it to the regulation of skilled movement (Amassian et al., 1989). However, MC stimulation of the cerebello-frontal cortical projection does not lead to a conscious sense of limb movement (Amassian et al, 1992b). Given the traditional role of the cerebellum in 'unconscious' regulation of skilled movement, it appears more likely that the projected sense of movement depends on the powerful connections of the frontal lobe to intralaminar (Amassian et al., 1991) and other higher level thalamic nuclei, and hence relates to the conscious sense of having "willed" the movement (Amassian et al., 1995).

The finding that powerful *local* MC pulses to parietal or occipital cortex do not elicit sensations, (although such stimuli clearly elicit movements from motor cortex) suggests that *briefly* exciting large numbers of cortical columns in primary cortical receiving areas is not a sufficient condition for sensations. Brindley and Lewin (1968) showed that focal repetitve electrical stimulation through a grid implanted over calcarine cortex of a blind person elicited a *spot* phosphene. Usually, several foci had to be stimulated simultaneously to elicit a line phosphene. Therefore, the finding that additional frontal lobe stimulation elicited a report of complex line phosphenes implies that the occipital stimulus must have stimulated many visual cortical, probably calcarine, columns without reaching consciousness, unless the frontal lobe was activated.

The diagram in Fig. 5 summarizes the findings. At the left, single localized electrical or MC pulses applied to the primary somatosensory or visual receiving areas do not readily elicit projected sensations. In the middle, repetitive stimuli have long been known to elicit projected sensations, possibly through opening an input or output gate related to cortical projections to intralaminar and other higher level thalamic nuclei. At the right, a frontal lobe stimulus, through powerful connections with these nuclei, opens the gate to responses to, for example, single occipital stimuli. The localized, projected somatosensory sensations elicited by frontal lobe stimulation present a problem, because Corkin et al, (1970) clearly showed the permanent loss of fine somesthesis after postcentral gyrectomy. By analogy with the dual stimulation of frontal and visual cortex, the frontal cortical stimulus probably both opens the thalamic gate and activates transynaptically the parietal lobe (dotted line). The diagram does not imply that the normal flow of afferent input with retinal or somatosensory stimulation must transit the frontal lobes as a necessary condition for perception. Patients with temporary akinetic mutism following bilateral frontal lesions, after recovery can report accurately sensory experiences occurring while they were mute.

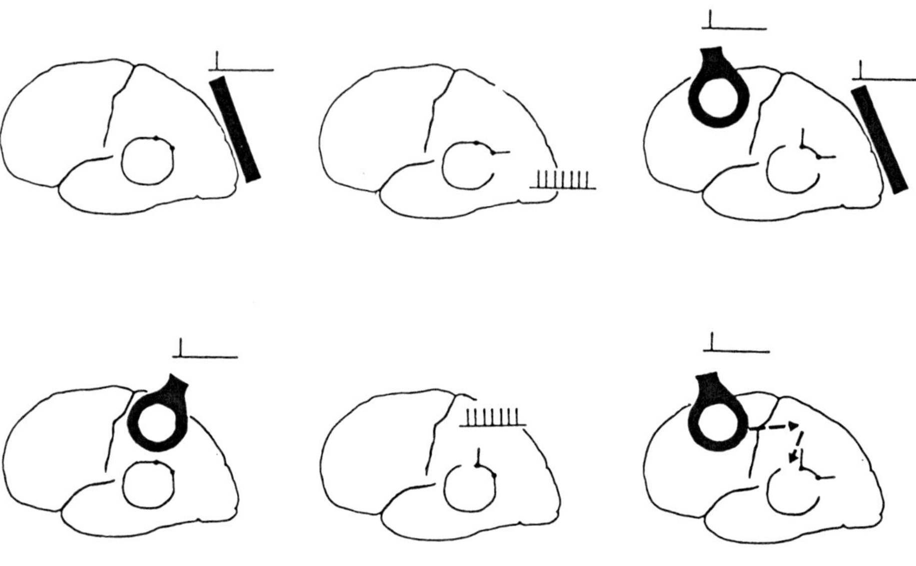

Figure 5. The diagram contrasts the effects on a hypothetical thalamic gate of single (left) and repetitive (middle) MC stimuli to primary visual (above) and somatosensory (below) areas. At right, single MC stimuli to frontal and primary receiving areas are combined. Thalamic gate is "open" in the middle and at right.

While a powerful, but brief activation of VI neurons is not a sufficient condition for visual perception, are any aspects of visual perception related closely in time to VI activity? The perception of an "A" when rapidly flashed is presumably related to a higher language area rostral to VI. However, the subject can 'deconstruct' the "A" into lines situated in a particular part of the eyefield and with a particular orientation, i.e., to VI type receptive fields, but not to spots. We suggest that VI activity is directly related to such perceptual deconstruction. More direct evidence is provided by the increased metabolic activity in VI associated with visual imagery, where there is no afferent visual stimulation (Kosslyn et al., 1993; Menon et al, 1996). Similarly, subjects previously repeatedly stimulated tactually on the tip of the index finger showed an increased flow in the contralateral somatosensory finger area when they only focused their attention on the tip of the finger without peripheral stimulation (Roland, 1981). Thus, both in the visual and the somatosensory system, activities in the primary cortical receiving areas are immediately related to some aspect, even imagined, of the percept. However, such localized activities hardly account for the common perceptual experience that when viewing the external world, one is aware of the texture of the seat of the chair upon which one is seated, despite there being no evidence of visual activity in the postcentral gyrus or somatosensory input to VI. An all-encompassing perceptual experience requires a near simultaneous combination of sensory modalities, which can plausibly be subserved by reverberation between cortex and thalamus (Llinas and Ribary, 1993; Joliot et al, 1994).

2. *The timing of perception*

Results

The parametric measurements of Libet et al. (1964) established that repetitive electrical stimulation of the exposed postcentral gyrus had to last at least 0.3-0.5 sec before the patient reported a projected sensation. This delay was taken to be a *minimum* delay for conscious perception, which could clearly take longer. Others have attempted to deal with the philosophical implications of these findings (for example Dennett, 1991; Penrose, 1990; Glynn, 1990). However, because *single* MC pulses to frontal lobe can access consciousness and lead to somatosensory sensations, the evidence of *minimum* train duration with postcentral stimulation is invalid as a measure of the minimum delay for perception. While the somatosensory responses to frontal lobe stimulation do not directly yield the time delay of perception, they open the possibility of much shorter delays than 0.3-0.5 sec.

We approached the problem of timing perception by recording the time flow of information from a flashed linguistic symbol to its vocalization. Fig. 6 summarizes the delays at the output end from visual cortex, and the motor output from frontal lobe subserving vocalization, with an intervening time gap requiring further analysis. The linguistic symbols, for example, 3 alphabetic letters, or a numeral are flashed on a 1/60 sec trace and individually subtend a visual angle of 0.4-1.0°. The earliest arrival at V1 is estimated at approximately 60 ms. When a single stimulus delivered through a round MC (9.8 cm, o.d.) was delayed 120-140 ms, the letters were recognized, implying that their representation had been transmitted from V1 (and perhaps V2) within about 130 ms (Amassian et al., 1989; 1993a).

Turning to the frontal cortical output subserving vocalization, the latency of extrinsic laryngeal muscle responses, specifically contralateral Sternohyoid and Sternothyroid muscles, is a function of which frontal area is excited. When stimulated focally by the MC during facilitation by vocalization of a linguistic symbol, 4 frontal areas can be differentiated (Fig. 9 in Amassian et al., 1995). Brief latencies as early as 6-8 ms were elicited from motor cortex, but latencies were 13-20 ms from presumed Broca's Area, SMA and the foot of the precentral gyrus, which is cytoarchitecturally Area 6 (Campbell, 1905). The difference in latency is illustrated in the superimposed upper and lower laryngeal EMGs (Fig. 6, lower middle). An average delay of 10 ms is allowed for this portion of the motor pathway. Finally, an average delay of 75 ms is allowed for the delay between activation of the laryngeal and abdominal expiratory muscles and the sound production, a delay which is significantly increased if the subject is not warned against inspiring just before the visual stimulus. Subtracting (130 + 10 + 75) = 215 ms from the mean latency of 345 ms for vocalization, yields an intervening delay of 130 ms (cf slightly differing values among groups; Amassian et al, 1993b; Cracco et al. 1996).

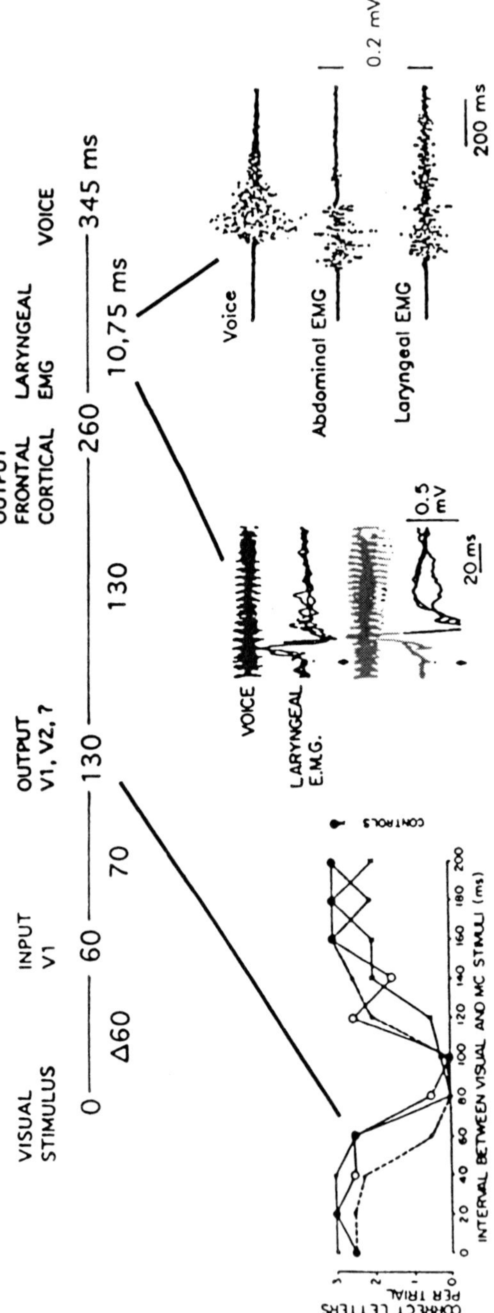

Figure 6. The diagram shows the timing of some events between the visual stimulus and its rapid vocalization (above) combined with illustrative recordings (below). Above: explained in text. Below: at left, suppression of responses to 3 flashed letters as a function of delay of the MC occipital pulse (reproduced from Amassian et al, 1989c); in middle, paired laryngeal muscle EMGs and voice recordings of responses elicited by motor cortical (top) and higher level, frontal cortical MC stimulation (bottom) while voicing "Aaaah" (reproduced from Amassian et al, 1995); at right, timing of recordings of abdominal expiratory and laryngeal EMGs compared with voice.

Does the intervening delay include routing of the representation through the traditional intermediary pathway of Wernike's Area, dominant Supramarginal and Angular gyri to Broca's Area? Posner et al. (1988) demonstrated with PET scanning a route to frontal lobe that appeared to bypass the intermediary structures. We used the following argument: If the visual cortical output to frontal lobe follows a direct route, then the frontal lobe output to laryngeal (and facial) muscles should be synaptically facilitated soon after visual cortical output has occurred. When the oval MC (5.5 x 6 cm, o.d.) was used for left frontal cortical stimulation, facilitation of the laryngeal and lower facial muscles was first detected 120-140 ms after the flashed visual stimulus (Fig. 7). An important practical detail in preventing non-specific facilitation was to adjust the MC stimulus intensity just below threshold when it was delayed 60 ms, i.e., given at an interval too brief to allow for the visual stimulus to have affected frontal cortex (Amassian et al., 1993b). While supporting a direct route from occipital to left frontal lobe, the above findings do not imply that the traditional structures subserving language functions are irrelevant to the task; it seems very unlikely that a massive lesion of such structures would permit a patient to understand the task, much less execute it swiftly. Thus a distinction must be drawn between dynamic routing of the earliest representation and a steady-state influence by traditional structures, which maintain the optimal functioning of the frontal lobe (cf, the role of frontal lobe output in maintaining segmental reflexes). It may be noted that early facilitation of laryngeal responses could not be elicited by right frontal lobe stimulation (Amassian et al., 1995).

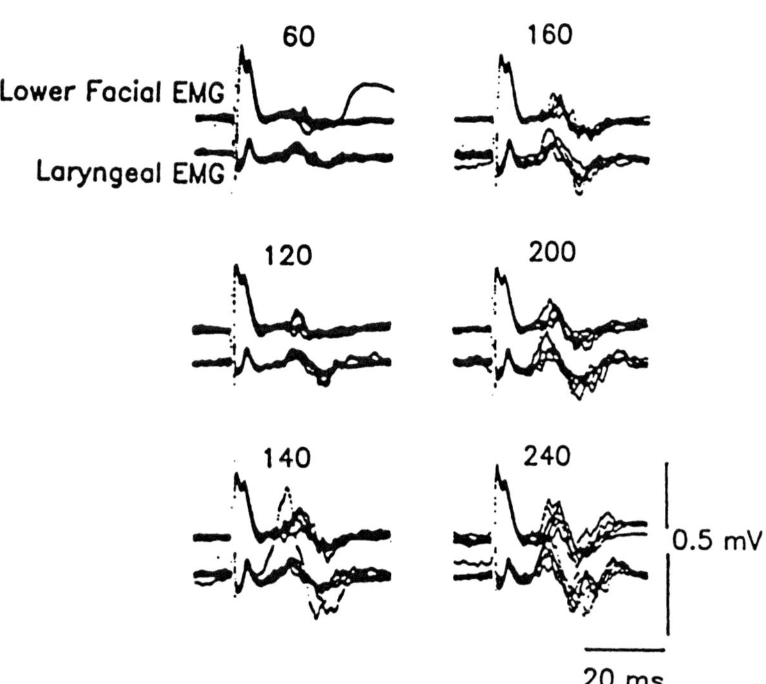

Figure 7. Facilitation of MC elicited lower facial and laryngeal EMG responses to frontal cortical stimulation by antecedent visual stimulus. Superimposed EMG traces shown at the indicated MC pulse delays. Facilitation only slight at 120 ms, but marked by 140 ms.

Further study of the facilitation of laryngeal responses disclosed that the occipito-frontal influence is delayed if the task is restricted to responding to a subclass only of numerals, i.e., to 'odd' or to 'even' numerals only. Such condition adds approximately 70 ms to the latency of the behavioral response and similarly delays the onset of detectable laryngeal response facilitation. Thus, visual cortical output does not automatically facilitate the frontal lobe but is behaviorally gated most likely in frontal rather than occipital cortex.

Fractionating the intervening 130 ms was attempted by giving subjects (4 Spanish speaking students) the following tasks to be performed at maximum speed: 1) Make a noise whatever digit is flashed; 2) Blurt out without first attempting to perceive the flashed numeral; 3) Perceive the number, then vocalize it. As expected, making a noise entailed the least latency, 218 ± 8 ms (mean, S.E.M.). Blurting out the numeral increased the latency, whose value was related to whether the answer was correct (332 ±8 ms), or incorrect (261 ±8 ms). Finally, perceiving the numeral, then saying it (346 ±15 ms) led to few if any errors and only a small difference in latency from that of *correct* blurted responses (Fig. 8). We interpret the latency difference between the blurted *incorrect* response less that of the noise response, i.e., (261-218) = 43 ms as an approximate measure of the *average* motor programming time. By "motor programming time" is meant that needed to initiate the sequence in the frontal cortical output that produces the correct sequence of muscle activations which lead to the phonemes characterizing a particular numeral. The remaining delay (130-43) = 87 ms is associated objectively with great accuracy in reporting and subjectively with having first perceived the numeral (Amassian et al., 1996). We refer to the 87 (rounded to 85) ms as the 'A' process.

Similar tests on *English* speaking colleagues revealed a shorter mean delay of the 'A' process (approximately 70 ms), but this may reflect the larger number of tests on our departmental faculty. (An important source of error identified in one subject blurting the response was an indeterminate noise immediately preceding (for example by 67 ms) the phoneme, which characterized the start of the correct numeral. This leads to an under estimate of the true delay for blurting the correct response).

Another approach to conscious intervention stems from *error* correction. Two types were identified: (a) Vocalizing initially with the wrong phoneme. For example, a '3' was flashed, but the subject started with "F" at 277 ms but switched 72 ms later to "REE" at 344 ms. (b) Vocalizing when the subject should have been silent, for example, responding to an even number instead of responding only to odd numbers. The correction was manifested by abrupt truncation of the external oblique muscle activity 72 ms after it commenced, externally visible as a halt in expiration.

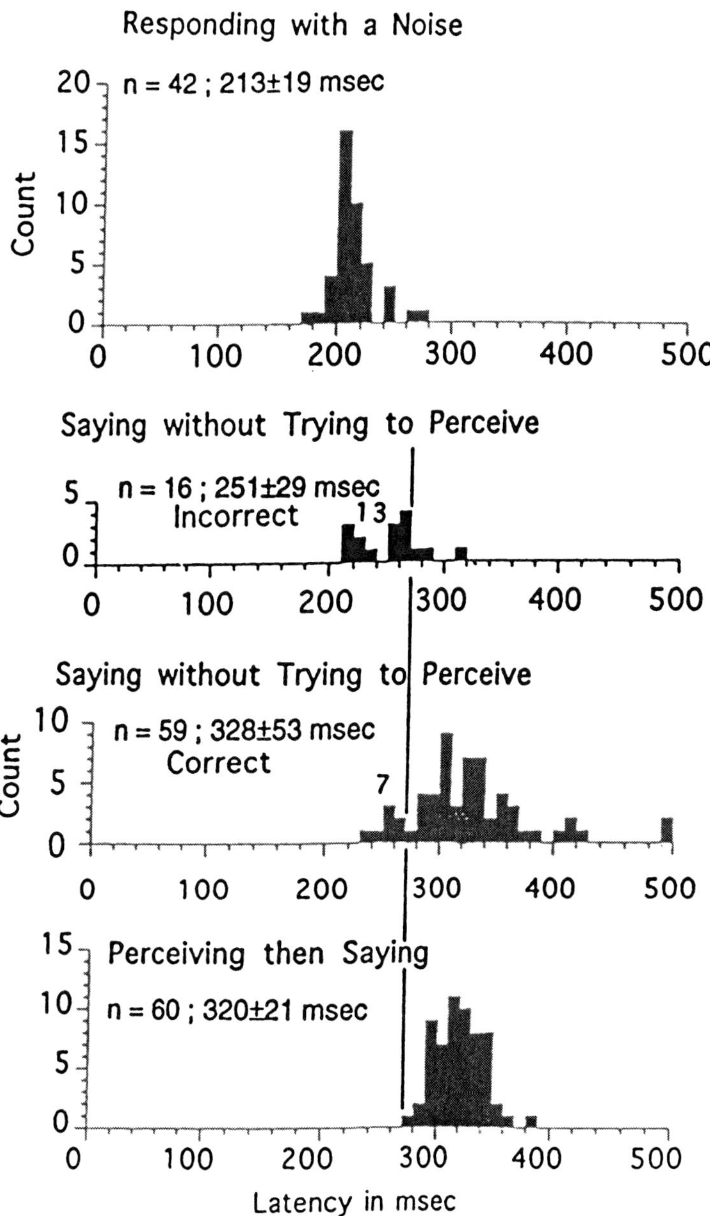

Figure 8. Distributions of latencies of vocalization to a flashed numeral in same subject performing various tasks. From above downwards: (1) responding with a noise regardless of what was flashed; (2) incorrect responses when not trying to perceive it; (3) correct responses when not trying to perceive it; (4) first perceiving, then responding. Other details in text.

Discussion of the perceptual delay

Introspection can clearly be unreliable in defining causal relationships. A naive subject withdrawing a limb from an injurious stimulus would likely attribute the withdrawal to the pain felt, a causal relationship easily refuted by observing the spinal human. Is the introspective sense that perception of a linguistic symbol precedes its *accurate* vocalization a similar type of error? First, it must be emphasized that the visual stimulus is a randomly selected linguistic symbol, i.e., a member of a *large* set. Subsequently, an appropriate motor response must be selected from a correspondingly large set; the pattern of muscle activations related to vocalizing a succession of specific phonemes that define the sound of a particular numeral is clearly more complicated than a finger tap, as used in classical reaction time experiments, or a limb withdrawal. Preprogramming of the linguistic responses to random presentations is very unlikely. It can readily be investigated by having subjects vocalize the same numeral, regardless of what was flashed. Such stereotyped vocal responses added only 6 ±5.5 ms to the latency of the noise response, implying that motor pattern for vocalizing a *predetermined* numeral had been preprogrammed, unlike the responses to a random presentation.

We point also to the similarity of the 'A' delay to correction delays. Furthermore, *driven* repetitive arithmetic calculations yield limiting values of 88 ms and 98 ms for addition and subtraction of 2 digits, respectively (Amassian et al., 1993c). Thus, a series of different mental activities, which are all introspectively consciously controlled have delays of 70-100 ms. The convergence of these separate measurements makes likely but does not *prove* that the 'A' process is the delay for conscious perception, or that mental arithmetic delay reflects the delay for conscious processing. Clearly, many brain operations, for example in tracking an accelerating target involve sophisticated, *rapid* computations of which the subject is consciously totally unaware. However, when inputed through linguistic symbols, except in human 'lightning' calculators, the simplest arithmetic operations require far more time.

The question arises whether the 'A' process can be bypassed in answering correctly. In Fig. 8, vertical lines define vocalized, blurted responses occurring earlier than the earliest vocalized after perception. Only 7 in 59 correct responses fall into the early latency category. The total number of correct and incorrect fast responses is (7 + 13) = 20. The proportion of fast, correct response is 7/20 instead of that expected by chance (1/9), permitting rejection of the null hypothesis (proportionality test; P < 0.05). In the distributions of the other 3 subjects similarly analyzed, the null hypothesis could not be rejected. Thus, without the 'A' process, not only is the probability of a correct answer much less than 1, but in 3 out of 4 subjects, the answer was only correct by chance. We interpret the correct, blurted out responses with mean latency similar to that of 'perceive then vocalize' as reflecting an inability to perform the task, i.e., vocalizing was postponed *until* perception had occurred. Indeed, one colleague, characteristically thoughtful, could not perform the experiment; no errors occurred with blurting, and latencies were similar in the two tests.

Vocalizing accurately a flashed numeral *before* its perception poses the following discontinuity. Presumably, it is not in doubt that a numeral can be perceived and its vocalization arbitrarily postponed. Suppose now the delay for vocalization is halved successively until a minimum delay is reached between the visual stimulus and accurate vocalization. Does a crossover occur with perception of the numeral now significantly following its vocalization? That is, does introspection become misleading? We think it more likely that the introspective ordering of events, correct for long and intermediate delays, is maintained. In the interest of efficiency, the 'A' process or perception would precede the motor programming for expression of the recognized numeral. Conceivably, motor programming for all possible answers commences first, the 'A' process eventually selecting the correct program. Such sequence would lengthen the time delay for the 'A' process and perception, but appears very inefficient compared with perception followed by selective motor programming.

The neural substrata for consciously vocalizing a flashed numeral are not restricted to the cerebral cortex. Hunter and Jasper (1949) have emphasized the role of the intralaminar thalamic nuclei in consciousness. Lesions in the walls of the third ventricle have long been known to be associated with stupor or coma, and are clearly incompatible with fast linguistic responses to visual linguistic input (Plum and Posner, 1990). In the first part of this report, we emphasized the connections of frontal lobe with the intralaminar and higher thalamic nuclei in subserving its various roles in perception. Clearly, these connections with thalamus would be expected to play a role also in the perceptual delays described in this section.

3. Temporary relief of induced pain by repetitive magnetic stimulation of parietal lobe

Results

Repetitive electrical stimulation of the precentral cortex was shown in several centers to relieve chronic, central "deafferentiation type" pain (Tsubokkawa et al., 1993; Peyron et al., 1995). Our attention was drawn to the possibility that the Neglect Syndrome (Heilman and Van Den Abell, 1990), associated especially with nondominant parietal association cortical lesions, might also include a reduced sensitivity to induced pain. If so, the hypothesis to be tested was that repetitive transcranial magnetic stimulation, by extended inhibition of cortical function (Amassian et al., 1993a; Pascual Leone et al., 1994), would lead to diminution of the induced pain. The Cadwell Laboratories repetitive MC stimulator was used in all the experiments below.

Initial observations were made on a 62 yr old male patient, with a right-sided parietal lobe vascular lesion, clearly visible in the CT scan. Clinically, the patient had left-sided neglect and left-sided lower facial weakness, but normal motor functions bilaterally in both extremities. Simultaneous repetitive digit flexions after brachial artery occlusion in both arms (Lewis et al., 1931) disclosed a clear asymmetry in the number of contractions before the patient stopped contracting, the contralateral (left) side continuing for 40% more contractions rather than the right.

We chose ischemic muscle pain of exercising forearm muscles, because the pain is easily produced in normal subjects, can be self-induced to a distinct but tolerable level (arbitrarily designated as level 4) and is maintained after contractions are stopped. Five of us were subjects. Because no motor responses were elicited by repetitive MC stimulation at the posterior parietal sites used, it appeared necessary to assay physiologically the stimulation intensities so that those used in different subjects could be compared. The single pulse threshold intensity was determined for movement in the voluntarily contracting hand (TIVC), i.e., a slightly greater intensity was required than for minimal EMG responses. (With a background voluntary contraction, the MC threshold intensity was usually lower and more consistent than during relaxation).

In four of the subjects, stimulation through the ovoid (5.5 x 6 cm, o.d.) MC with 10 pulses at 20 Hz gave delayed, temporary relief of the ischemic pain when a number of posterior parietal sites were stimulated. With the handle of the MC lateral and the tip pointing medially, ischemic pain relieving sites were found when the *rostral* windings were located from 6-3.5 cm posterior to the line joining Cz to the external auditory meatus and with the MC tip 0-6 cm to the right of the midline. The effective intensities ranged from 1.05-1.4 x TIVC; 1.2 ±0.16 (mean, S.D.). The two subjects that provided precise timing of the diminution and later return of ischemic pain showed a delay in pain relief of 3-6 sec from the start of the (0.5 sec) train, with return of the pain 30-35 sec later. A 'rebound' of later enhanced pain occurred after some MC stimulations.

As described above, the parietal cortical region effective in reliefing pain could lie anywhere under the ovoid coil windings. The diminished efficacy when the rostral windings were moved 8 cm posterior to the interaural line implies that cortex under the caudal windings in the 6 cm MC location was less effective than under the rostral windings at the 6 cm location. This was confirmed by the efficacy of more focal stimulation with the junction of a double square MC (7 x 14 cm) at this location (Fig. 9). (Under the junction, the induced electric field intensity is 2x that under the lateral coils.) Also compared is the reproducibility of the pain relief at 60% stimulator output, with increased relief at 65% output (1.45 x TIVC with this MC). We estimate that the junction lay over the right posterior parietal lobe, probably close to the supramarginal and angular gyri.

Pain relief varied from being complete to about 50%, i.e. the subjective pain level fell to 0-2. Pain relief was not accompanied by numbness, or loss of sense of the existence of the arm, and some subjects reported a warm, pleasurable sensation replacing the pain.

No seizures were encountered with the parameters of repetitive magnetic stimulation used (cf Pascual-Leone et al., 1993). The fifth subject had no relief of pain and had a TIVC among the highest in the group. Utilizing 1.4x this value or more for repetitive stimulation in this subject was considered potentially hazardous with this MC and was not tested.

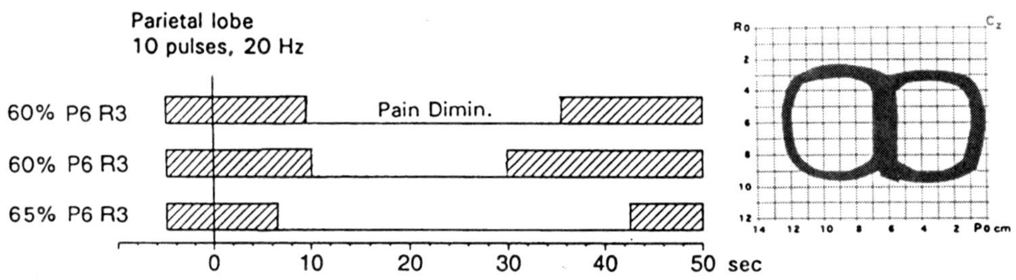

Figure 9. Diagram showing timing of pain relief at the indicated intensities of repetitive stimulation and position of the double square MC. The junction of the MC is orientated lateromedial and is 6 cm posterior to the interaural line, with its medial bifurcation 3 cm to the right of the midline. Subject is strongly right-handed. The intensities indicated on the left are the dial readings. The maximum output intensity is approximately 90% of the MES-10 single pulse model, i.e. a little less than 2 T. Measurement of induced pulses after the first pulse with a search coil disclosed a reduction by 10% at 20 Hz. Therefore, the average intensity of the 9 impulses in the train after the first at 65% was 58.5%.

The effect of parietal lobe stimulation was also tested on cutaneous pain. Two *shallow* indentations, 6 mm apart, were drilled in the left thumb nail and filled with electrode jelly. Two Ag ball electrodes were placed in the indentations and taped to the nail. An electric pulse of for example, 1.25 mA at 1 Hz elicited a repeated, uniformly intense pain with a clear later 'hot' component. Using a potentiometer to signal pain level, clear delayed temporary diminution of the pain was observed at various parietal sites stimulated 1.4-1.6 x TIVC (Fig. 10).

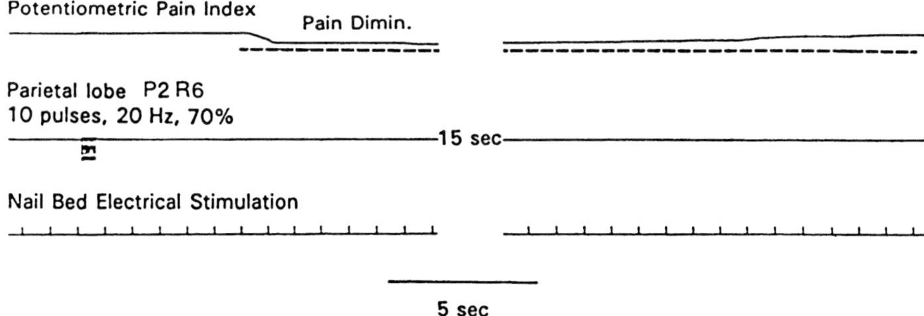

Figure 10. Potentiometic recording of timing of relief of nail-bed pain after repetitive parietal lobe stimulation by the MC. Subject strongly right-handed. Nail bed electrical stimulation at 1.25 Hz. Although each stimulus elicited a discrete pain sensation, the pain is represented as a steady level until it changed.

The above account deals exclusively with relief of acute, induced pain. One of us had severe pain in the *right* neck induced most probably by prolonged exposure to a cold airjet. Stimulation with the ovoid MC of either the right (non-dominant, ipsilateral), or the left parietal lobe with 9 pulses at 20 Hz gave delayed temporary relief of the pain (intensity 1.6 x TIVC); 5 pulses gave no relief. Stimulation of either the left or the right prefrontal cortex with 9 pulses at 1.6x TIVC afforded no relief. Finally, it was noted that at the end of repeated stimulations in the session, the steady pain level had diminished. Although admittedly anectodal, this finding does raise the question of whether the therapeutic value of parietal lobe stimulation should be investigated.

Discussion of relief of induced pain by parietal lobe stimulation

Although this study was prompted by the phenomenon of the Neglect Syndrome, the eliciting of positive, pleasurable sensations in the ischemic limb following repetitive MC stimulation of parietal lobe, implies that the pain relief did not reflect classical neglect. The delayed timing of the relief clearly differs from the early timing of visual suppression, even when repetitive occipital MC stimuli are used (Amassian et al., 1993a). Thus, it is unlikely that production of parietal IPSPs that are delayed for many seconds is responsible for the relief. Release of endorphins is a possibility and should be tested by pretreating the subjects with Naloxone.

Acknowledgement

We thank F. Monje, F. Cardenas, E. Rey and M. Lamphrea for assisting with the vocalization reaction time experiments.

Plenary discussion

Wall P.: Could you relate your parietal cortex stimulation effect to the installed neglect seen with parietal cortex lesions and their alteration with vestibular stimulation?

Amassian V.: A clear possibility is that transcranial magnetic stimulation of the parietal lobe produces a temporary "neglect" of the induced pain, as I think you suggest. Somewhat against this is that several subjects did not merely have reduction of the ischemic pain, but pleasant sensations in the limb.

Seltzer Z.: Have you been studying "split brain" subjects to test whether the contralateral cortex contributes to the gating efficacy of the frontal lobe. Have you tried to train subjects with repeated sensory stimulation of one target in the body, and then tried to remap the area in the cortex where stimulation elicits a motor output?

Amassian V.: No, we haven't studied split brain patients. This would be very interesting in relation to the transfer of perceptual enhancement. I have been in contact for future collaboration at UCLA with the neurosurgeon David Bogen, who did many callosotomies. However, this was in relation to differential left versus right hemisphere effects on lymphocyte subsets.
Concerning your second question, the NIH group have evidence that experience increases the cortical area related to the sensory input provoking motor output.

Apkarian V.: Regarding your comment about the details of somatosensory representation, we have now evidence with fMRI showing that across a population of subjects finger tip representation looks random, but not in single subjects. We are very interested in TEA for pain relief. Since our fMRI data show that in acute pain parietal cortex is important while in chronic pain prefrontal cortex may be crucially involved. What is your experience of stimulating the prefrontal cortex for pain relief?

Amassian V.: The first question implies that it is not easy to transfer data from magnetic stimulation to fMRI and uptake techniques. I may point out that if representations of digits were really separate, cortical lesions might be expected to lead to clear deficits in individual digits early in the evolution of the lesion.
The second question relates to the very interesting difference you showed between acute and chronic lesions. My own experience, admittedly anecdotal, when suffering from an acute right shoulder muscle spasm brought on by an air jet, was that a few days later, it was temporarily reduced by right and left parietal lobe stimulation, but not by right or left prefrontal stimulation even at increased strength.
A later thought: Could the increased flow in fMRI in prefrontal areas in chronic pain be related to depression or anxiety? It would be interesting to look for correlations between bloodflow and susceptibility to drugs acting on depression and anxiety.

References

Amassian VE, Cracco RQ, Maccabee PJ (1989a) A sense of movement elicited in paralyzed distal arm by focal magnetic coil stimulation of human motor cortex. Brain Res 479: 355-360.

Amassian VE, Cracco RQ and Maccabee PJ (1989b) Focal stimulation of human cerebral cortex with the magnetic coil: A comparision with electrical stimulation. Electroenceph clin Neurophysiol 74:401-416.

Amassian VE, Cracco RQ, Maccabee PJ, Cracco JB, Rudell A and Eberle L (1989c) Suppression of visual perception by magnetic coil stimulation of human occipital cortex. Electroenceph clin Neurophysiol 74:458-462.

Amassian VE, Quirk G and Stewart M (1990) A comparison of corticospinal activation by magnetic coil and electrical stimulation of monkey motor cortex. Electroenceph clin Neurophysiol 77:390-401.

Amassian VE, Somasundaram M, Rothwell JC, Britton T, Cracco JB, Cracco RQ, Maccabee PJ and Day BL (1991) Paraesthesias are elicited by single pulse, magnetic coil stimulation of motor cortex in susceptible humans. Brain 114:2505-2520.

Amassian VE, Eberle L, Maccabee PJ and Cracco RQ (1992a) Modelling magnetic coil excitation of human cerebral cortex with a peripheral nerve immersed in a brain-shaped volume conductor: The significance of fiber bending in excitation. Electroenceph clin Neurophysiol 85:291-301.

Amassian VE, Cracco RQ, Maccabee PJ and Cracco JB (1992b) Cerebello-frontal cortical projections in humans studied with the magnetic coil. Electroenceph clin Neurophysiol 95:265-272.

Amassian VE, Maccabee PJ, Cracco RQ, Cracco JB, Rudell AP and Eberle L (1993a) Measurement of information processing delays in human visual cortex with repetitive magnetic coil stimulation. Brain Res 605:317-321.

Amassian VE, Cracco RQ, Maccabee PJ, Cracco JB, Somasundaram M, Eberle L and Rudell A (1993b) The transfer time of symbolic visual information through human frontal cortex. J Physiol (Lond) 459:453P.

Amassian VE, Cracco RQ, Maccabee PJ, Cracco JB, Eberle L and Rudell A (1993c) The time cost of mental arithmetic and its relationship to conscious awareness. J Physiol (Lond) 467:97P.

Amassian VE, Hassan N, Cracco JB, Maccabee PJ, Cracco RQ and Henry K (1994) Combined magnetic stimulation of human frontal and calcarine cortex facilitates awareness of phosphenes. J Physiol (Lond) 477:57-57P.

Amassian VE, Cracco RQ, Maccabee PJ, Cracco JB and Henry K (1995) Some positive effects of transcranial magnetic stimulation. 79-106 In: Advances in Neurology:67, Negative Motor Phenomena (Fahn S, Hallett M, Lüders HO and Marsden CD, eds) Raven Press, New York

Amassian VE, Cracco RQ, Maccabee PJ, Cracco JB, Hassan N, Vergara M and Eberle L (1996) Does human perception of a visual symbol precede its correct vocalization? J Physiol (Lond) 491:74P.

Barker AT, Freeston IL, Jalinous R, Merton PA, Morton HB (1985) Magnetic stimulation of the human brain. J Physiol (Lond) 369:3P.

Barker AT, Freeston IL Jalinous R, Jarratt JA (1987) Magnetic stimulation of the human brain and peripheral nervous system: an introduction and the results of an initial clinical evaluation. Neurosurgery 20:100-109.

Barker AT, Garnham CW and Freeston IL (1991) Magnetic nerve stimulation: The effect of waveform on efficiency, determination of neural membrane time constants and the measurement of stimulator output. Electroenceph clin Neurophysiol, Suppl 43:227-237.

Brindley GA,and Lewin WS (1968) The sensations produced by electrical stimulation of the visual cortex. J Physiol (Lond) 196:479-493.

Campbell A W (1905) Histological studies on the localization of cerebral function. Cambridge University Press, Cambridge 360 pp.

Cole JD and Sedgwick EM (1992) The perceptions of force and movement in a man without large myelinated sensory afferents below the neck. J Physiol (Lond) 449:503-515.

Corkin S, Milner B and Rasmussen T (1970) Somatosensory thresholds: contrasting effects of postcentral gyrus and posterior parietal-lobe excisions. Arch Neurol 23:41-58.

Cracco RQ, Amassian VE, Maccabee PJ and Cracco JB (1996) Flow of symbolic visual information from retina to vocalization; Excepta Medica Int Congr Series 1101, Elsevier Science in press.

Damasio H (1981) Cerebral localization of the aphasias. In: Sarno MT, ed. Acquired aphasia. New York: Academic Press 27-50.

Dennett DC (1991) Consciousness explained. Little Brown, Boston pp 511.

Fuster JM The prefrontal cortex: Anatomy, physiology and neuropsychology of the frontal lobe. Raven Press, New York.

Gandevia SC Killiam K, McKenzie DK, Crawford M Allen GM. Gorman RB and Hales JP (1993) Respiratory sensations, cardiovascular control, kinaesthesia and transcranial stimulation during paralysis in humans. J Physiol (Lond) 470:85-108.

Glynn IM (1990) Consciousness and time. Nature 348:477-479.

Heilman KM, Van Den Abell T (1990) Right hemisphere dominance for attention: The mechanisms underlying hemispheric asymmetries of inattention (neglect). Neurol 30:327-330.

Hunter J and Jasper HH (1949) Effects of thalamic stimulation in unanesthetized animals. Electroenceph clin Neurophysiol 1:305-324.

Joliot M, Ribary U and Llinas R (1994) Human oscillatory brain activity near 40 Hz coexists with cognitive temporal binding. Proc Nat Acad Sci 91:11748-11751.

Kosslyn SM, Alpert NM, Thompson WL, Maljkovic V, Weise SB, Chabris CF, Hamilton SE, Rauch SL and Buonanno FS (1993) Visual mental imagery activates topographically organized visual cortex: PET investigations. J Cognit Neurosc 5:263-287.

Levy WJ, Jr, Amassian VE, Traaad M and Cadwell J (1990) Focal magnetic coil stimulation reveals motor cortical system reorganized in humans after traumatic quadriplegia. Brain Res 510:130-134.

Levy WJ, Amassian VE, Schmid UD and Jungreis C (1991) Mapping of motor cortex gyral sites non-invasively by transcranial magnetic stimulation in normal subjects and patients. Electroenceph clin Neurophysiol Suppl 43:51-75.

Lewis T Pickering GW and Rothchild P (1931) Observations upon muscular pain in intermittent claudication, Heart 15:359-383.

Libet B, Alberts WW, Wright EW, Delattre LD, Levin G and Feinstein B (1964) Production of threshold levels of conscious sensation by electrical stimulation of human somatosensory cortex. J Neurophysiol 27:546-578.

Llinas R and Ribary U (1993) Coherent 40 Hz oscillation characterizes dream state in humans. Proc Natl Acad Sci 90:2078-2081.

Maccabee PJ, Amassian VE, Eberle LP and Cracco RQ (1993) Magnetic coil stimulation of straight and bent amphibian and mammalian peripheral nerve in-vitro: Locus of excitation. J Physiol (Lond) 460:201-219.

Mari Z, Sagliocco L, Maccabee PJ, Cracco RQ Bodis-Wollner I and Amassian VE (1996) Magnetic stimulation of anterior frontal lobe can facilitate and distort human perception of language symbols. J Physiol (Lond) 495:131-132P.

Menon V, Desmond JE, Lim KO Demb JB, Spielmann D, and Pfefferbaum A (1996) Activation of primary visual cortex underlying visual imagery. Cognit Neurosc Soc Abstr, vol. 3.

Meyer B-U, Diehl R, Steinmetz H, Britton TH and Benecke R (1991) Magnetic stimuli applied over motor and visual cortex: influence of coil position and field polarity on motor responses, phosphenes, and eye movements. Electroenceph clin Neurophysiol Suppl. 43:121-134.

Pascual-Leone A, Houser CM, Reese K, Shotland LI, Grafman J, Sato S, Valls-Sole J, Brasil-Neto JP, Wasserman EM, Cohen LG, Hallett (1993) M Safety of rapid-rate transcranial magnetic stimulation in normal volunteers. Electroenceph clin Neurophysiol 89:120-130.

Pascual-Leone A, Gomez-Tortosa E, Grafman J Alway D, Nichelli P, Hallett M (1994) Induction of visual extinction by rapid-rate transcranial magnetic stimulation of parietal lobe. Neurol 44:494-498.

Penfield W and Boldrey E (1937) Somatic motor and sensory representation in the cerebral cortex of man as studied by electrical stimulation. Brain 60:389-443.

Penfield W and Roberts L (1959) Speech and brain mechanisms. Princeton University Press, Princeton.

Penrose R (1990) The Emperor's new mind. Oxford University Press, New York.

Peyron R, Garcia-Larrea L, Deiber MP, Cinotti L, Convers P, Sindou M, Mauguiere F and Laurent B (1995) Electrical stimulation of precentral cortical area in the treatment of central pain: electrophysiological and PET study. Pain 62 (3):275-286.

Plum F and Posner JB The diagnosis of stupor and coma. 3rd edition, Davis, Philadelphia.

Posner MI Petersen SR, Fox PT and Raichle (1988) ME Localization of cognitive operations in the human brain. Science 240:1627-1631.

Reilly JP (1989) Peripheral nerve stimulation by induced electric currents: exposure to time-varying magnetic fields. Med Biol Eng Comput 27:101-110.

Roland PE (1981) Somatotopical tuning of postcental gyrus during focal attention in man. A regional cerebral blood flow study. J Neurophysiol 46:744-754.

Rosenthal J, Waller HJ and Amassian VE (1967) An analysis of the activation of motor cortical neurons by surface stimulation. J Neurophysiol 30:844-858.

Roth BJ and Basser P (1990) A model of the stimulation of a nerve fiber by electromagnetic induction. IEEE Trans Biomed Eng 37:588-597.

Rothwell JC, Thompson PD, Day BL, Boyd S and Marsden CD (1991) Stimulation of the human motor cortex through the scalp. Exp Physiol 76:159-200.

Rothwell JC, Day BL and Amassian VE (1992) Near threshold electrical and magnetic transcranial stimuli activate overlapping sets of cortical neurones in humans. J Physiol (Lond) 452:109P.

Tasaki I Conduction of the nerve impulse. In: J. Field (Ed.), (1959) Handbook of Physiology. Amer. Physiol. Soc., Washington, DC; I (1):75-121.

Tsubokawa T, Katayama Y, Yamamoto T, Hirayama T and Koyama S (1993) Chronic motor cortex stimulation in patients with thalamic pain. J Neurosurg 78:393-401.

Willis WD, Jr and Grossman RG (1981) Medical neurobiology, neuroanatomical and neurophysiological principles basic to clinical neuroscience. Mosby, St. Louis.

Pharmacology

Design of Novel Nicotinic Acetylcholine Receptor Agonists with Potential Antinociceptive Activity

G.P. Basmadjian*, S. Singh*, K. Avor*, B. Pouw*, and T.W. Seale[+]
**Department of Medicinal Chemistry and Pharmaceutics*
College of Pharmacy
[+]Department of Pediatrics, Psychiatry and Behavioral Science
College of Medicine
University of Oklahoma Health Sciences Center
Oklahoma City, OK, USA

Introduction

Opioids are the major class of clinically available centrally-acting analgesics. However, the morphine-like antinociception of this class of drugs is not free from side effects and liability of abuse. The non-opioid analgesics have the inherent advantage of lacking opioid-related side effects. Epibatidine (Fig. 1), isolated in trace amounts by Daly et al. in 1992 from the Ecuadorian poison frog, *Epipedobates tricolor*, belongs to the non-opioid class of drugs, and has been shown to mediate its antinociceptive action through the nicotinic cholinergic system (Spande and Garraffo, 1992).

As with the $GABA_A$ receptor, much remains to be learned regarding exactly which nicotinic acetylcholine receptor (nAChR) subtypes are associated with particular central effects and behavioral responses. Medicinal chemistry research in the area of nicotinic agonists as therapeutic entities has been limited because of the negative connotations associated with the recreational use of (-)-nicotine in tobacco products. Nicotinic acetylcholine receptors are pentameric, ligand-gated ion channels belonging to a family of receptor complexes including the glycine (Betz,1990), $5\text{-}HT_3$ (Maricq et al. 1991) and $GABA_A$ (Wisden and Seeburg, 1992) receptors. The receptor creates a transmembrane ion channel (the gate), and acetylcholine (the ligand) serves as gatekeeper by interacting with the receptor to modulate passage of sodium, potassium and, in some cases, appreciable calcium ions through the channel. Unlike the muscle nAChRs, which are comprised of a, b, g (or e), and d subunits arranged as pentamer (with two a subunits), neuronal nAChRs are assembled from only two classes of subunits, a and b, and in some cases only an a subunit (Couturier et al. 1990). The two best characterized nAChR subtypes in mammalian brain are those that are assembled from a combination of a4 and b2 subunits (Flores et al. 1992) (ratio 2a:3b) (Anand et al. 1991 and Cooper et al. 1991) and those composed of a7 (Couturier et al. 1990). However, ganglionic nAChRs contain a3 in combination with b2 or b4 and possibly α5 (Lukas, 1993). Although molecular biology of the nAChRs suggests the potential for extensive nAChR diversity, the radioligand binding techniques have thus far defined only three major neuronal nAChR subclasses in the brain: 1) those that have high affinity for (-)-nicotine, (Kd = 0.5-5 nM) and are labeled by [^{3}H]-acetylcholine (Schwartz et al. 1982), (-)-[^{3}H]-nicotine (Marks et al. 1986), (-)-[^{3}H]-cytisine (Pabreza et al. 1991) and [^{3}H]-methylcarbamylcholine (Pabreza et al. 1991); 2) those that recognize α-bungarotoxin (αBgT) with high affinity (Kd = 0.5 nM) (Clarke et al. 1985); and 3) a population of receptors that display marked selectivity for neuronal bungarotoxin (n-BgT) (Schulz et al. 1991). Even with the currently limited selection of ligands selective for the different nAChR subtypes, the pharmacology of these receptors is complex.

Analgesic or antinociceptive effects of nicotine have been known for more than two decades (Phan et al. 1973, Sahley and Bernston, 1979 and Tripathi et al. 1982), but the mechanism of this action is unclear. However, the antinociceptive effect of nicotine in a variety of species is attenuated in animals pretreated with the neuronal nicotinic cholinergic receptor channel blocker, mecamylamine, which by its ability to cross the blood-brain barrier blocks nicotinic function in brain as well as in peripheral autonomic ganglia, but not with the bisquaternary nicotinic receptor antagonist, hexamethonium, which does not cross the blood-brain barrier, implying a central mechanism (Tripathi et al. 1982). Iwamoto postulated that (-)-nicotine may activate nAChRs located on cell bodies in subcortical areas resulting in release of ACh and ultimately pain modulation via activation of descending pain inhibitory pathways (Iwamoto, 1991). Damaj and co-workers, however, speculated that (-)-nicotine stimulates nAChRs in the spinal cord resulting in intracellular calcium increase and thus activating mechanisms responsible for its antinociceptive effects (Damaj et al. 1993). An isoxazole analog of nicotine, ABT-418 (Fig. 1) is a potent nAChR ligand with selectivity for a4b2 binding site (Ki = 4.5 nM) (Arneric et al. 1994), whereas 2,4-dimethoxybenzylidene anabasine (DMXB) binds with similar affinity at both neuronal a4b2 and a7 binding sites. This suggests that a7 nAChR subtypes are not particularly important for analgesia. However, 3-(4)-dimethylaminocinnamylidine (DMAC), which is more potent at a7 than at a4b2 subunit combinations, also has some analgesic activity (Decker et al. 1995). Tropane backbone containing compound, (R)-(+)-hyoscyamine has antinociceptive activity resulting from an increased acetylcholine release secondary to antagonism of central muscarinic receptors (Gualtieri et al. 1994a and Gualtieri et al. 1994b). Related 2-phenoxypropionic acid has also been found to possess potent antinociceptive and cognition-enhancing properties, possibly by antagonizing presynaptic M_2 receptors (Gualtieri et al. 1994b). Epibatidine is the most potent nicotinic cholinergic agonist yet reported (Ki = 0.04 nM and 230 nM for [^{3}H]-cytisine and [^{125}I]-a-bungarotoxin binding sites, respectively), which produces potent antinociception that is not blocked by the opioid antagonist, naloxone or by hexamethonium, but is attenuated by pretreatment with nicotinic cholinergic antagonist, mecamylamine (Qian et al. 1993, Badio and Daly, 1994 and Damaj et al. 1994). Apart from its analgesic effects, epibatidine induces several other effects consistent with potent actions at neuronal nicotinic receptors. It lowers body temperature in mice and decreases their locomotor activity (Damaj et al. 1994 and Sullivan et al. 1994). It is approximately 80- and 300-fold more potent than morphine and nicotine, respectively. It is also at least 3000 times more potent than (-)-nicotine in activating ^{86}Rb$^+$ cation flux (IC$_{50}$ = 7 nM) in IMR32 cells, a cell line rich in a3 subunits (Sullivan et al. 1994). Unfortunately, epibatidine has potent effects on autonomic nervous system function via an action on ganglionic nAChRs (Fisher et al. 1994). Finally it is highly toxic and produces convulsions and death at doses of 40-80 mg/kg (~0.2-0.4 mM/kg) (Sullivan et al. 1994 and Bonhaus et al. 1995). Similar effects are observed with nicotine and other nAChR agonists, although not with such high potency. The unique pharmacological profile of activity of (±)-epibatidine makes this agent a useful prototype ligand to investigate central nervous system functions regulated by nAChRs, particularly in pain control. The discovery of epibatidine has rekindled interest in nAChR mediated analgesia. Separation of side-effect liabilities of epibatidine from its efficacy at nAChR, to mediate analgesia could be a major breakthrough in the field of analgesia therapy.

In this publication, we describe the design of novel neuronal nAChR agonists in three series of 8-azabicyclo[3.2.1]octane/6-azabicyclo[2.1.1]hexane-containing nicotine/epibatidine analogs, a new structural class of agents not heretofore reported. Our choice of structures for these compounds is based on both molecular modeling and consideration of the chemical structures of other known nAChR agonists, and it combines the chemical attributes of epibatidine, nicotine, ABT-418, A-85380 and cocaine/hyoscyamine. Preliminary pharmacological evaluation of nicotine/epibatidine and analog #13 (see table 1) *in vitro* for their binding affinity to cortical nAChR as well as functional selectivity as judged by the potency ratio for neuronal/ganglionic nAChR-gated ion channel activity is presented. We are in the process of identifying potent novel analgesics of known pharmacological selectivity. The analgesic activities of such compounds will be reported in future publications.

Design of novel nAChR agonists

Structural features: Recent advances in the search of novel nAChR agonists indicate that activity is associated with such structures as ABT-418, an isoxazole analog of nicotine (Arneric et al. 1994 and Decker et al. 1994) currently in development for treatment of AD; epibatidine (Damaj et al. 1994 and Sullivan et al. 1994), a potent analgesic with high affinity for nAChRs; A-85380, a 3-pyridyl ether derivative of azetidine (Abreo et al. 1996) with subnanomolar affinity for central neuronal nAChRs and such compounds as ferruginine, a simple 2-substituted tropane derivative. (Davies et al. 1991, Caldwell et al. 1993 and Davies and Saikali, 1994). The tropane ring is also a key structural feature found in cocaine and its analogs (Carroll et al. 1994). Therefore, the designed series of compounds encompass the structural features present in nicotine, epibatidine, cocaine/hyoscyamine, ABT-418, and A-85380 (Fig. 1). The characteristic structural features of the novel epibatidine analogs are as follows:

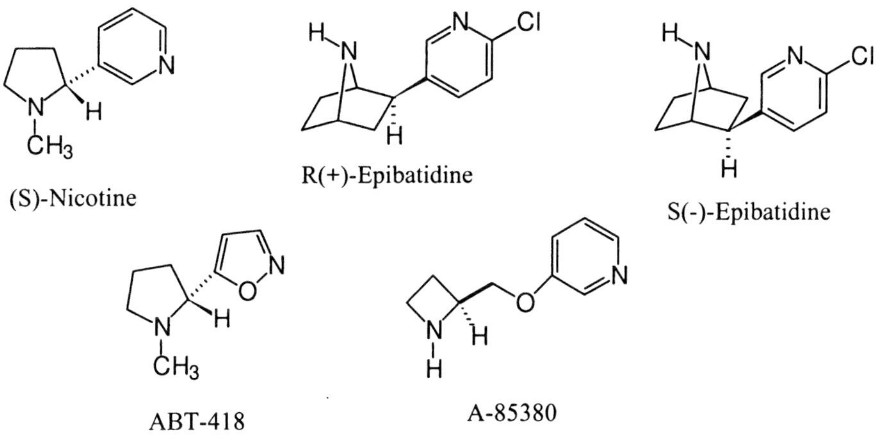

Figure 1. Structures of some nicotinic acetylcholine receptor agonists

1) The 7-azanorbornane (7-azabicyclo[2.2.1]heptane) ring in epibatidine is replaced with the tropane (8-azabicyclo[3.2.1]octane) or 6-azabicyclo[2.1.1]hexane ring structure. The tropane ring structure is present in cocaine, the phenyltropane analogs of cocaine which have been shown to have strong affinity at the dopamine reuptake site (Carroll et al. 1994, Carroll e al. 1992, Carroll et al. 1991, Boja et al. 1994, Davies et al. 1994 and Newman et al. 994), and in ferruginine and anhydroecgonine methyl ester, two compounds claimed as nAChR agonists with potential usefulness in the treatment of neurodegenerative diseases (Caldwell et al. 1993 and Davies and Saikali, 1994). The 6-azabicyclo[2.1.1]hexane ring system (pyrrolidine-azetidine) is novel. However, structurally and stereochemically it combines the structural features present in some known nAChR agonists, e.g., nicotine/ABT-418 (pyrrolidine), epibatidine (pyrrolidine-pyrrolidine), A-85380 (azetidine). The 7-azanorbornane ring is retained in some of the analogs due to its known nAChR agonist activity in epibatidine (Figs. 2-4).

2) The pyridine ring structure in epibatidine/nicotine is retained in these structures and is attached to C-2 or C-3 of the tropane, or C-2 of the 6-azabicyclo[2.1.1]hexane/7-azabicyclo[2.2.1]heptane ring either directly (Fig. 2) or through an ester bond (Fig. 3) or an ether bond (Fig. 4).

3) The pyridine ring structure in epibatidine/nicotine is replaced with a bioisostere, an isoxazole ring, which is attached to C-2 or C-3 of the tropane, or C-2 of the 6-azabicyclo[2.1.1]hexane/7-azabicyclo[2.2.1]heptane ring either directly (Fig. 2) or through an ester bond (Fig. 3) or an ether bond (Fig. 4).

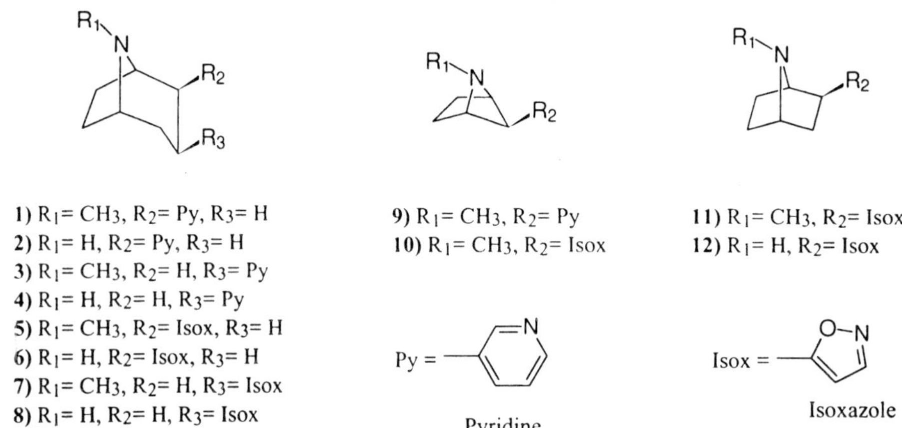

Figure 2. Novel rigid analogs containing the tropane/6-azabicyclo[2.1.1]hexane/7-azabicyclo[2.2.1]heptane and pyridine/isoxazole ring structures.

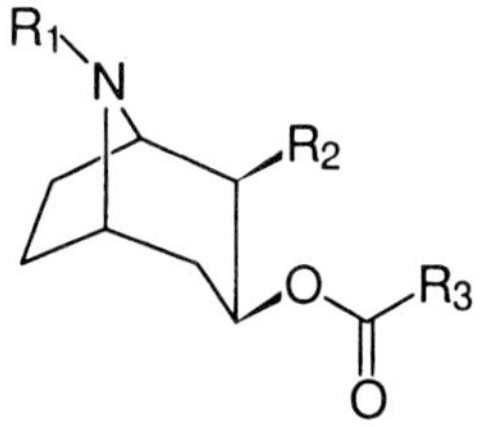

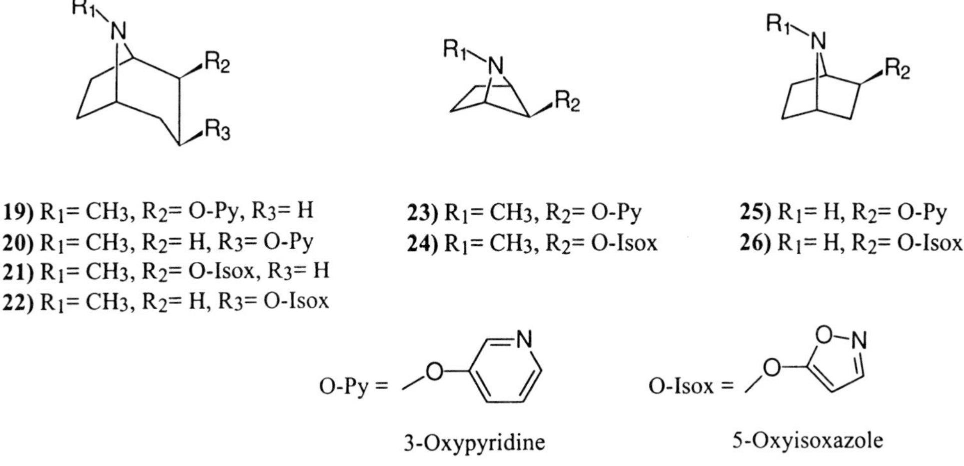

13) R_1= CH3, R_2= COOCH3, R_3= Py
14) R_1= CH3, R_2= H, R_3= Py
15) R_1= CH3, R_2= COOCH3, R_3= Isox
16) R_1= CH3, R_2= H, R_3= Isox

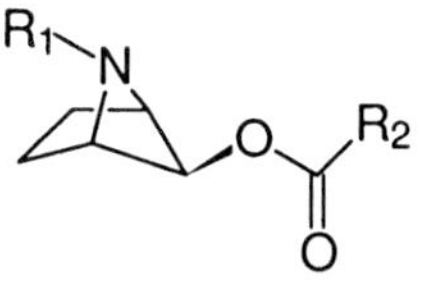

17) R_1= CH3, R_2= Py
18) R_1= CH3, R_2= Isox

Isox = 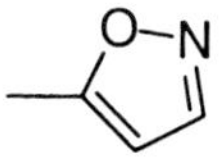 Isoxazole

Py = 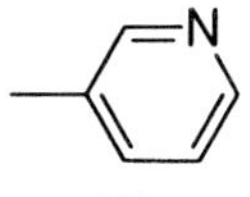 Pyridine

Figure 3. Tropane/6-azabicyclo[2.1.1]hexane substituted esters containing pyridine/isoxazole ring structures.

19) R_1= CH3, R_2= O-Py, R_3= H
20) R_1= CH3, R_2= H, R_3= O-Py
21) R_1= CH3, R_2= O-Isox, R_3= H
22) R_1= CH3, R_2= H, R_3= O-Isox

23) R_1= CH3, R_2= O-Py
24) R_1= CH3, R_2= O-Isox

25) R_1= H, R_2= O-Py
26) R_1= H, R_2= O-Isox

O-Py = 3-Oxypyridine

O-Isox = 5-Oxyisoxazole

Figure 4. Tropane/6-azabicyclo[2.1.1]hexane/7-azabicyclo[2.2.1]heptane substituted ethers containing pyridine/isoxazole ring structures.

Rationale: The following rationale was used to design the above compounds.

1) Compared to the chemical structures of other known nAChR agonists, e.g. quaternary amines (acetylcholine and methylcarbamylcholine), piperidine (lobeline, arecoline, and isoarecoline), pyrrolidine-pyridine (nicotine), piperidine-pyridine (cytisine, anabasine), piperizine (DMPP), pyrrolidine-isoxazole (ABT-418), isoquinolines (bridged nicotines), tropidine (ferruginine), 9-azabicyclo[4.2.1]non-2-ene (anatoxin-a), azetidine-pyridine (A-85380), and 7-azabicyclo[2.2.1]heptane (7-azanorbornane)-pyridine

(epibatidine), the proposed 8-azabicyclo[3.2.1]octane/6-azabicyclo[2.1.1]hexane/7-azabicyclo[2.2.1]heptane-pyridine/isoxazole represent a new class of drugs (Figs. 2-4).

2) Based on the Beers and Reich (1970) and the Sheridan et al. (1986) pharmacophore models, and subsequently expanded by Abreo et al. (1996), in nicotine, epibatidine and A-85380 (a potent nAChR agonist), the internitrogen distance (the N- in the 7-azanorbornane/azetidine rings and the pyridine -N) was shown to be 4.8, 5.6 and 6.3 A° respectively. Using the Biosym Molecular Modeling software, our measured values were: 4.85, 5.54 and 6.29 A° respectively corresponding to the lowest energy conformers. Our series of compounds bracket these distances and have N-N distances of 4.05 - 7.91 A° (Table 1).

3) Cognitive-enhancing (Gualtieri et al. 1994, Davies et al. 1991, Caldwell et al. 1993 and Davies and Saikali, 1994) and analgesic (Gualtieri et al. 1994 and Schuelke et al. 1996) properties have been associated with compounds bearing the tropane ring structure. Compounds bearing the tropane ring structure e.g. esters like atropine and cocaine, phenyltropane cocaine analogs and simple structures like ferruginine and anhydroecgonine methyl ester, have much reduced toxicity compared to epibatidine/nicotine. Thus if the toxicity is eliminated or reduced and the cognitive-enhancing properties and/or antinociceptive activities are retained, then these compounds could be therapeutically valuable agents.

Molecular Modeling Studies: The molecular visualization was performed using the QUANTA 4.1 suite of programs provided by Molecular Simulations Inc., Burlington MA. The energy minimizations were performed using the CHARMM package from the same company.

The analogs shown in Figs. 2-4 were originated after our molecular modeling studies searched for those compounds that could adopt the conformation of epibatidine in the nicotinic receptor. Since both nitrogens in the structures seem to be important for binding (in nicotine, epibatidine and ABT-418, Fig.1), we chose the N-N distance as a discriminator for activity. The conformation of the molecule was mostly determined by rotations of the linker between the tropane and the pyridine/isoxazole rings, since the later groups are mostly rigid. We performed a full scan of the conformational space of these linkers using QUANTA suite of programs. The angular window grid was set to 30°. After every rotation of one of the bonds joining both rings, 200 steps of energy minimization was performed using CHARMM suite of programs. The energy minimization protocol used was the steepest descent method. The top ten lowest energy conformers were then collected and their N-N distances were determined, and are presented in Table 1. Those compounds that have a range of N-N distances bracketing those of nicotine/epibatidine and A-85380 were identified. Further checks on the molecular conformations were carried out on the putative agonists by superimposing the lowest energy conformers of each molecule over epibatidine using Quanta. The targets for the superimposition were the tropane/6-azabicyclo[2.1.1]hexane/7-azabicyclo[2.2.1]heptane and the pyridine/isoxazole rings. Those molecules with the lowest RMS (root mean square) deviation with respect to epibatidine deviation were identified. Some of these RMS values are also presented in Table 1.

Table 1. Computational parameters of novel epibatidine analogs (#1 – 26) containing tropane/6-azabicyclo[2.1.1]hexane/7-azabicyclo[2.2.1]heptane and pyridine/isoxazole biophores.

Compound name/no.	Potential energy (kcal)	N-N distance (A°)	RMS deviation
Nicotine	17.28-19.40	4.21-4.92	
Epibatidine	41.50-42.10	4.50-5.54	
N-Me-epibatidine	47.50-48.59	4.76-5.72	
A-85380[31]	46.52-48.26	6.29-6.47	
1	43.15-44.06	5.07-6.00	0.42
2	36.99-38.66	4.90-5.89	0.38
3	40.71-41.20	4.48-5.81	
4	39.66-40.31	4.36-5.47	0.61
5	64.79-66.45	4.89-5.63	0.41
6	61.59-62.61	4.96-5.45	0.43
7	56.79-58.73	4.73-4.89	0.40
8	55.14-58.00	4.05-4.89	0.40
9	63.07-63.24	4.15-4.65	
10	76.86-77.92	4.63-4.91	
11	67.61-69.81	4.51-5.16	
12	68.87-70.05	4.47-5.26	0.10
13	36.02-38.63	7.56-8.30	1.54
14	34.48-38.45	7.91-8.46	
15	52.97-54.82	6.17-6.90	1.08
16	50.14-51.20	6.27-6.97	1.08
17	56.81-57.72	5.66-6.61	
18	68.83-71.31	6.39-6.84	
19	50.12-51.42	5.91-6.74	
20	41.37-42.93	6.57-7.12	
21	43.73-46.73	5.62-6.16	
22	45.96-47.78	6.25-7.04	
23	63.53-65.13	5.66-6.07	0.55
24	63.97-66.91	5.43-5.89	
25	56.57-58.58	5.46-6.35	0.66
26	54.26-58.47	5.50-5.80	

Note 1. The N-N distance refers to the distance between bicyclic ring system N and pyridine/isoxazole N.
Note 2. The side chain (spacer) C-C (or C-O) bonds were rotated one by one. The torsion angle was 300 and 200 energy minimization steps were used.
Note 3. RMS deviation were calculated by superimposing epibatidine on to the different analogs.

The molecular modeling studies led to the identification of three distinct series of compounds:

1) Rigid analogs of tropane/6-azabicyclo[2.1.1]hexane/7-azabicyclo[2.2.1]heptane with a pyridine or with a bioisostere isoxazole ring, with the N-N distances of 4.05-5.07 A° within the N-N distances in nicotine (4.85 A°), epibatidine (5.54 A°), N-methyl epibatidine (4.79 A°) and A-85380 (6.29 A°). (Table 1).

2) Pyridine/isoxazole esters of 6-azabicyclo[2.1.1]hexane/7-azabicyclo[2.2.1] heptane, analogs of cocaine and β-tropanol esters with the benzene ring in cocaine and the tropic acid moiety in hyoscyamine, replaced by the pyridine/isoxazole rings. The N-N distances of 5.66-7.91 A° in these compounds were higher than the N-N distances in nicotine/epibatidine but because they are flexible molecules, other conformations with energies higher than the minimum exist with shorter N-N distances.

3) Ether analogs of 6-azabicyclo[2.1.1]hexane/7-azabicyclo[2.2.1]heptane and 2- or 3-β-tropanol with an ether linkage between the tropane/6-azabicyclo[2.1.1]hexane/7-azabicyclo[2.2.1]heptane ring and the pyridine/isoxazole rings. The N-N distances in these compounds were 5.43-6.57 A°.

Pharmacological evaluations

[³H]-cytisine binding and displacement evaluations in vitro: The method of Pabreza et al.(1991) was used to determine the relative binding potency of novel compounds for neuronal nAChR using rat cortical membranes. Figure 5 shows the relative potency of epibatidine, cytisine, nicotine and **13**, for displacement of [³H]-cytisine specific binding. IC$_{50}$ values were respectively 0.3±0.1 , 1.1±0.1, 9.2±0.2 nM for the control compounds and 900±20 nM for **13**. **13** exhibited low potencies for [³H]-WIN 35,428 displacement from rat striatal dopamine transporter (10±0 μM) whereas the control nAChR ligands had IC$_{50}$ values >100 μM.

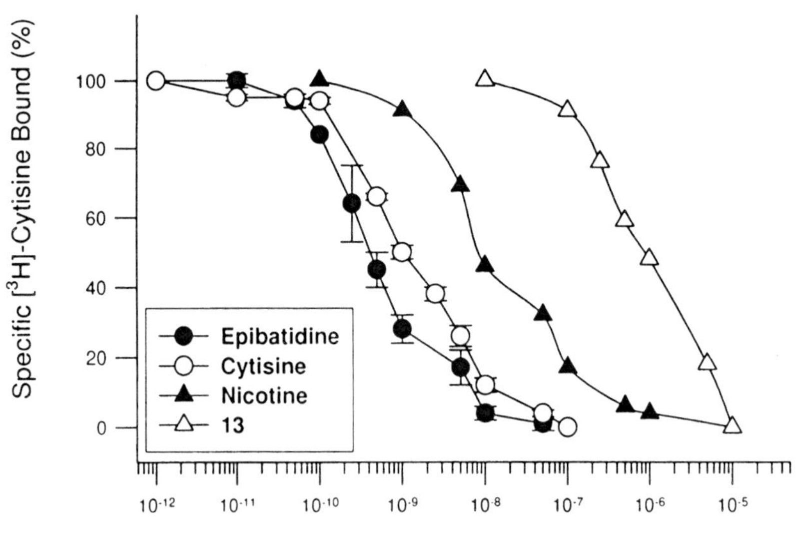

Figure 5. Displacement of [³H]-cytisine binding to rat cortical membranes.

Functional assessment of nAChR activation in vitro; Thallium-201 efflux from cell lines expressing nAChR subtypes: The ^{86}Rb$^+$ efflux method of Lukas (Lukas and Cullen, 1988) was modified to facilitate the use of this assay with the large number of compounds to be tested. Cells of the IMR-32 line were maintained in a log phase of growth in Minimum Essential Medium (GibcoBRL) containing 10% Fetal Bovine Serum and L-glutamine, NEAA, NaPyruvate and Penn-Strep, in flasks in a humidified atmosphere of 5% CO_2 in air at 37°C. Cells were seeded at a density of 2.5 - 5 x10^4 cells/well into a 96-well tissue culture dish. The plated cells were allowed to proliferate for at least 18-24 h before being loaded with ^{201}Tl$^+$, thallous chloride. Each well received 1-2 µCi of ^{201}Tl$^+$, in 0.5 ml of MEM. The cells were incubated at 37°C from 4 h to overnight. The loading medium was removed, cells rinsed three times with 200 µl of fresh medium and then exposed to 200 µl of medium containing the ligands of choice for 5 min at 37°C. After exposure to the drugs, radioactivity in the assay medium was aspirated (100 µl) and counted in a gamma counter. The EC$_{50}$ values for stimulation of ^{201}Tl$^+$ efflux were determined by nonlinear least-squares regression analysis. Figure 6 shows the concentration dependent efflux of ^{201}Tl$^+$ from IMR-32 human neuroblastoma cells after exposure to epibatidine, nicotine and **13**. The EC$_{50}$ values for epibatidine and nicotine were 13 nM and 18 µM respectively, very close to what was reported by Sullivan et al. (1994) (7 nM and 21 µM respectively). In addition, we found that **13**, a cocaine analog with the benzoyl group replaced by a nicotinoyl group, had an EC$_{50}$ of 220 µM, about 12 times less potent than (-)-nicotine but with an efficacy higher than (-)-nicotine, 150% but lower than epibatidine, 239% (Fig. 7). The antagonist mecamylamine at a concentration of 100 µM completely inhibited the actions of epibatidine and nicotine at their maximum effective concentrations, 100 nM for epibatidine and 100 µM for nicotine.

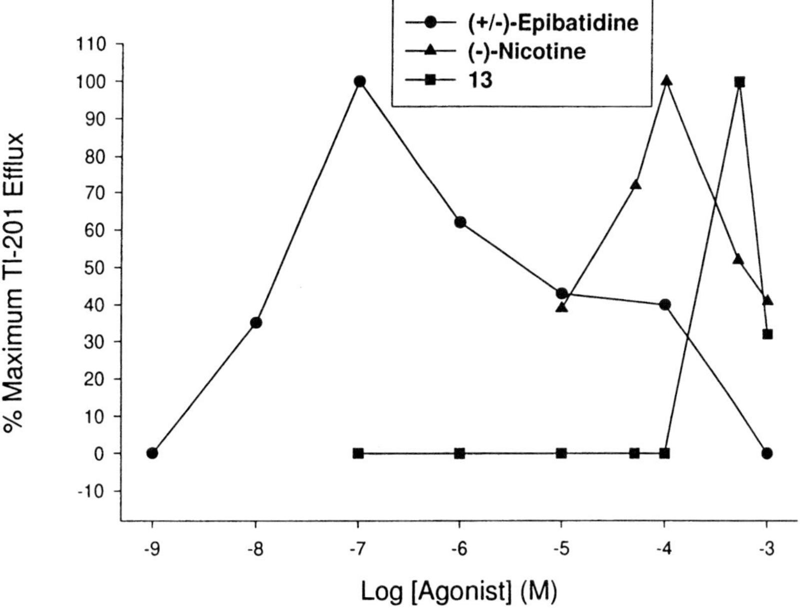

EC$_{50}$ values: (+/-)-epibatidine = 13 nM; (-)-nicotine = 18 uM; **13** = 220 uM

Figure 6. Effect of epibatidine, nicotine and **13** to stimulate TI-201 efflux from IMR-32 cells.

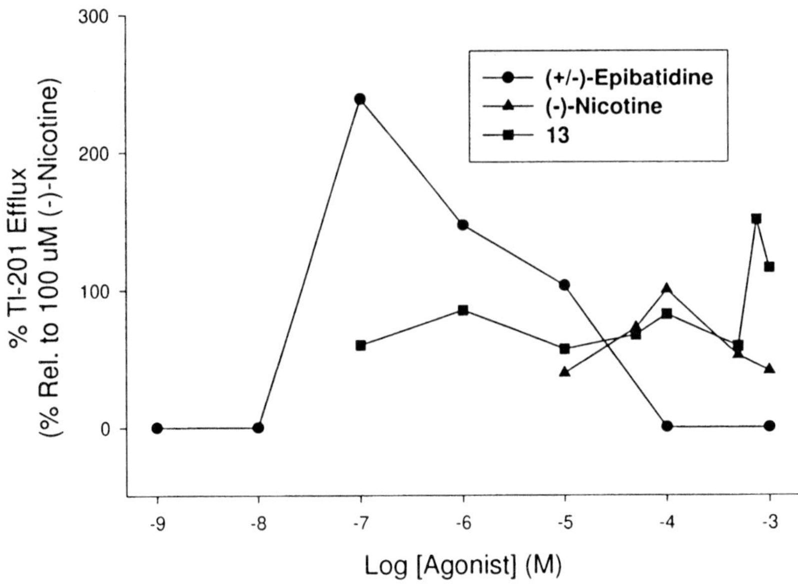

Figure 7. Effect of epibatidine, nicotine and **13** to stimulate Tl-201 efflux from IMR-32 cells.

Antinociceptive action of test compounds on the intact mouse; Choice of mouse strain: Nicotine's acute analgesic effects were determined by the tail-flick test. The tail-flick response time (sec) was measured with a Columbus Instruments tail-flick analgesia meter at an intensity setting of 10. The effect of vehicle treatment on tail-flick latency in CD-1 and CF-1 outbred mice was the 33999999same (3.6±0.2 and 3.3±0.2 sec, respectively). The overall effect of nicotine dosage on tail-flick response time was significant in CD-1 mice (p<0.0001) but not in mice of CF-1 strain (p= 0.08). Nicotine doses ≥0.5 mg/kg ip significantly increased tail-flick response time in CD-1 mice but not in CF-1 mice (Fig. 8). The lowest tested dose of nicotine which significantly increased analgesia in CD-1 mice was 0.5 mg/kg ip. Nicotine's ED_{50} for analgesia induction was 3 mg/kg ip. The maximal increase in tail-flick response time in CD-1 mice (to 9±0.8 sec) occurred at a dose of 5 mg/kg ip, the highest dose tested. (higher doses of nicotine caused seizure prodrome and tremor which may have interfered with the tail-flick assay.) These observations identify the inherent hyporesponsiveness of CF-1 mice to the analgesic action of nicotine as measured by the tail-flick method and the use of CD-1 mice as the choice of mouse strain for testing the compounds for their antinociceptive action.

Acute behavioral measures of undesirable side effects/toxicity in the mouse: Both the CD-1 and CF-1 mice were equally responsive to the acute convulsant and lethal action of nicotine. The non-overlapping dosage dependent behavioral responses to nicotine in CF-1 mice is illustrated in Fig. 9. From these dose effect curves the ED_{50} values were calculated (here respectively 5, 12.5 and 25 mg/kg ip for induction of locomotor inhibition, convulsions and lethality).

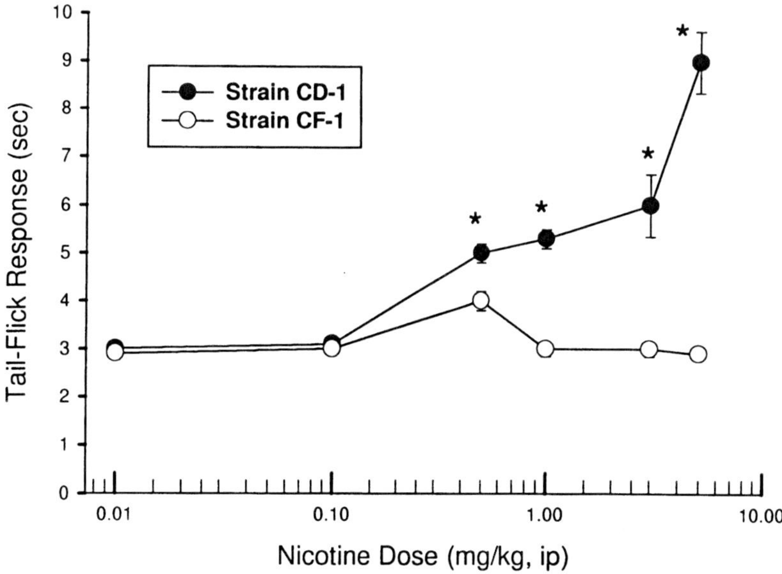

(*) - indicates p<0.05 for increased response time compared to vehicle treated control mice.

Figure 8. Non-identical responsiveness of CF-1 and CD-1 mice to nicotine-induced analgesia in the tail-flick assay.

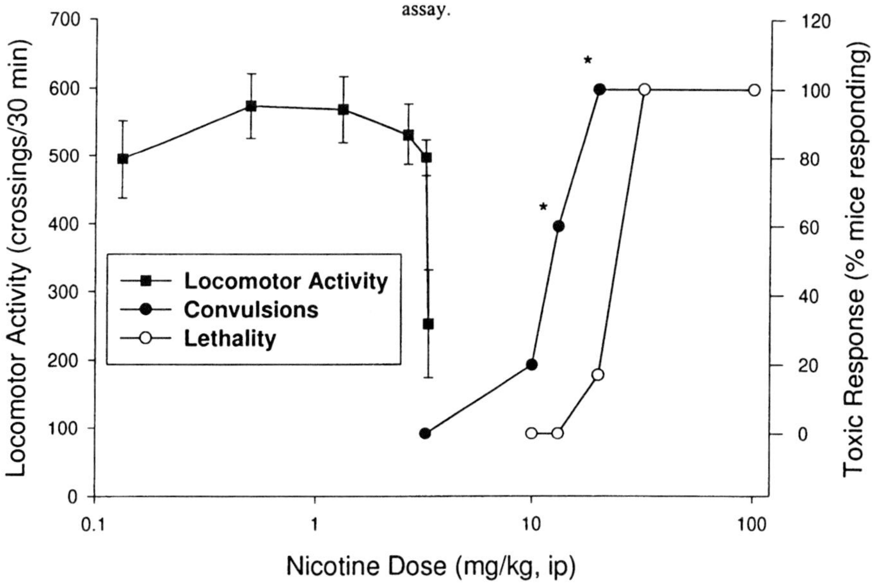

* Convulsant action of nicotine doses of 13.2 and 20 mg/kg is significantly greater than its lethal action.

Figure 9. Locomotor activity and toxic effects of nicotine administration in CF-1 mice.

Discussion

High-resolution 3-D structures of nicotinic receptors located on cell membranes are not yet known; therefore, docking studies using different conformations of each proposed structure in the binding site are not possible. However, both the Beers and Reich (1970) and the Sheridan (Sheridan et al. 1986) models have proposed two essential elements of the nicotinic pharmacophore: a hydrogen bond acceptor (i.e. pyridine lone pair of nicotine) and a charged species, e.g., a protonated or quaternary nitrogen. These models suggested an internitrogen distance of around 4.8 A° in nicotine. The subsequent discovery of epibatidine as an exceptionally high-affinity ligand for nAChR has suggested that the optimal internitrogen distance for high-affinity ligand may be close to 5.5 A° (Glennon et al. 1994). Recently, a compound (A-85380) with higher internitrogen distance (6.3 A°) has been found to possess subnanomolar affinity for nAChRs (Abreo et al. 1996). Given the importance of the distance between both binding sites, we determined the most probable N to N distances of our putative agonists (Figs. 2-4) by carrying out a molecular mechanics based modeling. The N to N distances fall within the range proposed by models given above. We are in the process of performing a full iterative search of the most probable torsion angles for the linkers, although this restricted search mentioned above has provided us with an initial guideline for scoring of our drug leads.

Both nicotine and epibatidine contain two pharmacophores: Nicotine contains a pyrrolidine and a pyridine while epibatidine contains a nitrogen-containing bicyclic ring, 7-azabicyclo[2.2.1]heptane and a pyridine. The systematic design of nAChR agonists using nicotine/epibatidine as the model compound could be performed by modifying one pharmacophore at a time. In our approach, we used two strategies, i.e., changing one or both the pharmacophores at a time. In the first approach we decided to change pyrrolidine/7-azabicyclo[2.2.1]heptane pharmacophore present in nicotine/epibatidine, respectively, with 8-azabicyclo[3.2.1]octane/6-azabicyclo[2.1.1]hexane pharmacophore. Since both nicotine and epibatidine contain a pyridine ring, the choice of pyridine as the other pharmacophore was obvious. In choosing the two different nitrogen containing bicyclic ring systems several factors were taken into consideration. The most important factor of them all was to see if there was any biological activity associated with 8-azabicyclo[3.2.1]octane ring system. In addition to precedent reports of biological activity, the 8-azabicyclo[3.2.1]octane ring was chosen because it gave more options to connect the pyridine pharmacophore, e.g., attachment at carbon C-2, which is equivalent to C-2 of 7-azabicyclo[2.2.1]hexane of epibatidine, or carbon C-3. The 6-azabicyclo[2.1.1]hexane ring system is novel and there is no mention of its synthesis or any biological activity associated with this ring system in the literature. Nevertheless, the 6-azabicyclo[2.1.1]hexane ring system is unique from its chemical structure point of view. For example, 6-azabicyclo[2.1.1]hexane (pyrrolidine-azetidine) ring system is complementary to the 7-azabicyclo[2.2.1]heptane (pyrrolidine-pyrrolidine) and the 8-azabicyclo[3.2.1]octane (pyrrolidine-piperidine) ring systems. Besides, the 6-azabicyclo[2.1.1]hexane ring system could allow for the introduction of additional functional groups without essentially hurting the nitrogen to nitrogen distances between the two pharmacophores because of its relatively smaller size. The 7-azabicyclo[2.2.1]heptane ring was chosen in some of the analogs because of its known potent biological activity at the nAChRs. In the second approach both the pharmacophores present in epibatidine were changed at the same time. As given above, the 7-azabicyclo[2.2.1]heptane pharmacophore was replaced with 8-azabicyclo[3.2.1]octane or 6-azabicyclo[2.1.1]hexane, however, the pyridine pharmacophore was replaced with an isoxazole pharmacophore. The choice of isoxazole was based on the finding that ABT 418, currently in development for treatment of AD McDonald et al. 1995), is a nAChR agonist equipotent to nicotine in displacing [^{3}H]-cytisine and has an isoxazole ring instead of the pyridine ring as in nicotine. The choice of the esters was supported by the fact that R-(+)-hyoscyamine and related 2-phenoxy, 2-(phenylthio)- and 2-(phenylamino) alkanoic acid esters of (-tropanol show analgesic activities comparable to morphine as well as nootropic properties as a consequence of increased central presynaptic ACh release (Gualtieri et al. 1994b). In addition Shuelke et al. (1996) conducted an *in vivo* structure-activity study of cocaine; its metabolites and 17 phenyltropane analogs injected intracerebroventricularly in rats, and showed that these tropane containing compounds have analgesic properties. The choice of ether analogs was supported by the work of Abreo et al. (1996) who showed that pyridyl ethers of pyrrolidine/azetidine have subnanomolar affinity for central neuronal nAChR. Furthermore, as shown in epibatidine and in the pyridyl ether analogs by Abreo et al. (1996) the N-methylation of these compounds was not detrimental to their binding affinity to the nAChR.

The potency and selectivity for binding to particular receptors (e.g. cortical nAChR) and other binding sites (e.g. the cocaine binding site on the dopamine transporter) is conveniently measured by displacement of selective radiolabeled ligands from membrane preparations derived from isolated brain regions. Binding potency determined by displacement of [^{3}H]-cytisine from cortical membranes provides limited information about the functional effect of a new compound as agonist, partial agonist or antagonist at nAChR. The nAChR form ligand-gated cation channels whose activation by agonists can be assessed by measuring efflux of radioisotopically labcled cations such as ^{86}Rb$^+$ from cultured cells expressing selected nAChR subtypes Sullivan et al. 1994 and Gopalakrishnan et al. 1996). Thus both functional potency and efficacy should be assessed and compared to binding potency. The availability of cell lines selectively expressing neuronal or ganglionic type nAChR provides an opportunity to determine *in vitro* selectivity of new compounds for these receptor subtypes, a parameter expected to be of value in predicting receptor-mediated toxic potency of nicotinic ligands. Our intention was to avoid the use of the ^{86}Rb$^+$ cation and to use ^{201}Tl$^+$ cation because this isotope has several technical advantages over ^{86}Rb. Thallium is a monovalent cation of which ^{201}Tl$^+$ is an isotope that is presently used in nuclear pharmacies and nuclear medicine as a "mimic" for K$^+$ ions in evaluating myocardial tissue and has long replaced rubidium and cesium isotopes previously used for the same purpose, and thus could be substituted for ^{86}Rb$^+$ without detriment to the assay. ^{86}Rb($t_{1/2}$=18.65 days, β=1.77; γ=1.07 MeV) is not an ideal isotope either for counting in a gamma counter, Cerenkov counting in liquid scintillation counters (26% efficiency) or with regard to radioactive waste management. In addition researchers must be well protected because of the high energy gamma emitted by ^{86}Rb. ^{201}Tl$^+$ has a $t_{1/2}$ of 73 h, with low energy x-ray gamma radiation of 0.135 and 0.167 MeV is much better suited for gamma counting and radioactive waste management. In fact, it was found that using the cells of IMR-32 human neuroblastoma and ^{201}Tl$^+$ as the isotope, the results obtained by Sullivan et al. (1996) with ^{86}Rb$^+$ were reproducible with epibatidine and nicotine as controls.

In summary, molecular mechanics based modeling has led to the identification of new drug leads which might have reduced toxicity associated with the structure of epibatidine and therefore, reduced propensity to elicit side effects. The synthesis and pharmacological evaluation of the compounds proposed in this publication is currently under way in our laboratory.

Plenary discussion

Wall P.: Cocaine analogues also led to the development of local anesthetics. Does your approach to nicotine relate to the development?

Basmadjian G.: We are aware of this fact, and justified the use of this tropane ring structure agonist by mentioning that cocaine, atropine and other tropane analogs do have analgesic activity. The site of this analgesic activity is not known.

References

Abreo MA, Lin N-H, Garvey DS, Gunn DE, Hettinger A-M, Wasicak JT, Pavlik PA, Martin YC, Donnelly-Roberts DL, Anderson DJ, Sullivan JP, Williams M, Arneric SP, Holladay MW (1996) J Med Chem 39, 817-825.

Anand R, Conroy WG, Schoepfer R, Whiting P, Lindstrom J (1991) J Biol Chem 266, 11192-11198.

Arneric SP, Sullivan JP, Briggs CA, Donnelly-Roberts D, Anderson DJ, Raszkiewicz JL, Hughes ML, Cadman ED, Adams P, Garvey DS, Wasicak JT, Williams MJ (1994) Pharmacol Exp Ther 270, 310-8.

Badio B, Daly JW (1994) Mol Pharmacol 45, 563-9.

Beers WH, Reich E (1970) Nature 228, 917- 922.

Betz H (1990) Neuron 5, 383-92.

Boja JW, Kuhar M, Kopajtic T, Yang E, Abraham P, Lewin AH, Carroll FI.(1994) J Med Chem 37, 1220-1223.

Bonhaus DW, Bley KR, Broka CA, Fontana DJ, Leung L, Lewis R, Shieh A, Wong EH (1995) J Pharmacol Exp Ther 272, 1199-1203.

Caldwell WS, Davies HML, Lippieollo PM (1993) US Patent 5,227,385.

Carroll FI, Gao Y, Rahman MA, Abraham P, Parham K, Lewin AH, Boja JW, Kuhar MJ (1991) J Med Chem 34, 2719-2725.

Carroll FI, Lewin AH, Boja JW, Kuhar MJ (1992) J Med Chem 35, 970-981.

Carroll FI, Mascarella SW, Kuzemko MA, Gao Y, Abraham P, Lewin AH, Boja JW, Kuhar MJ (1994) J Med Chem 37, 2865-2873.

Clarke PB, Schwartz RD, Paul SM, Pert CB, Pert A (1985) J Neurosci 5, 1307-15.

Cooper E, Couturier S, Ballivet M (1991) Nature 350, 235-238.

Couturier S, Bertrand D, Matter J, Hernandez M, Bertrand S, Millar N, Valera S, Barkas T, Ballivel M (1990) Neuron 5, 847-856.

Damaj MI, Creasy KR, Grove AD, Rosecrans JA, Martin BR (1994) Brain Res 664, 34-40.

Damaj MI, Welch SP, Martin BR (1993) J Pharmacol Exp Ther 266, 1330-8.

Davies HML, Saikali E (1994) US Patent 5,288,872.

Davies HML, Saikali E, Huby NJS, Gilliatt VJ, Matasi JJ, Sexton T, Childers SR (1994) J Med Chem 37, 1262-1268.

Davies HML, Saikali E, Young WB (1991) J Org Chem 56, 5696-5700.

Decker MW, Brioni JD, Bannon AW, Arneric SP (1995) Life Sci 56, 545-70.

Decker MW, Brioni JD, Sullivan JP, Buckley MJ, Radek RJ, Raszkiewicz JL, Kang CH, Kim DJ, Giardina WJ, Wasicak JT, Williams M, Arneric SP (1994) J Pharmacol Exp Ther 270, 319-28.

Fisher M, Huangfu D, Shen TY, Guyenet PG (1994) J Pharmacol Exp Ther 270, 702-707.

Flores CM, Rogers SW, Pabreza LA, Wolfe BB, Kellar KJ (1992) Mol Pharmacol 41, 31-7.

Glennon RA, Herndon JL, Dukat M (1994) Med Chem Res 4, 461-473.

Gopalakrishnan M, Monteggia LM, Anderson DJ, Molinari EJ, Piattoni-Kaplan M, Donnelly-Roberts D, Arneric SP, Sullivan JP (1996) J Pharmacol Exp Ther 276, 289-297.

Gualtieri F, Conti G, Dei S, Giovannoni MP, Nannucci F, Romanelli MN, Scapecchi S, Teodori E, Fanfani L, Ghelardini C, Giotti A, Bartolini AJ (1994a) Med Chem 37, 1704-1711.

Gualtieri F, Bottalico C, Calandrella A, Dei S, Paola G, Mealli S, Romanelli MN, Scapecchi S, Teodori E, Galeotti N, Ghelardini C, Giotti A, Bartolini AJ (1994b) Med Chem 37, 1712-1719.

Iwamoto ET (1991) J Pharmacol Exp Ther 257, 120-33.

Lukas RJ (1993) J Pharmacol Exp Ther 265, 294-302.

Lukas RJ, Cullen MJ (1988) Anal Biochem 175, 212-218.

Maricq AV, Peterson AS, Brake AJ, Myers RM, Julius D (1991) Science 254, 432-7.

Marks MJ, Stitzel JA, Romm E, Wehner JM, Collins AC (1986) Mol Pharmacol 30, 427-36.

McDonald IA, Cosford N, Vernier J-M (1995) Ann Reports Med Chem 30, 41-50.

Newman AH, Allen AC, Izenwasser S, Katz JL (1994) J Med Chem 37, 2258-2261.

Pabreza LA, Dhawan S, Kellar KJ (1991) Mol Pharmacol 39, 9-12.

Phan DV, Doda M, Bite A, Gyorgy L (1973) Acta Physiol Acad Sci Hung 1, 85-93.

Qian C, Li T, Shen TY, Libertine-Garahan L, Eckman J, Biftu T, Ip S (1993) Eur J Pharmacol 250, R13-4.

Sahley TL, Bernston GG (2979) Psychopharmacology 65, 279-283.

Schuelke GS, Terry C, Powers RH, Rice J, Madden J, (1996) A Pharmcol Biochem Behav 53, 133-140.

Schulz DW, Loring RH, Aizenman E, Zigmond RE (1991) J Neurosci 11, 287-97.

Schwartz RD, McGee R Jr, Kellar KJ (1982) Mol Pharmacol 22, 56-62.

Sheridan RP, Nilakantan R, Dixon JS, Venkataraghavan RJ (1986) Med Chem 29, 899-906.

Spande T, Garraffo H, Edwards M, Yeh H, Pannell L, Daly J (1992) J Am Chem Soc 114, 3475-3478.

Sullivan JP, Decker MW, Brioni JD, Donnelly-Roberts D, Anderson DJ, Bannon AW, Kang CH, Adams P, Piattoni-Kaplan M, Buckley MJ, Gopalkrishnan M, Williams M, Arneric SP (1994) J Pharmacol Exp Ther 271, 624-31.

Tripathi HL, Martin BR, Aceto MD (1982) J Pharmacol Exp Ther 221, 91-6.

Wisden W and Seeburg PH (1992) Curr Opinion Neurobio 2, 263-9.

Pain Mechanisms and Management
S.N. Ayrapetyan and A.V. Apkarian (Eds.)
IOS Press, 1998

Low and High Molecular Compounds from Plants and Animals with Antiinflammatory Activity - A Survey of Results from a 10 Year Screening Program

H. Wagner
Institute of Pharmaceutical Biology, University of Munich
Munich, Germany

Since chronic pain is often associated with chronic inflammation (Dray, 1995) the search for safer and more potent antiinflammatory drugs lacking adverse effects is of the greatest importance. This review summarizes the results obtained mainly in the author's laboratory during ten years of screening for antiinflammatory acting constituents from plants (Wagner, 1989).

Prostanoids (prostaglandines, leukotrienes and hydroxy fatty acids) are among the most important mediators of inflammatory hyperalgesia. Since they are generated from arachidonic acid by cyclooxygenase (COX) and 5-lipoxygenase (5-LO), we have concentrated our screening program on plant constituents with potential inhibitory effect on these two enzymes.

We used a cyclooxygenase microsome preparation from sheep seminal vesicles (Wagner et al., 1986; 1987), and for the 5-lipoxygenase test porcine leukocytes (Wagner and Fessler, 1986). For some compounds (i.e. triterpenoids and polysaccharides) the classic alternative complement test (guinea pig and human serum) has also been applied. In some cases the *in vitro* results could also be confirmed in the rat paw edema model (Wagner, 1989).

A retrospective evaluation of all tested compounds with potential antiinflammatory activity shows that we can divide them into two major subclasses: phenolic compounds, e.g. flavonoids, simple phenols, polyphenols, coumestans, phenolcarboxylic acids, acetophenones (class A) and arachidonic acid analogues, e.g. alkylamides, arylheptanoids, thiosulfinates, sulfinyldisulfides (class B). The antiinflammatory activities of a third group of natural products including some triterpenoic acids, sesquiterpenlactones and polysaccharides (class C), may be primarily due to their immunomodulating activities, although some of them, such as boswellic acid from incense (*Boswellia carteri*), also turned out to act as dual inhibitors of the complement system, as well as 5-LO.

Class A

Following the introduction of acetylsalicylic acid as a classic nonsteroidal anti-rheumatic agent, innumerable structural analogues have been synthesized, however, no essential improvement of activity has been achieved. Since many plants, such as *Salix spp.*,

Populus spp., Filipendula ulmaria, Gaultheria procumbens, Betula spp., Viola tricolor and *Primula spp.*, contain salicylic acid and/or salicyl alcohol-derivatives, it is surprising that most of the corresponding extracts did not exhibit any effect in either *in vitro* enzyme tests (Wagner, 1989). Nevertheless, free salicylic acid, formed *in vivo* in the gut by hydrolysis, and in the liver by oxidation of salicyl alcohol, exerts an antiinflammatory activity similar to that of acetylsalicylic acid. We isolated 4- and 5-methoxy salicylic acid esters from *Primula spp.* (Wagner and Reger, 1987), and found the 4-methoxy-salicylic acid methylester to be the most potent COX inhibitor (50% inhibition at 250 µM). Among the simple phenolic phenyl(iso)propan derivatives eugenol (1) thymol (2), and carvacrol from *Syzygium aromaticum, Thymus vulgaris* and *Ledum palustre* can be regarded as structural analogues of salicylic acid and its derivatives. The IC_{50} values of these compounds were found to be of the same order of magnitude as that of indomethacin (IC_{50} : 1.2 µM). It is interesting to note that acetyleugenol exhibits a stronger inhibitory effect than eugenol, suggesting that the mechanism of action is similar to that of aspirin: inhibition of the enzyme by an irreversible binding of the transferred acetyl group to the enzyme.

Among the flavonoids investigated the 5,7-dihydroxy flavone galangin (3) (IC_{50} of 5.5 µM) was found to be the most potent COX-inhibitor. Flavonoids with an ortho-dihydroxy substitution pattern in ring A or B were stronger inhibitors than those with a free 3-hydroxy group. In comparison to the flavonoids the flavan catechin exhibited only a weak inhibitory effect (IC_{50}: 130 µM). The lichen constituent 4-0-Methyl cryptochlorophaeic acid (4), which is biosynthetically related to flavonoids, showed an IC_{50} of 0.3 µM.

Tannins have repeatedly been reported to possess antiphlogistic properties (Kimura et al., 1986), but since this is due to a non specific binding, a gallotannin mixture consisting of tetra-, penta- and oligo-galloylglucose exhibited in our COX-test an inhibitory effect of ~ 10 µM: tannins must be removed from plant extracts before screening for the presence of other potent COX-inhibitors.

The flavonoids quercetin, cirsiol, baicalein (5) and the coumarin esculetin (6) are among the most potent 5-LO inhibitors with IC_{50} values between 0.1 and 5 µM. The presence of a catechol structure appears to be essential for a high 5-LO inhibitory effect, which can suggest that they act via an oxygen radical scavenger mechanism. Therefore, it was not surprising that wedelolactone (7) from *Eclipta alba* and *Wedelia calendulacea* (Wong et al., 1988) was found to have nearly the same inhibitory activity as the most potent 5-LO inhibitor nordihydroguaretic acid (NDGA; IC_{50} : 1.5 µM).

It is feasible to suggest that most of the lipoxygenase inhibitors also act as strong oxygen radical scavengers, or nitric oxide (NO) inhibitors, and thus antagonize pain sensations. As far as the therapeutic usefulness of phenolic compounds is concerned, it can be suggested that they have beneficial effects if applied topically or inhaled, e.g. for the treatment of respiratory tract inflammations and hyperreactivities, gastric inflammations, neurodermitis or psoriasis. When used systemically, however, an adequate blood level can only be achieved under exceptionally favourable conditions (high doses), since most phenolic compounds will be conjugated and eliminated very fast.

Class B

In this class, powerful COX inhibitors have been found among the diarylheptanoids and phenylalkanols, e.g. gingerols (8) isolated from members of the Zingiberacee family. The alkylcatechols of *Toxicodendron radicans*, a group of compounds structurally related to the phenylalkanoids possessing C_{17} or C_{15} side chains with varying degrees of unsaturation, collectively known as urushiols, produced a dose-dependent COX inhibition with IC_{50}-values in the range of 1.5 - 2.5 µM. Urushiol also inhibits 5-LO and therefore belongs to a group of dual inhibitors of the arachidonic metabolism which could be of therapeutic advantage over only COX inhibitors, since it is suggested that such compounds can prevent the so-called "substrate shift." The allergenic potential of urushiol, however, will make it necessary to search for other nonallergenic alkylcatechols. Of the aliphatic and aromatic amides, spilanthol of *Spilanthes oleracea*, a dodeca-tetraenoic acid amide of *Echinacea purpurea* and the pungent capsaicin of *Capsicum annunum* are the most potent 5-LO-inhibitors. Capsaicin (9), known for its skin irritating activity, has dual inhibitor potential. The antiinflammatory activity of Capsaicin is explained by the so-called "counter-irritant effect," which might be due to a liberation of corticoids and/or an increased production of cytoprotective prostaglandin E_2 (Atkinson and Hicks, 1975; Dearden and Nicholson, 1984). The additional analgesic effect of Capsaicin can be explained by a depletion of substance P from primary sensory neurons associated with the transmission of thermal noxious stimuli (Yaksh et al., 1979). It is interesting to note that constituents of garlic, such as the disulfide E/Z-ajone (10) also exert inhibitory effects on COX and 5-LO with IC_{50}-values of about 5.0 µM (Sendl et al., 1992).

In this context it is worth mentioning that N-(2-hydroxyethyl) hexadecanamide, an arachidonic acid analog involved in inflammatory processes, was found recently in peripheral tissues of animals. The compound is suggested to act as an endogenous ligand for the Δ^9-tetrahydrocannabinol (THC) receptor (the peripheral CB2 subtype of cannabinoid receptor), which is expressed on mast cells (Facci et al., 1995; Mazzari et al., 1996).

Another amide, the anandamide (N-arachidonoylethanolamine)(13) was identified as the putative endogenous ligand for the CNS type cannabinol receptor (CB1). It is believed that the ethanolamide and its close derivatives are potent antiinflammatory agents acting specifically on mast cell activation. Following oral administration in rats this compound has been shown to improve the nociceptive changes (hyperalgesia) resulting from chronic sciatic nerve constriction. These interesting results may, at least partly, explain the well known applications of cannabis in the treatment of muscle spasm, rheumatism and generalized pain (Jack, 1996). There is no question that these surprising findings will stimulate the search for new antiinflammatory drugs derived from anandamides.

While selecting plants for our screening program we, in most cases, followed the ethno-pharmacological strategy, i.e. we primarily investigated plants which have gained great medicinal reputation in traditional medicine. In this context, we also investigated the fat and oil of badger, mink and the alp-marmot (Wagner and Nusser, 1988, 1989) which are widely used for the topical treatment of rheumatism and arthritis in Asia and Europe.

In the fat of alp-marmot and badger, eight corticoids--cortison, hydrocortison, dehydrocorticosterone, corticosteron, Reichstein substances, deoxycorticosteron, 17-α-OH-progesteron and progesteron--were identified and quantified (at a total concentration of 30-80 mg/kg in free and conjugated form). The mink oil was found to be composed of C19 steroids (androsterone, etiocholanolone and 5-α-dihydrosterone,) and two C21-steroid metabolites (5-α-pregnane-3α-ol-20-one and 5-α-pregnane-3α, 21-diol-20-one in addition to usual and unusual fatty acids). The amount of corticosteroids ranges from 3.0 to 11.0 mg/kg, the amount of C19-steroids from 14 to 160 mg/kg, and the amount of C11 steroid-metabolites from 6.0 to 660 mg/kg. Even though these concentrations are relatively low, there can be no doubt that the well-documented analgesic and antiinflammatory effect of remedies prepared using these fats must be, at least partly, due to the content of these steroidal compounds. Surprisingly, hibernating animals were found to have a relatively high content of these steroids, and one can speculate that these compounds are produced as thermoregulating or CNS-damping agents during hibernation (Wünnenberg et al., 1974; Majewska et al., 1986).

Class C

The resin of *Boswellia carteri* (incense), used in India for the treatment of arthritis, contains the triterpenoid boswellic acid (11) a dual inhibitor of 5-LO (Ammon, 1996) and of the classic alternative complement cascade (Knaus and Wagner, 1996). From *Tanacetum parthenium* (syn. *Parthenium integrifolium* = feverfew), claimed as an effective agent against migraine and rheumatoid arthritis, the sesquiterpenlactone parthenolide (12) has been isolated. Extract and parthenolide seem to mitigate migraine attacks through a serotonin and histamin inhibitory effect (Heptinstall et al., 1985; Hayes and Foreman, 1987) and/or suppressive effects on the release of inflammatory mediators from leukocytes (Fessler, 1988). Similar effects have also been described for a series of other sesquiterpen lactones (Hall et al., 1980).

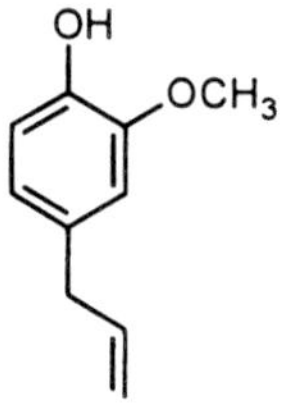

(1) Eugenol 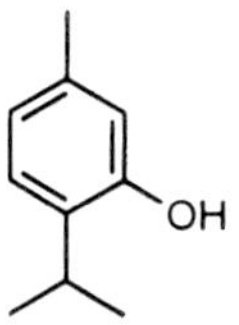   (2) Thymol 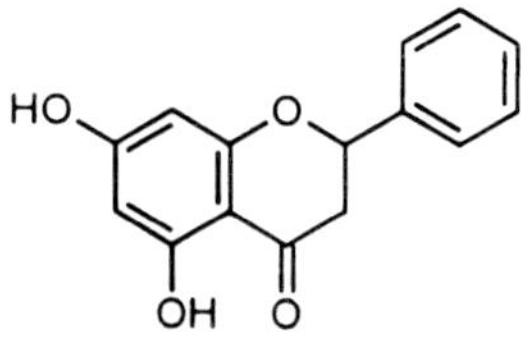   (3) Galangin

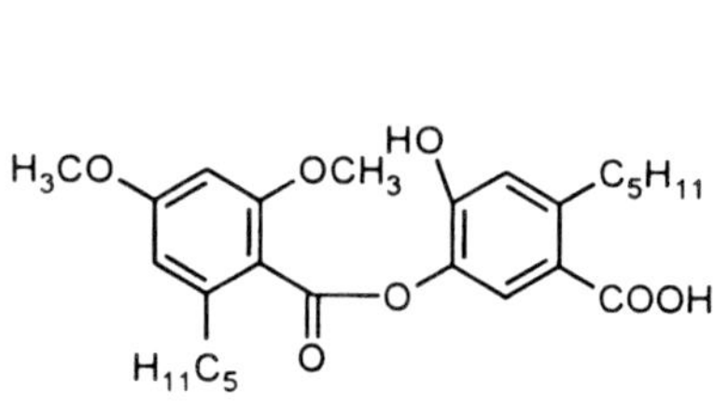

(4) 4-O-methylcryptochlorophaeic acid 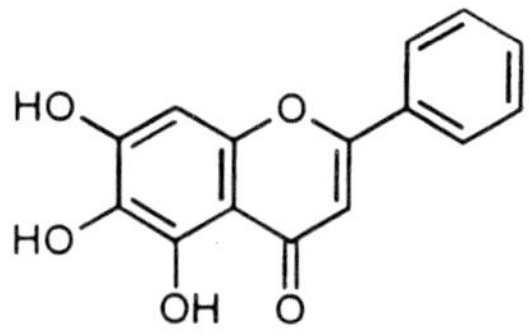   (5) Baicalein

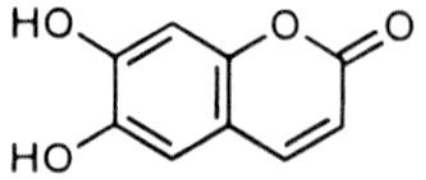

(6) Esculetin 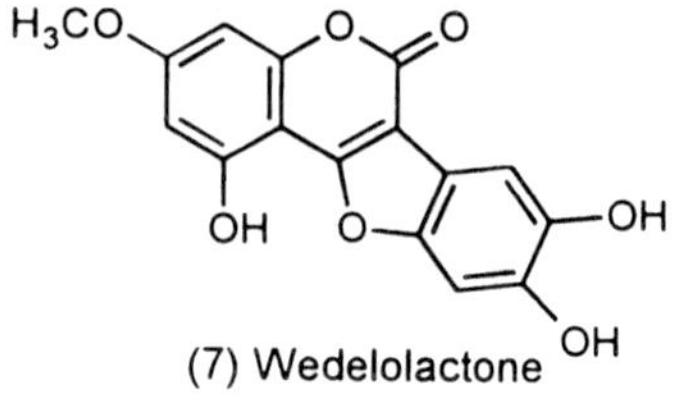   (7) Wedelolactone

Figure 1.

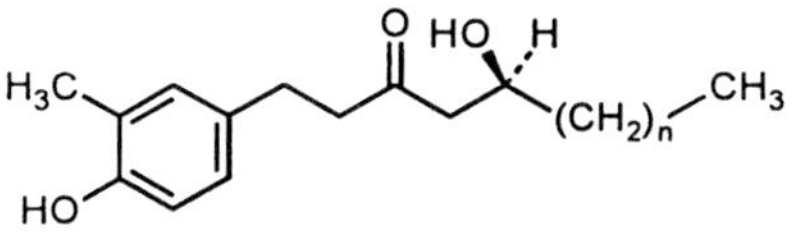

(8) Gingerols (n = 4,5,8)

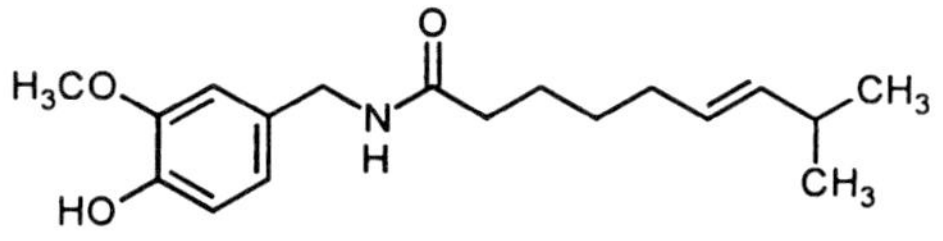

(9) Capsaicin

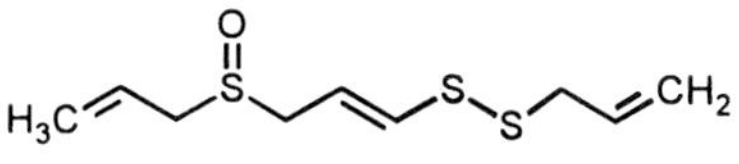

(10) (*E*,*Z*)-ajoene

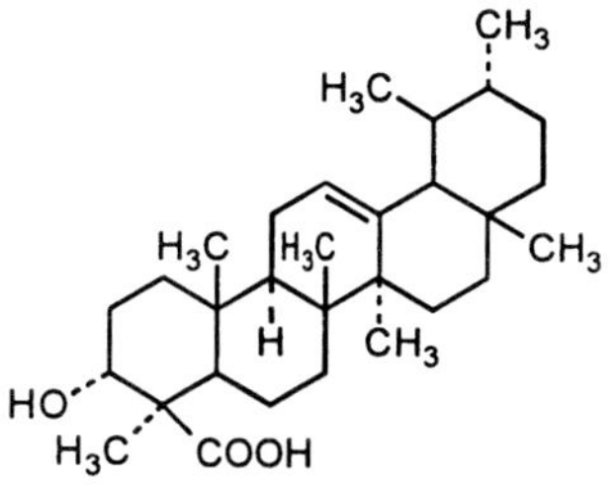

(11) *β*-Boswellic acid

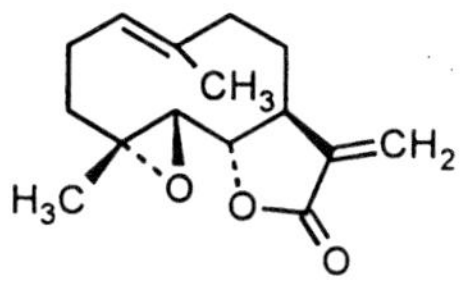

(12) Parthenolide

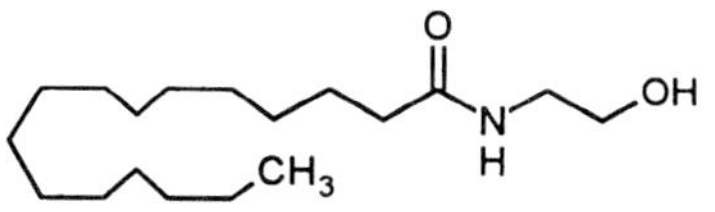

(13) N-(2-hydroxyethyl) hexadecanamide

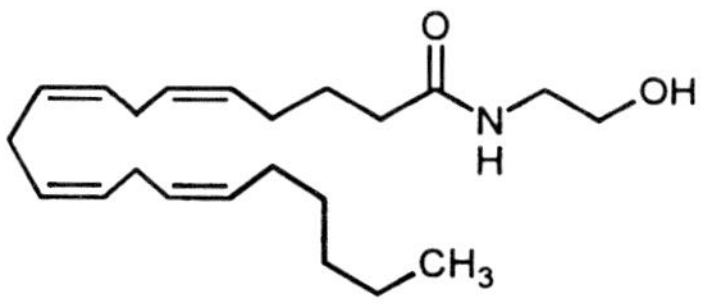

(14) Anandamide

Figure 2.

Plenary discussion

Lebrun Ph.: What is the mode of action of piperine at the molecular level?
Wagner H.: Piperin is structurally analogous to Capsaicin. It is an irritant and might exert its antiinflammatory activity in a way which is similar to Capsaicin.

Amassian V.: Given the extraordinary ability of chromatographic analysis to characterize old and new chemical compounds, I wonder what would be a good strategy to find out if they are therapeutically effective? Clinical trials are now so elaborate and expensive, it appears that some strategy is needed.

Wagner H.: Antiinflammatory or analgesic compounds in plant extracts can be found only by screening the extracts or fractions using some *in vitro* or *in vivo* models followed by a bioguided fractionation of the extract.

Morpurgo C.: We are looking for drugs with local activity, where the tissues are damaged by traumatic events, which can mimic the action of ice-therapy on the blood vessels and of some drugs active in modulating the reaction of the mesenchymal elements. Do you have any news?

Wagner H.: I know only of the topical application of extracts of Chamomil, Arnica or onion.

Trifaro J.-M.: You mentioned in your talk that canabis acts on CB_2 receptors to produce a downregulation of mast cells. Could you be more specific on the effects of canabis on mast cells?

Wagner H.: In the literature it is described that Cannabis may exert its antiinflammatory effect via a downregulation of mast cell activation in a way that differs from established steroidal and nonsteroidal antiinflammatory agents.

References

Ammon HPT (1996) Phytomedicine 3: 67.

Atkinson DC and Hicks R (1975) Agents and Actions 5: 239.

Dray A (1995) Br J Anaesth 75: 125.

Dearden JC and Nicholson RM (1984) J Pharm Pharmacol 36: 713.

Facci L, Dal Toso R, Remanello S, Buriam A and Pionello D. (1996) Arachidonic acid in cell signalling, Chapter 6, Springer, Heidelberg, Germany.

Fessler B (1988) Thesis, Munich, Germany.

Hall IH, Starnes CO, Lee KH and Waddel TG (1980) I Pharm Sci 69: 537.

Hayes MA and Foreman JC (1987) J Pharm Pharmacol 39: 466.

Heptinstall S, White A, Williamson L and Mitchell JRA (1985) Lancet 1071.

Jack DB (1995) Drug News and Perspectives 9 (2): 93.

Kimura Y, Okuda H, Okuda T and Anichi S (1986) Planta Med 54: 337.

Knaus U and Wagner H (1996) Phytomedicine 3: 77.

Mazzari S, Canelia R, Peurelli L, Marcologno G and Leon A (1997) Eur J Pharm (in press)

Majewska MD (1980) Science 232: 1344.

Sendl A, Elbl G, Steinke B, Redl K, Breu W and Wagner H (1997) Planta Med 58: 1.

Shaper SD and Leon A (1995) Proc Natl Acad Sci, USA 92: 3376.

Wagner H (1989) Planta Med 55: 235.

Wagner H and Fessler B (1986) Planta Med 54: 343.

Wagner H and Nusser D (1988) Dtsch Apoth Ztg 128: 1921.

Wagner H and Nusser D (1989) Dtsch Apoth Ztg 129: 2099S.

Wagner H and Reger H (1987) Dtsch Apoth Ztg, 126: 2613.

Wagner H, Wierer M and Bauer R (1986) Planta Med 54: 184.

Wagner H, Wierer M and Fessler B (1987) Planta Med 55: 305.

Wong SM, Antus S, Gottsegen A, Fessler B, Rao GS, Sonnenbichler I and Wagner H (1988) Arzneimittel-Forsch (Drug Res) 38: 661.

Wünnenberg W, Merker G and Brück K (1974) Pflügers Arch 352: 11.

Yaksh TL, Farb DH, Leemann SE and Jesell TM (1979) Science 206: 418.

Pain Mechanisms and Management
S.N. Ayrapetyan and A.V. Apkarian (Eds.)
IOS Press, 1998

Arachidonic Acid Release and Metabolism Associated Mode of Action of Some Plant Immunomodulators

A. G. Panossian[1], E. Gabrielian[1] and H.Wagner[2]
[1]*C.Guelbenkian Research Laboratories of the Drug Agency*
National Academy of Science
Yerevan, Armenia
[2]*Institute of Pharmaceutical Biology of the LMU*
Munich, Germany

Abstract. Capsaicin, the pungent principle of red hot pepper, is known for its reversal effects on the tracheobronchial system depending on the treatment: acute capsaicin treatment induces pro-inflammatory effects, whereas chronic treatment has an inflammatory protective effect. The dual nature of capsaicin treatment is obviously associated with its dose dependent reversal effects on cell membranes, and the accumulation of capsaicin in the body during chronic treatment. In the present study of the mechanism of the action of capsaicin, an attempt has been made to determine the dose dependent effects of capsaicin on the early intracellular events after binding of capsaicin to membranes--arachidonic acid metabolism followed by production of inter-leukin 1α and nitric oxide in human immunocompetent cells. We found that capsaicin stimulates IL-1α production at low concentrations 10^{-8} to 10^{-5}M, and inhibit it at the concentration 10^{-4}M. A possible explanation of this dual reversal effects of capsaicin could be that capsaicin in high concentrations stimulates the release of AA from isolated human PMNL. As a result of activation of AA release production of PGE_2 an nitric oxide is also increased, thus leading to an inhibition of IL-1α production (antiinflammatory effect). Both NO and PGE_2 are known as potent vasodilators. Our finding could also explain the beneficial effects of capsaicin on tracheobronchial system during chronic treatment, when capsaicin is accumulated in the organism. In acute treatment with capsaicin (low concentrations) an increase IL-1α production could induce inflammatory effects.

Introduction

Normally, when high intensity stimuli induces little or no tissue damage, transient pain is induced and serves as physiological warning. However, during inflammation produced by mild tissue damage or infection, the pain produced differs in quality and may be more persistent. A number of events can be considered as a physiological protective response; the nociceptive system reverting back to normal state once the underlying injury has healed.

In chronic pain conditions associated with chronic inflammation, physiological relevance of the nonciptive signals is less clear and the protective function of afferent activity is obscure. Chronic pain is symptomatic of numerous conditions including rheumatoid arthritis, cancer neuropathic pain etc. The mechanisms of chronic pain are still poorly understood, and pain is difficult to ameliorate. It is likely, however, that in pain conditions, whether inflammatory or neuropathic, there is an associated phase of inflammation in which a variety of chemical mediators are able to alter the functions of peripheral afferent fibers. These factors produced during tissue damage include reactive oxygen species, such as NO, eicosanoids, kinins, protons, serotonine and histamine, cytokines. Inhibition of the formation of these mediators of inflammation can have beneficial effect and is associated with pain relief.

In our studies we have investigated effects of various natural compounds which are recognized as active principles responsible for antitumoral and antiinflammatory activity on the release of key mediators of activation of immune system in activated leukocytes: leukotriene B4, hyperalgesic mediator of inflammation, an activator of neutrophils, and a modulator in the immune system which induce prostaglandin E2 (which induces the release of substance P from sensory neurons nitric oxide, which induces a delayed burning pain upon intradermal injection, and activates cerebral sensory fibers directly), and IL-1α, which is released from variety of immune cells and induces powerful hyperalgesia, affecting indirectly via several mechanisms including prostanoid release.

Capsaicin (8-methyl-*n*-vanillyl-6-nonenamide), the pungent principle of red hot pepper, is known for its irritating properties. It has reversal effects on the tracheobronchial system depending on the treatment. Acute capsaicin treatment induces proinflammatory effects (i.e. airway smooth muscle contraction, tracheal plasma extravasation, an increased submucosal secretion and bronchoconstriction in animals). Chronic capsaicin treatment, on the other hand, has inflammatory protective effect, preventing cigarette smoke induced tracheal dye extravasation, and desensitizes the respiratory tract mucosa against a variety of chemical and mechanical irritants. It also protects rat lungs from damage induced by free radicals [Buck and Burks, 1986; De and Ghosh, 1988 -1991; De et al., 1992; Lundberg and Saria, 1983; Papka et al.,1984].

The mechanism of action of capsaicin is not fully elucidated. It has been demonstrated that it is associated with alterations in cell membrane lipids, calcium homeostasis, antioxidant enzyme defense system, lysosomal leakage and the release of neuropeptides from sensory neurons [Buck and Burks, 1986; De and Ghosh, 1988 -1991; De et al., 1992; Papka et al.,1984].

Treatment with low doses of capsaicin produces a significant increase in UV-induced peroxidation of liposomal membranes, while high doses causes a decrease. It has been suggested that these pro-oxidant and antioxidant activities of capsaicin on liposomal lipid peroxidation may be attributed to activation, followed by desensitization, of the membrane lipid systems [De et al., 1992; Mandal et al., 1995].

The dual nature of capsaicin treatment is obviously associated with its dose dependent reversal effects on cell membranes and the accumulation of capsaicin in the body during chronic treatment.

Usually membrane receptor activation by various stimuli is followed by certain receptor specific intracellular events, which ultimately may induce the release of arachidonic acid from membrane phospholipids and thus leukotriene biosynthesis. During inflammation, products formed by arachidonic acid oxidation act in concert with numerous additional mediators including cytokines, PAF, nitric oxide, and histamine, which are important mediators of the immune response.

In the present study, an attempt has been made to determine the dose dependent effects of capsaicin on the early intracellular events after binding of capsaicin to membranes--arachidonic acid metabolism followed by production of interleukin 1α and nitric oxide in human immunocompetent cells in order to examine if the dual effects of capsaicin are associated with the production of these modulators of the inflammatory response.

Material and methods

AA, LTB$_4$, 6E-LTB$_4$, 5S, 6E-LTB$_4$, ωOH-LTB$_4$, ωCOOH-LTB$_4$, 5S,6S-DHETE, 5S,6R-DHETE, 5-,12-,15-HETEs, PGB$_2$, PGE$_2$-ELISA-Kits and LTB$_4$-ELISA Kits were obtained from Cascade Biochem Ltd.; IL-1α EIA Kits and Nitrate/Nitrite Assay Kits from Cayman Chemical; [5,6,8,9,11,12,14,15- H^3]-AA (213 Ci/mmol) was purchased from Amersham Int.; Ionophore A-23187 from Boehringer Mannheim Biochemica, TPA; and 12-HHT from ICN Biomedicals, Inc.; Ficoll (n=1.077 g/ml) from Gibco; BSA from Sigma; Hank's medium solutions from Biochrom KG.

Human granulocytes, mononuclear cells and lymphocytes were isolated by means of dextran sedimentation, hypotonic lysis of erythrocytes and density gradient as described by Boyum [Boyum, 1987]. Granulocyte preparations contained 85-95% neutrophils, viability greater than 95% as determined by trypan blue exclusion.

Release of AA and AA-metabolites from human PMNL (Phospholipase test)

For the prelabeling of cells, 40 ml suspension of PMNL was incubated for 60 min at 37°C (100x10^6 cell/ml in Hank's buffer solution containing Ca^{+2} and Mg^{+2}) with 30 ml ethanolic solution of [^{3}H]$_8$-AA (30 mCi) [Walsh et al., 1983]. The cells were then sedimented by centrifugation (300 x g, 10 min), washed twice in Hank's and Dulbecco's phosphate buffer (PBS) solution containing 0.1% BSA (without Ca^{+2} and Mg^{+2}), in order to remove free [^{3}H]$_8$-AA bound to the cells. The resulting washed pellet was suspended in PBS to a concentration of 40x10^6 cells/ml and radioactivity of the cell suspension was measured (55-65% incorporation of [^{3}H]$_8$-AA into the cells).

^{3}[H]$_8$-AA prelabeled cells were incubated for 15 min at 37°C with capsaicin in the presence of BSA. Reaction mixtures were centrifuged at 400 x g for 10 min at 4°C, and supernatants were assayed for ^{3}H labeled compounds (released from the cells) using Beckman LS 1801 beta scintillation counter.

1 ml of labeled cells (100-120 $\cdot$10^3 cpm) was added to 10 ml of capsaicin ethanolic solution (final concentration 10^{-8} - 10^{-4} M) and incubated for 15 min at 37°C. All samples were run in triplicate. To control samples only solvent was added. After 30 min of incubation the reaction mixture was centrifuged at 400g, 10 min, 4°C. Supernatants were collected, and radioactivity measured in duplicate (0.2 ml solution in 2 ml of scintillation cocktail "Biofluor").

ELISA for LTB$_4$ and PGE$_2$

Suspensions of isolated human granulocytes (1 ml) were incubated for 10 min at 37°C in PBS containing capsaicin, reaction mixtures were centrifuged at 400g for 10 min at 4°C, supernatants were diluted and assayed for LTB$_4$ and PGE$_2$ (released from the cells) using ELISA test kits as described in instructions supplied with the assay kits. In another series of experiments, incubation reactions were terminated by the addition of 1.5 ml MeOH, followed by centrifugation at 400g for 10 min. 100 ml of aliquots from supernatants were evaporated in vacuum, residues were dissolved in 1 ml of PBS and assayed for LTB$_4$ and PGE$_2$.

Measurement of LTB4: 50 ml of anti-LTB$_4$ antibody solution was added to wells pre-coated with anti-rabbit IgG antibody (96 well MaxiSorp Nunc microplate), followed by the addition of 50 ml of test solutions and LTB$_4$-enzyme (horseradish peroxidase) conjugate. After one hour of incubation at room temperature wells were washed with buffer solution containing Tween 20, and 150 ml of K-blue substrate (stabilized 3,3',5,5'-tetramethylbenzidine with hydrogen peroxide) was added to each well. After 30 min incubation at room temperature absorbance (650 nm) was measured using Microplate reader SLT Spectra (SLT Labinstruments Deutschland GMBH) and concentrations of LTB$_4$ were calculated using a curve for absorbance of standard solutions of LTB$_4$.

Measurement of PGE2: 50 ml of test solutions and PGE$_2$-enzyme (horseradish peroxidase) conjugate solutions were added into wells pre-coated with PGE$_2$ antibody (96 well MaxiSorp Nunc microplate) and incubated for one hour at room temperature. Wells were then washed with buffer solution containing Tween 20, and 150 ml of K-blue substrate (stabilized 3,3',5,5'-tetramethylbenzidine with hydrogen peroxide) was added to each well. After 30 min of incubation at room temperature, absorbance (650 nm) was measured using a Microplate reader SLT Spectra (SLT Labinstruments Deutschland GmbH) and concentrations of PGE$_2$ were calculated using a curve for absorbance of standard solutions of PGE$_2$.

Metabolism of arachidonic acid in PMNL (Lipoxygenases pathway test)

To 10 ml of capsaicin solution (final concentrations 10^{-4} - 10^{-8} M, in triplicate) 1 ml PMNL suspension (40 ·10^6 cells/ml) was added. After 10 or 30 min of preincubation at 37°C 10 ml solutions of calcium chloride, calcium ionophore and arachidonic acid were added (final concentrations 2 mM, 5 mM and 33 mM respectively). Incubation was stopped after 5 min by the addition of 1.5 ml methanol containing PGB$_2$ ($25ng/10^3$ cells). The mixture was centrifuged (600g, 10 min), the supernatant diluted with water to 10 ml, acidified by 2N HCl to pH 3.0, and applied to a Chromabond C18 (100 mg, Machery-Nagel) cartridge, preliminary washed by methanol and water. Elution was performed with 3 ml methanol-water (15:85,v/v) followed by and 5 ml of acetonitril. The acetonitril fraction was evaporated to dryness, redissolved in 100 µl of acetonitril and analyzed by HPLC.

HPLC analysis: HPLC was performed using a "Lichro CART" HPLC cartridge with LiChrospher RP18, 5 mm reversed phase column (Merk, Darmstadt), linear gradient elution with a water-methanol solvent system containing 0.01% acetic acid (65% - 100% methanol, 35 min), flow rate 1.0 ml/min (Hewlett-Packard, HP liquid chromatograph Model 1090, with diode array detection at 235 and 270 nm).

Identification of eicosanoids was performed on the basis of R$_f$ values by comparison with authentic standards (Cascade Biochemical Ltd.).

Assays of IL-1 α and NO production in mononuclear cells

To 10 ml of capsaicin solution (final concentrations 10^{-4} - 10^{-8} M, in triplicate) 1 ml of suspension of monocytes (20×10^6 cells/ml) in RPMI 1640 MEDIUM (containing 0.1% BSA, 2 mM CaCl$_2$, 25 mM HEPES, 2 mM Glutamine, NaCl 5.5 g/l, NaHCO$_3$ 2.0 g/l, and phenol red 5 mg/l) or in balanced Hank's solution containing 0.1% BSA, Glucose, Ca^{+2} and Mg^{+2}) was added. After 30 min of preincubation in a laminar box with fluorescent light, 10 ml PBS solution LPS was added to a final concentration of 10 mg/ml. After 24 and 40 hours of incubation in the laminar box under UV light at room temperature, reactions were terminated by centrifugation at 300 g, 10 min.

Supernatants were assayed for IL-1α and Nitrite/Nitrate as described in instructions supplied with the assay kits.

Measurement of IL-1α: 100 ml of test solutions were added into wells pre-coated with the capture IL-1α antibody 96 well plate, then 100 ml of acethylcholieesterase:Interleukin-1α Fab' conjugate was added and incubated overnight at 4°C. Supernatants were discarded, wells washed with buffer solution containing Tween 20, and 200 ml of Ellman's Reagent {a mixture of acetyl-choline and 5, 5'-dithio-bis-(2-nitrobenzoic acid)} was added to each well. After 15, 30, 60, 90, 120 and 240 min of incubation at room temperature absorbance (415 nm) was measured using a Microplate reader SLT Spectra (SLT Labinstruments Deutschland GMBH). Concentrations of IL-1α were calculated using a curve for absorbance of standard solutions of IL-1α.

Nitric oxide: Nitric oxide production was determined by measurement of total nitrite and nitate anions concentration in a two-step process: conversion of nitrate to nitrite by nitrate reductase, and using Greiss reagent, {0.1% N-(1-Naphtyl)-etylendiamin dihydrochloride, 1% sulfanilamid, 5% phosporic acid }, which converts nitrite into a deep purple azo compound [Green et al., 1982], which have maximum of absorbance at 540 nm. 80 ml of tested solutions were added into each well, then 10 ml of Nitrate reductase and 10 ml of enzyme Co-factor were added. After incubation for two hours, 100 ml of Griess reagents were added, plate allowed to develop colour for 10 min. Absorbance was measured at 540 nm using Microplate reader SLT Spectra (SLT Labinstruments Deutschland GMBH) and concentrations of nitrite were calculated using a curve for absorbance of standard nitrite and nitrate solutions.

Statistical analysis: Statistical analysis was performed using unpaired two-tailed t-test ("t-EASE" ISI Software. version 2. 1987, H.J.Motulsky). The values were expressed as mean ± SE.

Results and discussion

In the first steps of activation of immune cells an activation of arachidonic acid release from membrane phospholipids occurs. In our test model we have used calcium ionophore for cell activation and, a tumor-promoting phorbol ester in concentrations which do not induce effect when they are used alone, but in combination act synergistically and induce the release of AA and eicosanoids from the cell (Figure 1). This activation is mediated by protein kinase C. The increased PKC activity represents a biochemical and functional marker of malignancy. Altering PKC enzyme activity by downregulation or direct inhibition reduces the tumor growth rate. In this regard, various inhibitors of PKC have been shown to inhibit tumor growth.

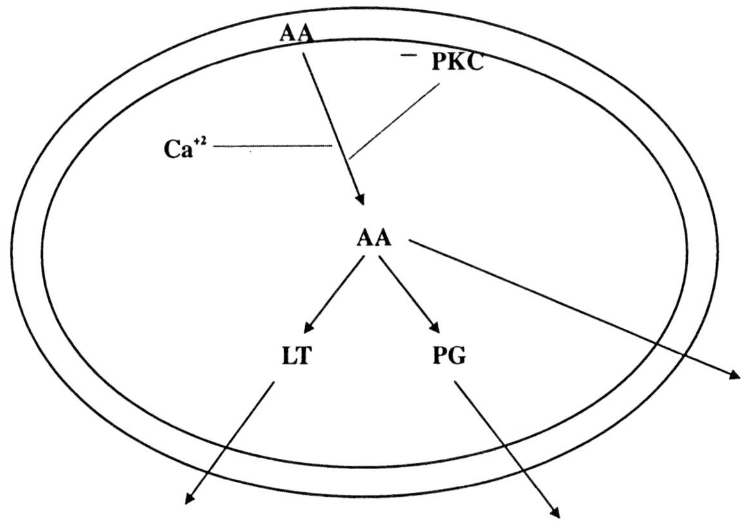

Figure 1.

Table 1. Effect of some natural immunomodulators on the release of arachidonic acid metabolites from stimulated (*) (TPA + A-23187) and non-stimulated (**) human PN

Compound	Activation**	Inhibition*	Compound	Activation**	Inhibition*
Carragenine	-	-	**Hypericin**	-	+
Echinaceae PS-VI	-	-	Apocinin	-	-
Rumex PS-III	-	-	Acetosyringin	-	-
Calendula PS-II	-	-	Syringin	-	-
Chamomillae PS-I	-	-	**Syringenine -DG**	-	+
Mistletoe Lectine I	-	-	Coniferin	-	
Bryostatin	+	+	Coniferyl-DG	-	+
Aristolochic acid	-	+	Rosmarinic acid	-	
Marchantin B	-	-	Caloptylic acid	-	-
Cheledonine	-	-	Inophyllum	-	-
Berberine	-	-	Plumbagin	-	-
Sanquinarine	-	-	**Capsaicin**	+	-
Scopoletine	-	-	Ajoene	-	-

Our further experiments were conducted with capsaicin.

In order to investigate an influence of capsaicin on IL-1α and nitric oxide production human monocytes were incubated with capsaicin for 24 hours. The dual dose dependent effect of capsaicin on IL-1α production can bee seen in table 2. Surprisingly, in low doses (10^{-8}-10^{-5} M) of capsaicin the IL-1α production is stimulated, whereas high dose (10^{-4} M) inhibits the production of IL-1α.

Table 2. Concentration dependence of the effect of capsaicin on IL-1α release from LPS stimulated human monocytes.

Capsaicin concentration (μM)	IL-1α, pg/106cells a	IL-1α, pg/106cells b	IL-1α, pg/106cells c
0 (control)	115 ± 9	75	145
0.1	310 ± 46 *	155	190
1	245 ± 31 *	72	155
10	209 ± 20 *	34	100
100	10 ± 5 *	0	10

a - incubation in balanced Hank's solution containing glucose, incubation for 40 hours
b - incubation in RPMI 1640 MEDIUM, incubation for 24 hours
c - incubation in RPMI 1640 MEDIUM, incubation for 40 hours
* significantly different from control experiments ($p < 0.05$). The results are the mean ± SE of three experiments.

In order to examine an effect of capsaicin on the production of eicosanoids in PMNL, $^3[H]_8$ arachidonic acid labeled human PMNL were incubated with capsaicin for 15 min and centrifugated. Supernatants were assayed for radioactive compounds (AA-metabolites) released from the cells. As can be seen in table 3. capsaicin stimulates the release of arachidonic acid from membrane phospholipids of human neutrophils in a dose dependent manner.

Table 3. Effect of capsaicin on $[^3H]_8$- arachidonic acid release from human PMNL.

Capsaicin concentration (μM)	$[^3H]_x$- arachidonic acid release (% of control, 100%)
0	100 ± 6
0.01	106 ± 2
0.1	106 ± 2
1	114 ± 4 *
10	109 ± 3 *
100	120 ± 4 *

* significantly different from control experiments ($p < 0.05$). The results are the mean ± SE of three experiments.

Table 4. Concentration dependence of the effect of capsaicin on PGE_2 and LTB_4 release from human PMNL.

Capsaicin concentration (μM)	PGE_2,pg/40x10^6cells	LTB_4,pg/40x10^6cells
0	21 ± 7	46 ± 12
0.01	10 ± 4	30 ± 10
0.1	30 ± 8	50 ± 25
1	30 ± 8	33 ± 3
10	110 ± 4 *	30 ± 15
100	190 ± 15 *	250 ± 28 *

* significantly different from control experiments ($p < 0.05$). The results are the mean ± SE of three experiments.

As shown in table 4, treatment with high doses of capsaricin significantly stimulates both LTB_4 and PGE_2 production of human granulocytes.

We found also that high doses of capsaicin activate NO production in isolated human leukocytes (Table 6).

Since capsaicin activates lipid peroxidation, it was important to investigate the proinflammatory effect of capsaicin on the metabolism of arachidonic acid and the biosynthesis of leukotrienes. Capsaicin was incubated in various concentrations with isolated granulocytes and exogenous arachidonic acid. No statistically significant effect was detected. Only at highest concentration of capsaicin (100 µM) biosynthesis of 12-HETE is increased and biosythesis of 5-lipoxygenase products decreased (Table 5a).

In another series of experiments the antiinflammatory effect of capsaicin was studied:

Cells were preincubated with capsaicin and then stimulated with calcium ionophore A-23187. No statistically significant effect was found. (Table 5b).

Table 5a. Effect of capsaicin on the metabolism of exogenous arachidonic acid from isolated human granulocytes, incubation with 33 mM AA.

Capsaicin conc. (µM)	LTB$_4$ ng/10^{6}cells	5-HETE ng/10^{6}cells	12-HETE ng/10^{6}cells	12-HHT ng/10^{6}cells
0	32 ± 18	190 ± 26	207 ± 64	80 ± 29
0.01	36 ± 19	104 ± 55	115 ± 67	43 ± 38
0.1	70 ± 17	275 ± 74	225 ± 54	80 ± 32
1.0	54 ± 18	170 ± 48	177 ± 65	62 ± 30
10	38 ± 21	120 ± 54	169 ± 55	58 ± 31
100	2 ± 13 *	66 ± 39 *	590 ± 74 *	30 ± 18 *

* significantly different from control experiments (p<0.05). The results are the mean ± SE of three experiments.

Table 5b. Effect of capsaicin on the metabolism of exogenous arachidonic acid from isolated human granulocytes, incubation with 33 mM AA, and 5 mM calcium ionophore A-23187

Capsaicin conc. (µM)	5-HETE ng/40 106 cells	LTB4 ng/40 106 cells	HO-LTB4 ng/40 106 cells	6E-LTB4 ng/40 106 cells	5S,6E-LTB4 ng/40 106 cells	5S,6S-DHETE ng/40 106 cells	12-HHT ng/40 106 cells	12-HETE ng/40 106 cells	15-HETE ng/40 106 cells
0	663±170	308±34	1005±39	256±43	245±40	87±21	76±19	201±35	105±26
0.01	520±85	322±46	902± 85	228±43	220±43	49±32	51±21	640±425	76±35
0.1	806±73	380±38	1312±233	216±54	190±35	55±29	88±21	552±355	58±48
1	727±62	352±44	1076±190	179±65	165±62	61±31	68±29	331±143	60±32
10	1180±121	435±8	1501±407	270±52	250±51	72±35	66±32	513±247	80±37
100	1062±175	448±62	771±231	162±72	145±75	75±29	8±6 *	365±164	82±29

The results are the mean ± SE of three experiments

IL-1α is known as a potent mediator of inflammation and immune response: it has pirogenic properties, induces acute-phase reaction, activates granulocytes, eosinophils, natural killers, T- and B-cells, reactive oxygen intermediate and nitric oxide production, etc. [Durum et al.,1985].

As shown at table 2 capsaicin stimulates IL-1α production at low concentrations 10^{-8} to 10^{-5}M, and inhibits it at the concentration 10^{-4}M. This observation is in accordance with other publications where it is shown that low doses of capsaicin have proinflammatory effects, and high doses reversal effects in various test systems [De et al., 1992; Mandal et al., 1995].

A possible explanation of this dual reversal effect of capsaicin could be that capsaicin, depending on concentrations (or doses) used affects various enzymatic systems associated with each other in a suppressive manner. We suggest that these systems could be arachidonic acid cascade, and eicosanoids which are known to interact with cytokins in a reversal manner [Cavaillon, Heaffner-Cavaillon,1990; Fenton et al., 1988; Lewis, 1990; Nakazato, 1991].

As it shown in table 3, capsaicin stimulates the release of AA. This effect could be due to alterations in cell membranes, induced by capsaicin, which has lipophylic carbohydrate chain and polar phenolic moiety attached to amide group.

As a result of activation of AA release, production of PGE$_2$ is also increased, table 4. We have not been able to find any effect of capsaicin on the biosynthesis of 12-HHT, a cyclooxygenase product formed upon incubation of AA acid with granulocytes. (table 5). PGE$_2$ is known to inhibit IL-1α production and therefore suppress certain immune reactions. Inhibition of lymphocyte activity is the main function of PGE$_2$ in the immune system, and PGE$_2$ may be viewed as a macrophage messenger transducing an inhibitory signal to lymphocytes [Goodwin, Webb, 1980].

In acute treatment with capsaicin (low concentrations) an increase IL-1α production is seen (the mode of action is still unknown). During chronic treatment capsaicin is accumulated in the body (high concentrations), the release of AA and the formation of PGE$_2$ is increased, thus leading to an inhibition of IL-1α production (antiinflammatory effect).

As shown in table 6, capsaicin induces NO production at 10^{-4}M concentration, whereas other concentrations are nonactive. We can only speculate that it could be a result of the increase of PGE$_2$ formation, since it is known that cyclooxygenase inhibitors (NSAID: aspirin, indometha-cin etc.) reduces NO formation in activated macrophages [Brouet, Ohshima, 1995].

Table 6. Effect of capsaicin on NO production in human monocytes.

Capsaicin concentration (μM)	Nitrite concentration (μM)
0	3
0.1	3
1	3
10	3
100	19

Both NO and PGE$_2$ are known as potent vasodilators [Moncada et al.,1991; Gabrielian and Amroyan, 1977]. An increase of their formation at high concentrations of capsaicin could be an explanation of the beneficial effects of capsaicin on tracheobronchial system during chronic treatment.

Abbrevations

PMNL	- polymorphonuclear leukocytes
AA	- arachidonic acid
LTB_4	- leukotriene B_4
PGB_2	- prostaglandin B_2
DHETE	- 5S,12S-dihydroxy-6,8,10,14(E,Z,E,Z)-eicosatetraenoic acid
5-HETE	- 5S-hydroxy-6,8,11,14(E,Z,Z,Z)-eicosatetraenoic acid
12-HETE	-12S-hydroxy-5,8,10,14(Z,Z,E,Z)-eicosatetraenoic acid
15-HETE	- 15S-hydroxy-5,8,11,13(Z,Z,Z,E)-eicosatetraenoic acid
12-HHT	- 12S-hydroxy-5,8,10(Z,Z,E)-hepta-decatrienoic acid
BSA	- bovin serum albumin
LO	- lipoxygenase
CO	- cyclooxygenase
IL	- interleukin
ELISA	- enzyme-linked immunosorbent assay

Acknowledgements

This work was supported by DFG. The authors are grateful to Mrs. S. Reiter and S. Berger for excellent technical assistance.

References

Boyum A (1987) Isolation of lymphocytes, granulocytes and macrophages. Scand J Immunol 5:9-15.

Brouet I and Ohshima H (1995) Curcumin, an anti-tumor promoter and anti-inflammatory agent, inhibits induction of nitric oxide synthase in activated macrophages. Biochem Biophys Res Commun 206: 533-540.

Buck HS and Burks TS (1986) The neuropharmacology of capsaicin. Review of some recent observations. Pharmacol Rev 38: 179-226.

Cavaillon JM and Heaffner-Cavaillon N (1990) Signals involved in interleukin I synthesis and release by lipopolysaccharide-stimulated onocytes/macrophages. Cytokine 2: 313-320.

De AK and Ghosh JJ (1988a) Inflammatory effects of chronic and acute capsaicin treatment on rat paw. Phytother Res 2: 175-179.

De AK and Ghosh JJ (1989) Capsaicin treatment protects free radical induced rat lung damage on exposure to gaseous chemical irritants. Phytother Res 3: 159-161.

De AK and Ghosh JJ (1988b) Short and long-term effects of capsaicin on the pulmonary anti-oxidant enzymes defense system. Phytother Res 3: 182-185.

De AK and Ghosh JJ (1990) Capsaicin treatment and pulmonary damage at the mitochondrial level. Eur J Pharmacol 183: 1693-1694.

De AK and Ghosh JJ (1991a) Effect of short-term capsaicin treatment on formalin and nitrogendioxide induced change in lipid peroxidation and anti-oxidant enzymes in rat lung. Phytother Res 5: 88-91.

De AK and Ghosh JJ (1991b) In vivo and in vitro studies on capsaicin and membrane bound calcium interactions in the rat lung using chlorotetracicline as a fluorescence probe. Phytother Res 5: 5-8.

De AK and Ghosh JJ (1991c) Effects of in vitro and in vivo capsaicin treatment on pulmonary lysosomal preparations in rat. Med Sci Res 9: 115-116.

De AK, Mandal TK and Ghosh JJ (1992) Ultraviolet radiation induced lipid peroxidation in liposomal membrane: modification by capsaicin. Phytother Res 7: 87-89.

Durum SK, Schmidt JA and Opperheim JJ (1985) Interleukin 1: an immunological perspective. Ann Rev Immunol 3: 263-287.

Fenton MJ, Vermeulen MW, Clark BD, Webb AC and Auron PE (1988) Human pro-IL-1 gene expression in monocytic cells is regulated by two distinct pathways. J Immunol 140: 2267-2273.

Gabrielian ES and Amroyan EA (1977) Influence of prostaglandins E1 and E2 on the adrenergic reactions of cerebral vessels. Pharmacol and Toxicol (Russ) 6: 698-703.

Goodwin JS and Webb DR (1980) Regulation of immune response by prostaglandins. Clinical Dermatology and Immunopatholigy 15: 106-122.

Green LC, Wagner DA and Glogowski J (1982) Analysys of nitrate, nitrite, and [^{15}N]nitrate in biological fluids. Anal Biochem 126: 131-138.

Lewis RA (1990) Interactions of eicosanoids and cytokines in immune regulation. In: Adv Prost Thrombox Leukotr Res (B Samuelsson et al. eds) Raven Press, New York, 20: 170-178.

Lundberg JM and Saria A (1983) Capsaicin induced desensitization of airway mucosa to cigarette smoke, mechanical and chemical irritants. Nature 302: 251-253.

Mandal TK, Chakraborty B and De AK (1995) Studies on the effects of capsaicin on leakage in egg lecithin (Phosphatidyl Choline) liposome membranes in vitro Phytother Res 9:425-428.

Moncada S, Palmer RMJ and Higgs EA (1991) Nitric oxide: physiology, pathophysiology and pharmacology. Pharmacol Rev 43: 109-142.

Nakazato Y, Simonson MS, Herman WH, Konieczkowski M and Sedor JR (1991) Interleukin 1a stimulates prostaglandin biosynthesis in serum-activated mesangial cells by induction of a non-pancreatic (type II) phospholipase A2. J Biol Chem 266: 14119-14127.

Papka RE, Furness JB, Della NL, Mutphy R and Costa M (1984) Time course of effect of capsaicin on ultrastructure and histochemistry of substance P immunoreactive nerves associated with the ardiovascular system of the guinea pig. Neuroscience 12: 12711 12792.

Walsh CE, Waite BM, Thomas MJ and DeChatelet LR (1981) Release and metabolism of arachidonic acid in human neutrophils. J Biol Chem 256(14): 7228-7234.

Pain Mechanisms and Management
S.N. Ayrapetyan and A.V. Apkarian (Eds.)
IOS Press, 1998

Review of the Medicinal Plants of Armenia and Karabagh

A.A. Charchoglian
Institute of Botany, Yerevan, Armenia

Throughout history, plants have been the most important source of medicines for human health. Many modern medicines are derived from plants, either extracted from the plants themselves or artificially synthesized to copy plant chemical compounds. Medicinal plants form an important part of the world's economy, and millions are used for medicine each year--leaves, bark, roots, stems, seeds, fruits and flowers.

The World Health Organisation estimated that up to 80% of the people of the world use plants for their primary health care. In China, for example, traditional medicine is largely based on some 5,000 plants and used to treat 40% of urban patients and 90% of patients in rural areas. In 1991, more than 700,000 tons of plant material was used in medicine in China, 80% collected from the wild.

Nowadays 600 different plants belonging to 120 families are used as raw material for pharmaceutical industry in Brazil.

In industrial countries, the use of plants for medicine has declined. But plants have contributed more than 7,000 different compounds in use today as heart drugs, laxatives, anti-cancer agents, hormones, contraceptives, diuretics, antibiotics, decongestants, analgesics, anaesthetics, ulcer treatments and anti-parasitic compounds. Worldwide, extensive pharmaceutical screening programs are being carried out to identify chemical compounds that may provide new treatments for human diseases.

Recently there has been a remarkable revival in the use of herbal medicine in many countries, partly as a result of rising interest in natural products. Plants have also contributed valuable drugs for modern medicine.

The floristic regions of Armenia and Karabagh have a rich diversity of plants and include about 115 families and 3,200 species. There are many species which have been known from ancient time as medicinal plants, and tribal communities whose knowledge about specific plant usage has been transmitted largely through word of mouth and tradition. Much of this ethnobotanical knowledge has therefore remained endemic to certain regions and needs to be systematically surveyed, documented and utilised. Ethnobotanical documentation provides an effective strategy for identification of promising leads from plants for development of new sources of drugs, edibles, oils, anti-fertility and therapeutic agents. It is very important to develop in Armenia ethnopharmacopoeia, which will be practised locally in traditional medicine, ethnoveterinary, and folk medicine. Recent ethnobotanical surveys have shown that there are about 400 wild species from various genera used for food, medicine, overages, contraceptives, and other uses: Achillea, Artemisia, Astragalus, Bryonia, Bidens, Carthamus, Centaurea, Capparis, Echinops, etc. Our studies will be aimed at exploration and survey of plants used in tribal societies; creating ethnobotanical repertories and database; establishing ethnobotanical herbaria, musea, and gardens; phytochemical, biological and pharmacological screening of important species.

Results of ethnobotanical research indicate that many species represent an important group of plants used in traditional medicine of Armenia and Karabagh. For example, as prophylactic remedy against different heart (cardiac) diseases, pain-weakness, coughing, headache, high blood pressure etc., it is very popular to use plants as medicinal teas. Tea from roots of *Acorus calamus* is used as sedative, antimicrobial, antipain, antialergic remedy. The flowers of *Armeniaca vulgaris* and *Crataegus ssp.* are used against hypertension, and sclerosis. The tea from *Hypericum perforatum* may be used as immunoadaptogene, sedative, antiviral agent. The population of these regions widely uses as medicinal teas the plants from genera *Mentha, Melissa, Sambucus, Thymus, Cornus, Betula, Morus, Rosa, Trifolium, Chamerion, Helichrysum, Berberis, Artemisia, Glycyrrhiza, Ribes, Cichorium, Quercus, Punica,* etc. People in Armenia and Karabagh are widely using forest resources as medicinal raw material. About 60 species from 24 genera and 10 families (18% of dendroflora of these regions) are used for medicinal purposes (*Rhamnus, Viburnuim, Sorbus, Hippophae, Elaeagnus, Juniperus, Tilia, Quercus, Populus, Rosa,* etc.). There are species with high antibiotic activity (*Rhamnus cathartica, Astragalus oleifolius*), phytoncide activity (representatives of *Populus, Ulmus, Clematis, Lonicera*), anti-cancer activity (*Hippophaea rhamnoides, Elaeagnus angustifolium*), antirheumatic activity (*Betula pendula*), and anaesthetic activity (*Amygdalus communis, Persica vulgaris*).

Many medicinal and industrial natural products are received from arid-adapted plants. *Capparis spinosa* is a representative species of Yerevan's flora and is used in food, flavour, pharmaceutical, chemical and other related industries. *Alhagi pseudoalhagi* is effective against hemorrhoides, disentery, ulcer of stomach and in the food industry, it is used as spice. Other respresentative species and their effects are: *Centaurea solstitialis*--antifever, gastric; *Centaurea depressa*--against neurasthenia; *Onopordum acanthium*--antitumor, antiseptic; *Centaurea behen, Serratula coriacea*--alkoloid producing; *Grossheimia macrocephala*--vitamin E producing species; *Acroptilon repens*--antimicrobial. It is important to note that the stock of the raw material of these species may supply the needs of the food and pharmaceutical industries.

Many important medicinal plants are in danger of disappearing as a result of natural habitat loss and over-harvesting from the wild. Urgent measures are needed to conserve these vital natural resources for the future. New strategies being developed include:

- cultivating medicinal plants as crops to take the pressure off the remaining wild stocks,

- conserving back-up collections in botanical gardens and seed banks,

- establishing special nature reserves to conserve wild stock,

- developing local programmes for the sustainable use and conservation of important medicinal plants,

- conserving the knowledge of local people and indigenous cultures on the use and value of plants for medicine,

- breeding and developing improved strains of medicinal plants to reduce the need for wild collecting,

- introducting various species of medicinal plants, especially endemics and rare ones, into isolated tissue culture. So far about 30 species of the Armenian flora have been introduced and they include: *Acorus calamus, Bryonia alba, Atropa belladonna, Salvia dracocephaoides, Hypericum perforatum, Ephedra procera,* etc.

Pain Mechanisms and Management
S.N. Ayrapetyan and A.V. Apkarian (Eds.)
IOS Press, 1998

Locust Poison (LP) as Pain Relieving Drug

A.A. Saghyan, A.Sh. Hunanian, S.N. Ayrapetyan and P. Usherwood*
Biophysics Center of Armenian National Academy of Sciences
Yerevan, Armenia
** Life Science Department*
Nottingham University, United Kingdom

Abstract. It was shown that Locust Poison (LP) has the following concentration-dependent effects on: neuronal membrane of Helix pomatia: 1) potential-independent inhibitory effect on neuronal membrane excitability 2) activation effect on electrogenic Na-K pump, 3) inhibitory effect on membrane chemosensitivity, 4) increasing effect on membrane resistance; Xenopus oocyte: 1) specific blocking effect on NMDA receptors without touching other receptor systems expressed in Xenopus oocytes previously injected with corresponding mRNA from rat brain.

Introduction

A number of biologically active substances from poisons of different insects are widely used in research and therapeutic practice. These poisons contain peptides, unsaturated fatty acids, and substances of a carbohydrate nature. The large family of locusts is widespread existing in different geographical regions of the world. All species of locusts exhibit buccal secretion (Locust poison LP) in extreme situations. In old Armenian folk medicine in the Nagorno-Karabagh Republic, LP was used as a pain relieving factor in case of skin surface injuries. The chemical composition of LP and the molecular mechanism of its biological effect are not clear yet, although it can serve as a good source for new drugs for pain relief.

According to the theory of metabolic regulation of membrane excitability (Ayrapetyan S.N.1996), pain could be considered as an abnormal excitation of nerve endings due to abnormal hydration (cell swelling). Na-K pump and Na:Ca exchange are seen as cellular protective mechanisms through which the metabolic regulation of cell hydration is realized (Ayrapetyan & Suleymanyan, 1979; Ayrapetyan, 1995). It was shown that membrane proteins having enzymatic, chemoreceptive and channel properties are functionally either in active or inactive state and that the ratio of these two groups of proteins depends on membrane surface area. Cell swelling leads to the increase of number of functional active molecules, while cell shrinking to the increase of reserved molecules in the membrane. Thus cell hydration is considered as a second messenger, through which external signals can modulate membrane functional activity. From this theory it can be predicted that any factor which has dehydration effect could have a pain relief effect too.

Methods

Electrical activity of single oocyte was recorded by a standard Voltage-Clump setup, using 2 separate glass microelectrodes filled with 2.5 M KCl solution. To express NMDA and kinate receptors, corresponding mRNA was injected in oocytes. These receptors were expressed in the membrane of oocytes in 7-10 days. For fast drug application on oocyte membrane, double perfusion technique was used. In addition to the basic perfusion of solution, which was a continuous flow of normal physiological solution through the whole experimental chamber, a thin (less than 2 mm2) tube was set up close to oocytes through which the drug-containing or normal solution was applied.

Stimulation of active transport of sodium ions from the cell was produced by increasing intracellular sodium concentration. This was done by preliminary incubation of the preparation for 15-20 min. in cold K-free Ringer's solution. The initial solution consisted of Ringer's solution for Helix with the following composition (in mM): NaCl 80, KCl 4,CaCl 27, MgCl 213,TrisHCl. The K ion concentration in the solution surrounding the cell was increased by equivalent substitution of Na ions by K ions.

Neurons of Helix pomatia and xenopus oocytes were used as experimental models. The standard microelectrode technique with VC and CC methods was used. (Ayrapetyan et al.,1986; Saghyan et al.,1987). Collected LP from Karabagh locusts and dried for 24 hours in a small Petry dish in a dry box at room temperature were used. The obtained crystals were dissolved in snail's Ringer solution. LP is easily dissolved in water solutions without causing any noticeable change in pH. The preliminary testing showed that all poisons from 10 species of locust had similar qualitative effect on neuronal membrane excitability and chemosensitivity. However, the highest potency LP is obtained from locust Leptophyes Albovittata. The data presented resulted from studies using mainly this LP, and the same LP is recommended for future investigations.

Results and discussion

In figure 1 presents the LP effect on membrane excitability. From the figure it can be seen that the blocking effect of LP on cell excitability is increased by the increase of LP concentration in medium. Complete blocking takes place in LP concentrations of $3x10^{-2}$ mg/ml. The I-V relation shows (Fig 2) that, in LP containing medium membrane, resistance increases as compared to control. In the next series of experiments, the effect of LP on Na pump activity was studied. Figure 3 shows that LP in concentration of $1x10^{-4}$ mg/ml leads to the increase of pump-induced hyperpolarization of neuronal membrane with beating activity. In the presence of LP, the amplitude of pump-induced hyperpolarization increased significantly as compared to the control. In the case of neurons with bursting activity (figure 4) the K-free solution with LP ($1x10^{-4}$ mg/ml) causes depolarization of the membrane which is not accompanied by the electrical pattern as in the case of beating neurons. It can also be seen that ouabain ($1x10^{-4}$M) completely inhibits this hyperpolarization.

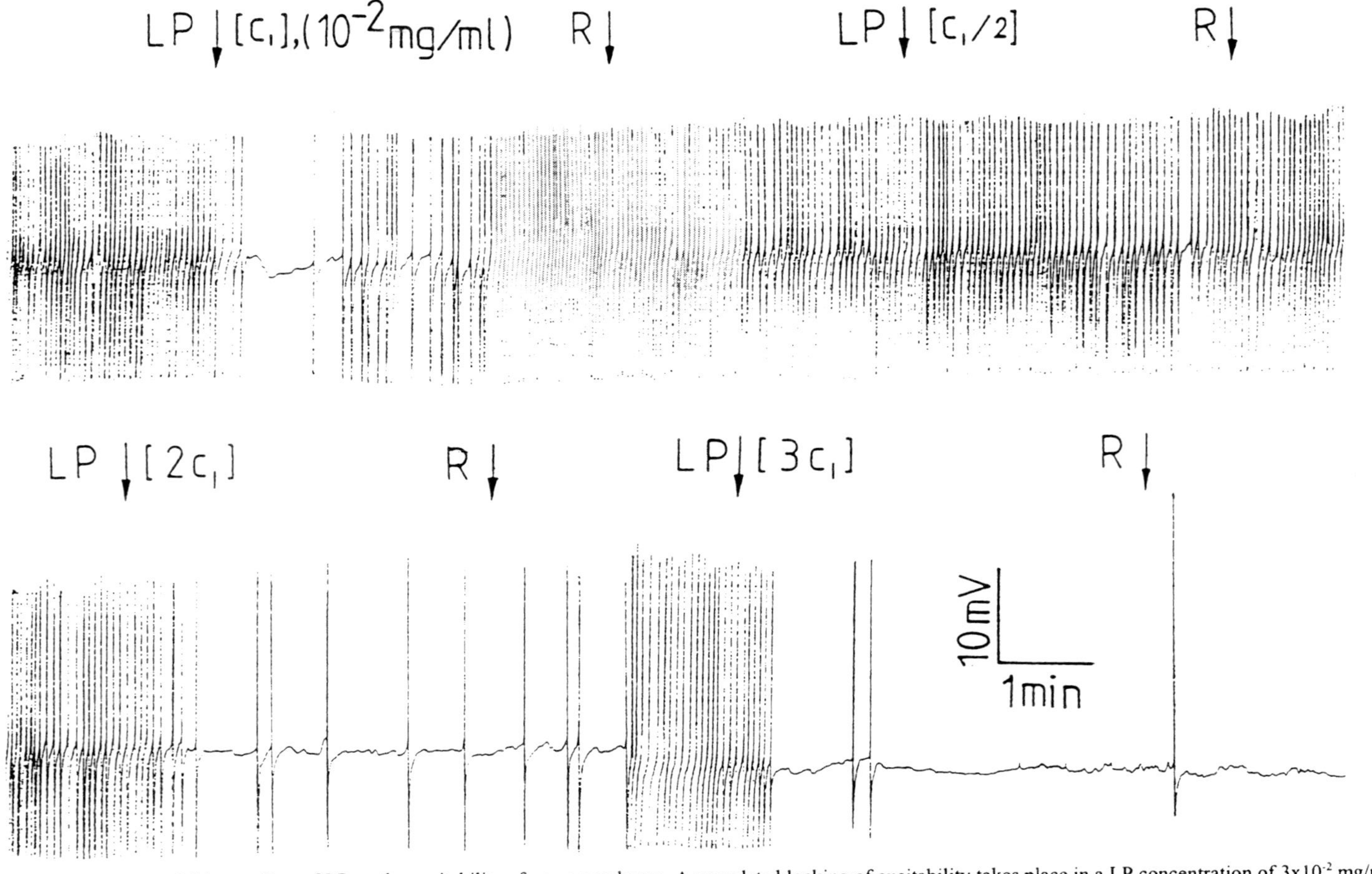

Figure 1. Dose-dependent inhibitory effect of LP on the excitability of neuromembrane. A complete blocking of excitability takes place in a LP concentration of 3×10^{-2} mg/ml in medium without further recovery of action potentials.

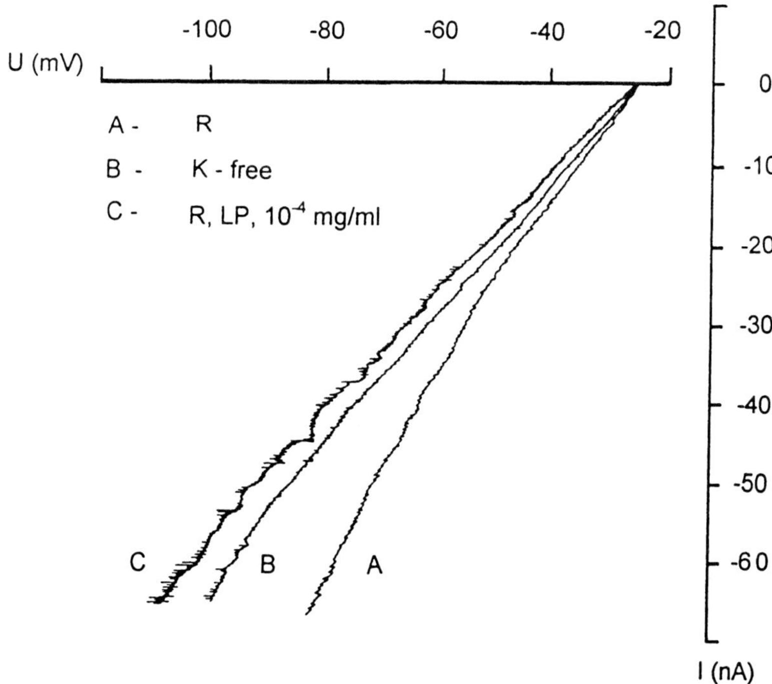

Figure 2. LP effect on membrane I-V relation. The membrane resistance is significantly increased upon LP application.

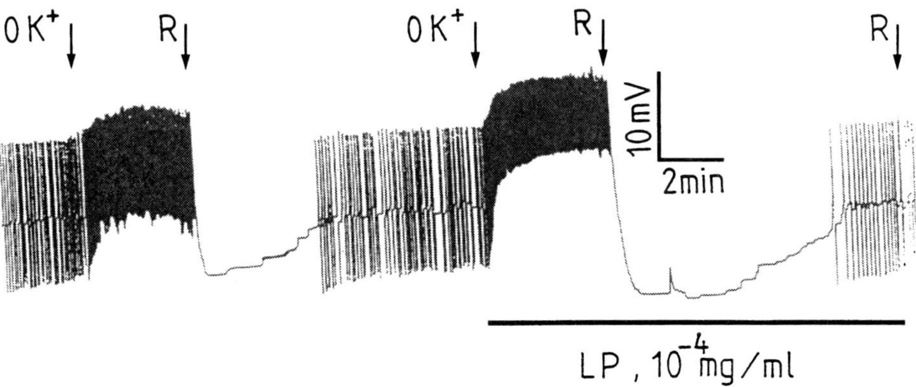

Figure 3. LP effect on pump-induced hyperpolarization of neuronal membrane. In the presence of LP in medium, the amplitude of the pump-induced hyperpolarization increased by more than two times compared to control.

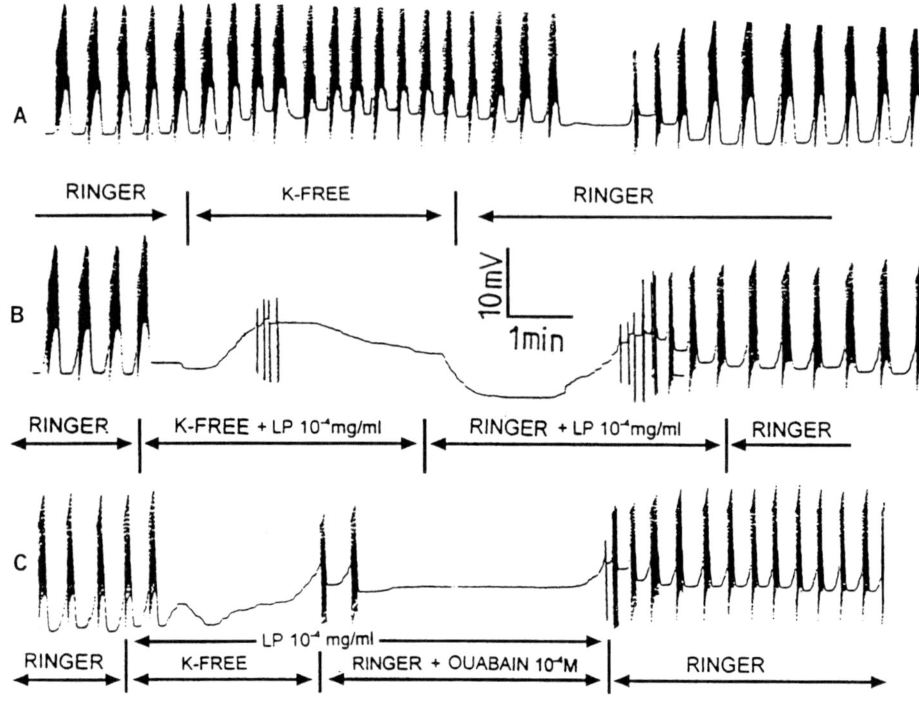

Figure 4. LP blocking effect on electrical activity of bursting pacemaker neuron.
A-Revealing of Na pump activation in control;
B-the effect of LP in K-free and normal physiological solutions;
C-the blocking effect of 1x10⁻⁴M ouabain on LP-induced activation of Na pump.

To study the LP effect on membrane chemosensitivity, the Ach-responses upon LP application were checked. Figure 5 shows that LP in concentration of 1×10^{-4} mg/ml decreases the Ach-induced ionic current in comparison to control for about 15%. However, after the washout of LP from medium the Ach-induced current is increased for about 15-20%. A similar but lesser effect is observed in concentration of LP lower than 10^{-4} mg/ml (date is not presented).

Earlier it was shown (Ayrapetyan, Suleimanian 1979) that Na pump activation leads to cell shrinking and, therefore, to the decrease in number of functional active receptors (Ayrapetyan, Arvanov 1979). These data suggest that this mechanism is responsible for LP effect on Ach-induced current. On the other hand, it was also shown (Ayrapetyan, Arvanov 1985) that Na pump modulates the affinity of Ach receptors to its ligands. The increase of Ach-induced current after the washout of LP from medium can be the result of Na pump-induced increased affinity of Ach receptors. As in the neuronal membrane different chemoreceptor systems are presented, the study of the specific effect of LP on chemosensitivity appears very complicated. For this purpose, the next series of experiments were performed on xenopus oocytes. It is known that this object has no endogenous receptors but, by injection of adequate mRNA from rat brain, corresponding receptor systems can be obtained.

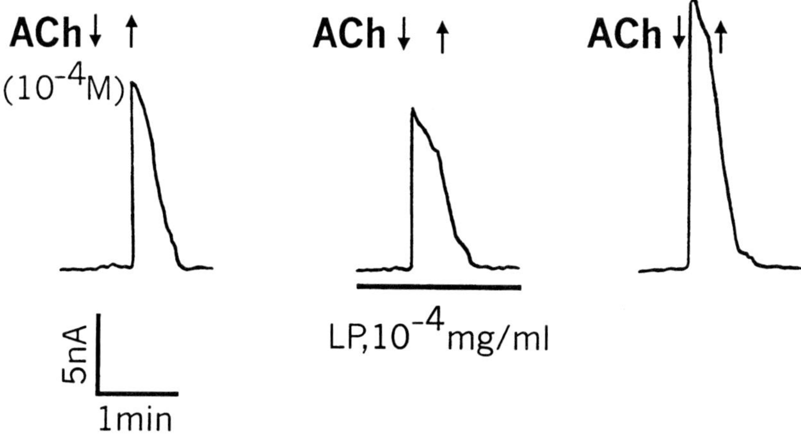

Figure 5. Effect of LP on ACh-induced ionic current after incubation of neurons in a LP-containing medium for 5 minutes and after its washout. The intervals between application of ACh were 10 minutes.

To express kainate or NMDA receptors corresponding mRNA was previously injected in oocytes. These receptors were expressed in the membrane of oocytes in 7-10 days.

Figure 6 shows that the kainate-induced inward current was insensitive to LP application. It also can be seen that LP in 10^{-5} mg/ml concentration had no effect on K-free induced depolarization reflecting the Na-pump inhibition. This fact suggests that Na pump in oocyte membrane is insensitive to LP.

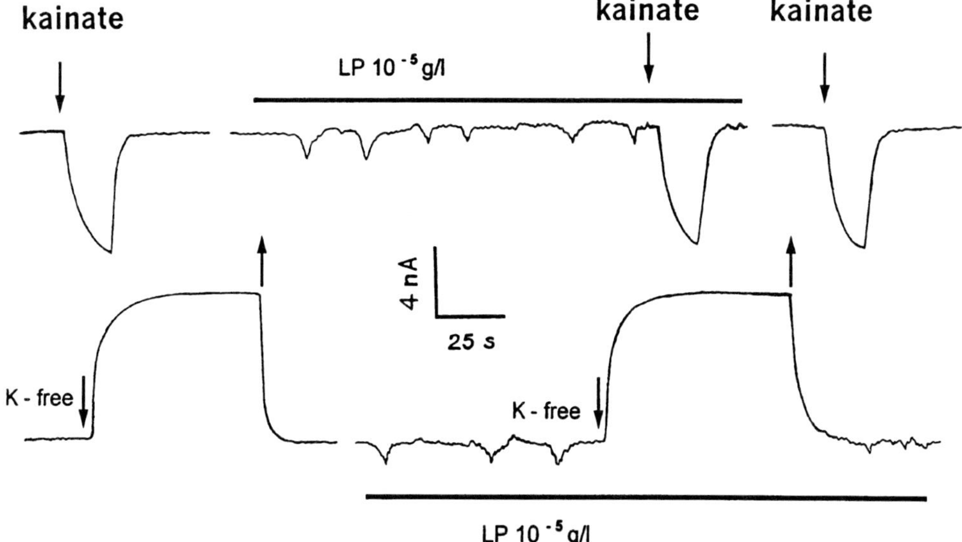

Figure 6. LP effect on kainate-induced inward current and the depolarization of oocyte membrane induced by K-free solution.

The study of LP on NMDA-induced current has shown that LP in low concentration (10^{-8} mg/ml) has a reversibly inhibitory effect on NMDA responses (figure 7). In the last concentrations, the irregular oscillation was so high that it was impossible to record NMDA responses. The fact that kainate responses are insensitive to LP allows us to suggest that, in this object, LP selectively affects NMDA receptors. By recent biochemical study, it was shown that total LP consists of a minimum 12 components. Which of them are (is) responsible for the obtained effects? This needs future investigation. Obtained data allow us to consider LP as a new important pain relieving drug(s), of which a more detailed investigation of biological activity and chemical nature seems important.

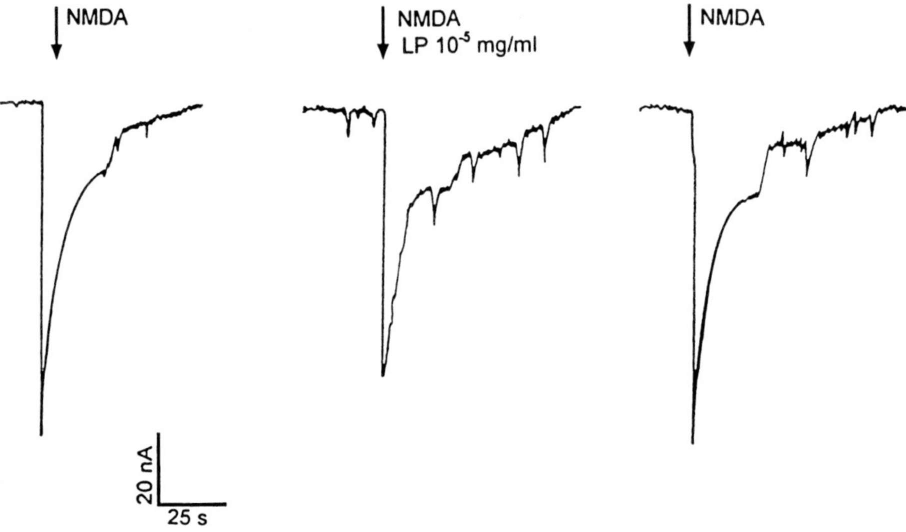

Figure 7. LP blocking effect on NMDA response of oocyte membrane.

References

Ayrapetyan SN (1995) Cellular Mechanism of pain. In "Pain-Clinical Aspects and Therapeutical Issues" (B Kepplinger, ed) Edition Selva Verlag Linz (in press).

Ayrapetyan SN (1996) The application of the theory of metabolic regulation to pain. Materials of Internat. Symposium "On the Application of the Theory of Metabolic Regulation to Pain," Stepanakert - Yerevan, Armenia (in press).

Ayrapetyan SN, Arvanov VL (1979) On the mechanism of electrogenic sodium pump dependence of membrane chemosensitivity. Comp Biochem Physiol 64A, 601-604.

Ayrapetyan SN and Suleymanyan MA (1979) On pump-induced cell volume changes. Comp Biochem Physiol 64A, 571-575.

Ayrapetyan SN, Arvanov VL, Maginyan SN, Azatian KV (1985) Further study of correlation between Na-pump activity and membrane chemosensitivity. Cell. Molec. Neurobiol 5: 231-243.

Saghyan AA, Avetisian TH, Ayrapetyan SN (1993) Effect of low ouabain on 22Na efflux, 86Rb and 45Ca influxes through the neuronal membrane of Helix pomatia. Biologicheskie membrany.

Saghyan AA, Ayrapetyan SN (1993) The correlation between Na-K pump and Na:Ca exchange in neurons of Helix pomatia. J Physiology.

Saghyan AA, Ayrapetyan SN (1993) The effect of high external K+ and Ca++ on active and passive properties of neuronal membrane of Helix pomatia. J Physiology.

Saghyan AA, Dadalyan SS, Takenaka T, Suleymanyan MA, Ayrapetyan SN (1986) The effects of short-chain fatty acids on the neuronal membrane functions of Helix pomatia. III. 22Na efflux from the cells. Cell Molec Neurobiol 6:397-405.

Pain Mechanisms and Management
S.N. Ayrapetyan and A.V. Apkarian (Eds.)
IOS Press, 1998

Halothane Anaesthesia in Molecular Mechanism of Oxidative Stress Pathogenesis

K.G. Karageuzyan
Institute of Molecular Biology of National Academy of Sciences
Yerevan, Armenia

Introduction

The expanded use of narcotic remedies in surgery leads to the need for detailed studies of the molecular mechanisms of origin, development and the generalisation of intracellular metabolic disturbances under their influence. Of special interest is the harmful effect of halothane on phospholipid (PL) metabolism and on the intensity of lipid free radical oxidation (FRO) reaction at different organisational levels of the cell structure which to some extent promotes cellular physiology.

Having close relation to the structural organisation and functional-metabolic peculiarities of the surfaces for cell and subcellular formations division, the state of separate PL fractions in normally functioning biological systems are characterised by status of phylogenetically strongly programmed constancy (Kreps, 1967 and Kreps, 1981), supplying in a whole the physiological level of the cell vital activity. In this aspect the main for membrane PL is based on their maintaining the necessary level of either liquidity, or fluidity of biological membranes formed due to the complex variety of PL-PL ratio, and formation of numerous complexes creating unique character for lipid surrounding of membrane proteins, and necessary level of hydrophobity for the given biological system as an element of regulation of its functional activity. It concerns more certainly to the membrane-bound, lipid-dependent enzymes catalysing reactions of transmembrane transfer of substances, transduction of outer signal (Karageuzyan et al., 1987 and Asatryan, 1993), as well as the constant maintaining of physiological level for ligand - receptor interrelations, and normal stereotype of cell functioning in a whole (Karageuzyan et al., 1980 and Karageuzyan and Hayrapetyan, 1997).

Thus, in the present work we have studied specific metabolic changes of PL in general brain homogenate (GBH) of mitochondrial and microsomal fractions (MCF, MSF) of animals brain being under halothane anaesthesia. It refers to the qualitative and quantitative changes of total PL (TPL), neutral PL (TNPL), acidic PL (TAPL), coefficients (C) of TNPL to TAPL ratio (C TNPL/TAPL), separate fractions of NPL, such as lisophosphatidylcholines (LPC), sphingomyelins (SPM), phosphatidylcholines (PC), phosphatidylethanolamines (PE), as well as APL - mono-, di-, and triphosphoinositides (MPI, DPI, TPI), phosphatidylserines (PS), phosphatidic acids (PA), cardiolipins (CL). Simultaneously there were investigated in details the peculiarities of changes of lipids FRO reactions intensity, results of which promoted principally new determination of mechanisms for PL metabolism products participation as pathogenic factors depending on the nature of halothane toxic effects.

Materials and methods

Investigations were carried out on white female rats weighing 180-200 g fed by general ration in vivarium. Experimental halothane anaesthesia was caused by putting the animals into the special glass camera enriched with oxygen and halothane vapour (1.0 - 1.5 v/%). Isolation of brain tissue MCF and MSF was made in medium containing 0,25 M saccharose solution and 0.01 M, Tris-HCl buffer solution using method of differential centrifugation and simultaneous determination of general protein concentration (Folch et al., 1957).

Measurement of intensity of the developing staining of malonic dialdehyde (MDA) in reaction with tiobarbituric acid and hydroperoxides with ammonium sulphocyanide of adequate concentrations of the mentioned compounds were made on spectrophotometer SP-26 at wave length 535 nm (Karageuzyan, 1969) and 480 nm (Han et al., 1989), respectively.

PL extraction from the studied materials (Chan and Fishman, 1978) has been made after their preliminary dehydration by acetone into acetone powder (Karageuzyan et al., 1987) with further fractionation by one-dimensional ascending thin layer chromatography in silicagel (CzSSR) in the solvents system: chloroform - methanol - concentrated ammonia (65:35:5). PL quantity was expressed in μg of mineralised lipid phosphorus (0.5 g dry residue).

Results and discussion

According to the results given in the Table 1, the experimental halothane anaesthesia at white rats is characterized by statistically certified changes of PL-PL ratio in GBH, MCF, and MSF of brain tissue dependent on qualitative and quantitative changes of the contents of individual representatives of PL.

The most acknowledged one is the decrease of PC quantity induced, perhaps, by the increase of phospholipase A_2 activity, which is testified by simultaneous output of high concentrations of LPC and non-etherified fatty acids (NEFA) of polyenic range, actively involved in FRO reactions, and promoting the formation of certain quantity of lipid peroxides which possess membranotoxic effect. The latter is considered at present as one of the main consistent of CNS complex pathogenic diseases (up to acute edema of brain) (Karageuzyan et al., 1986 and Chan and Fishman, 1978). On the other hand the decrease of PC was observed with parallel increase of PS in a result of probable carboxylation of PE. The formation of the latter from PC is possible as a result of activation of demethylation processes of PC.

The probability of the supposed mechanism of PS formation is apparent on our point of view, as under halothane toxic effect it obtains a real compensatory-adaptational character involving PS as stimulators for inhibited respiratory function of brain MCF.

It is of no less interest the lowering of SPM in MCF, which we are inclined to interpret as free response to the reactivity of myelin substance of brain tissue to halothane toxic effect.

Table 1. Changes in the contents of certain categories of phospholipids (μg lipid phosphorus/0.5 g dry residue of the studied material) in general homogenate (1), mitochondrial (2) and microsomal (3) fractions of white rat brain in control (4) and under halothane anesthesia (5).

PL GROUP	GBH		MCF		MSF	
	CONTROL	HALOTHANE	CONTROL	HALOTHANE	CONTROL	HALOTHANE
LPC	326.6±3.02	374.4±3.11*	28.8±2.81	120.8±4.03*	42.7±1.12	60.82±1.23*
SPM	129.0±2.01	12.9±1.09 •	93.3±2.16	52.0±1.99*	49.3±2.00	55.21±2.23$^{\otimes}$
PS	105.8±2.00	122.0±2.32$^{\otimes}$	47.1±3.11	84.1±3.03*	26.5±1.13	22.82±1.63$^{\otimes}$
MPI	246.8±3.07	191.5±2.22*	142.0±3.09	29.0±2.02*	95.0±2.03	74.80±2.91$^{\otimes}$
PC	607.7±6.01	54.2±4.13$^{\otimes}$	421.0±4.03	262.7±4.40*	239.8±2.01	204.21±2.01*
PE	553.8±3.00	493.0±3.01*	320.0±2.23	301.4±1.73$^{\otimes}$	152.0±2.00	140.02±1.97$^{\otimes}$
CL	106.8±0.32	108.2±0.91$^{\otimes}$	31.1±0.40	37.0±0.51*	-	-
TPL	2074.0±6.02	1950.4±4.00$^{\otimes}$	1085.0±6.04	884.0±5.00*	605.0±2.04	558.00±3.04*
TNPL	1616.0±6.09	1528.5±6.05•	863.1±4.02	734.0±3.07*	483.8±1.51	460.21±1.32*
TAPL	460.0±3.69	421.7±4.00•	220.0±4.05	50.1±4.16*	121.5±1.16	97.61±1.22$^{\otimes}$
C TNPL /TAPL	3.5	3.6	3.9	4.9	4.0	4.7

* - P< 0.001; # - P<0.01; $^{\otimes}$- P<0.02; •- P is unverified

In affirmation to the abovementioned ones it attracts our attention the fact of quantitative increase of CL in MCF. The formers are considered the main representatives of APL participating in the catalysing reactions of the cell respiratory function, especially at its inhibition.

At last, the significance of the mentioned PL, including MPI, under halothane anaesthesia, probably, is of more wide sense, namely phosphoinositide and phosphatidylcholine cycles are of the primary significance in transduction of outer signal into the cell, thus in supplying its activity in a whole (Karageuzyan et al., 1987, Karageuzyan et al., 1986 and Karageuzyan et al., 1988), which, perhaps, undergoes certain shifts under the effect of the studied anaesthetic remedy.

Interfractional changes of PL in GBH and intracellular brain formations under halothane effect defined by us , having various appearances, elucidate the understanding and interpretation of the obtained C TNPL/TAPL. It is interesting to note that in spite the developing shifts of TAPL to the increasement, their level in TPL is statistically certified for the decrease only in MSF, especially in MCF, but not in GBH, hence being less informative in the last case. Simultaneously the process of peroxide formation as in GBH, as well as in brain MCF and MSF according to Table 2 is noticeably activated, especially in enzymatic (NADP-H-dependent) system of lipids peroxidation.

Table 2. Changes in the contents of hydroperoxides (e_{480} / mg protein) and malonic dialdehyde (nm / mg protein) of general brain homogenate, mitochondrial and microsomal fractions in white rat brain non-enzymatic (1) and enzymatic (2) systems of lipid peroxidation in control (c) and halothane anaesthesia

	Control		Halothane Anaesthesia			
	1	2	1	% Changes from C	2	% Changes from C
MITOCHONDRIAL FRACTION						
Hydroperoxides	0.75±0.03	0.51±0.03	1.25±0.05*	67.0	0.99±0.05*	94.0
Malonic Dialdehyde	4.21±0.09	2.02±0.07	6.42±0.21*	52.5	4.67±0.06*	131.0
MICROSOMAL FRACTION						
Hydroperoxides	0.55±0.04	0.31±0.03	0.73±0.03•	33.0	0.58±0.02*	90.0
Malonic Dialdehyde	2.07±0.07	1.42±0.08	3.04±0.17*	47.0	2.07±0.11*	46.0
GENERAL BRAIN HOMOGENATE						
Hydroperoxides	0.42±0.06	0.29±0.05	0.65±0.03*	55.0	0.49±0.04*	68.0
Malonic Dialdehyde	1.66±0.02	0.81±0.07	1.86±0.02*	12.0	1.04±0.02$^{\otimes}$	29.1

* - P.0.001; • - P<0.002; -$^{\otimes}$ P<0.01)

It must be noted that comparatively high level of hydroperoxides output is an objective index of high rate of peroxide formation process which at a known extent is a testification of unique development and generalization of disease process. We must note also that the described regularity in the dynamics of quantitative changes of hydroperoxides and MDA in more expressed forms were observed in brain tissue MCF and MSF, and to some extent in GBH. Activation of processes of radicaloformation (which is compulsory, but it is not a specific index for pathogenic complex of different states of disease in the organism, including the states initiated at toxic effects of anaesthetic compounds) is accompanied both by PL deacylation with the release of NEFA involved in FRO reactions, and by sensitive changes of intermolecular fatty acid contents of PL, causing cardinal changes of their physical, chemical, functional and metabolic peculiarities, which will become the subject of our further special investigations.

Plenary discussion

Reeh W.: Activation of phospholipase A_2 results in production of more mediators than endoperoxides. What is your evidence that the loss of acetylcholine receptor affinity you reported is due to lipid peroxidation rather than to effects the eicosanoid mediators?

Karageuzian K.: The degradation of phospholipid-diglycerides - under the action of phospholipase A_2 activated by halothane - induced anesthesia accompanied by deacylation of high concentrations of non-esterified fatty acids predominantly of polyenic representatives of these compounds. Under the conditions of halothane induced anesthesia the most polyenic fatty acids participate in free radical peroxidation with the formation of pronounced quantities of hydroperoxies, malonic dialdehyde, dien conjugates, etc., which have membranotoxic and membranolytic effects. On the other hand the degradation of membrane phospholipids leads to the complete change of phylogenetically established phospholipid-phospholipid interrelations, which play an important role in changing membrane fluidity, membrane protein surroundings, which in turn lead to membrane protein confirmation changes (membrane-bound enzymes, receptor's proteins) and therefore the formation of abnormalities in their functional activity.

For example, 10 years ago in joint investigations carried out with Prof. S. Ayrapetyan's laboratory on the snail neuron membrane it was demonstrated that, when treated with phospholipase A_2 for 2 hours, the acetylcholine receptors lost their affinity to acetylcholine. We were able to explain this by changes of phospholipid surroundings of receptors mentioned. The affinity of acetylcholine receptor to its ligand was recovered when the membrane was washed by physiological solution. This phenomenon can explain the molecular mechanism of halothane anesthetic effect.

It was also shown by us that approximately 60-70% of fatty acids are involved in lipid peroxide formation reaction, and only 30-40% of these compounds participate in other biosynthesis processes.

References

Asatryan LYu (1993) Co-operation of processes for modification of lipid component of lymphocytes membranes at initiation of phosphoinositide cycle. Theses for obtaining a degree for cand biol sci, Yerevan.

Chan PH, Fishman RA (1978) Science v.201, p.358-360.

Folch J, Lees M, Sloane-Stane G (1957) J Biol Chem., v.226, p.497-509.

Han PH, Longer S, Chan S, Albert CH Yu, Hillerd L, Chu L, Imaisumi S, Bryan Pereira, Moore KL, Woolworth V, Fishman RA (1989) In: Arachidonic Acid Metabolism in the Nervous System. Physiological and Pathological Significance (AL Bakai and NG Bazan eds), NY Acad Sci, p.237-247.

Karageuzyan KG (1969) Probl Med Chem no.1, p.3-6.

Karageuzyan KG, Gevorgyan ES, Tadevosyan YuV, Yavroyan ZhV (1988) The Ukrainian Biochemical Journal v.60, No.4, p.81-83.

Karageuzyan KG, Hayrapetyan SN (1997) USSR-Switzerland Symp. on Biol. Membranes, Structure and Function Moscow, p75.

Karageuzyan KG, Hayrapetyan SN, Arvanov VL (1980) Proc Acad Sci USSR v.255, p.212-215.

Karageuzyan KG, Tadevosyan YuV, Batikyan TB (1986), Proc Acad Sci USSR v.286, No.2, p.465-467.

Karageuzyan KG, Tadevosyan YuV, Batikyan TB (1987) All-Union Symp. on Biochemistry of Lipids, Alma-Ata p.38-39.

Karageuzyan KG, Tadevosyan YuV, Batikian TB (1987) Proc Acad Sci USSR v.295, p.1254-1257.

Kreps EM (1967) XXII Bach readings, Nauka, Leningrad p73.

Kreps EM (1981) In: Lipids of Cell Membranes. Nauka Leningrad p340.

Kreps EM, Krasilnikova VI, Patrikeeva MV (1968) Evolutionary Biochemistry and Physiology No.4, p.211-23.

Cellular and Molecular Mechanisms of Nitric Oxide Effects

K.V. Azatian*, A.R.White, R.J.Walker and S.N.Ayrapetyan*
Biophysics Center of Armenian NAS
Yerevan 375044, Armenia
Department of Physiology and Pharmacology
of Southampton University, UK

Introduction

Nitric oxide (NO) is considered to be the retrograde messenger (Williams et al., 1993) and thus to participate in long-term potentiation (Schuman and Madison, 1993). Thereby NO is seen as a messenger in pain signaling.

According to the theory of metabolic regulation of membrane excitability (Ayrapetyan, 1996), pain could be considered as the abnormal excitation of the cell due to its abnormal hydration. Na-K pump and Na:Ca exchange are seen as cellular protective mechanisms through which the metabolic regulation of cell hydration is realized (Ayrapetyan and Suleymanian, 1979; Ayrapetyan, 1995). It's well known that NO production is elevated in hyperexcitable state of nerve endings. It is explained by the increase in intracellular Ca concentration and activation of Ca-calmodulline sensitive nitric oxide synthase (NOS) (Mayer, 1993).

The biological effect of NO in the literature is considered as a result of the elevation of intracellular cGMP level (Garthwaite, 1993). However major deficiency at present is in understanding of the physiological significance of the NO-cGMP pathways. It has been shown that NO causes the relaxation of smooth and heart muscles in vertebrates and invertebrates (Rand, 1992; White et al., 1996). Some investigators have suggested that cations channels are involved in the mechanisms of NO-caused relaxation of heart and smooth muscle (Bialecki R.A., Stinson-Fisher C.,1995). At the same time data obtained in our lab show that carrier-driving mechanisms (Na-K pump and Na:Ca exchange) are more sensitive to the external signals than channel-driving ones (Dadalian et al., 1988; Ayrapetyan & Carpenter, 1991; Ayrapetyan et al., 1992; Azatian et al.,1994). Thus, the study of NO effect on both Na-K pump and Na:Ca exchange seems to be of a great importance for the understanding of the cellular and molecular mechanisms responsible for NO induced modulation of membrane function.

The aim of present work is to investigate NO effects dependent on Na-K pump and Na:Ca exchange activities.

As the inotropic function of heart muscle depends on the intracellular Ca ions content its contractility was chosen as a model for the investigation of NO effects.

It's well known that nitrovasodilators are NO donors, one of which, S-nitroso-N-acetyl-penicillamine (SNAP) was chosen for present investigations.

Effect of SNAP on: a) heart muscle contractility ; b) ^{86}Rb uptake; c) cGMP content, depending on Na-K pump, Na:Ca exchange activities was studied.

Material and methods

Experiments were performed on Helix aspersa hearts.

Physiological experiments

The apparatus is shown on Fig.1. Removed hearts were cannulated and suspended in an organ bath with saline of composition (mM): NaCl (80), KCl (4), $CaCl_2$ (7), Tris-HCl (5), pH 7,5. Continually intra- and extra-heart perfusion with saline was applied. Heart contractions were recorded isotonically and displayed on a Harvard Oscillograph. Under these conditions heart continued to beat spontaneously for many hours. A one ml aliquot of SNAP was applied by the injection in intra-heart perfusing solution, and the response recorded on the pen recorder.

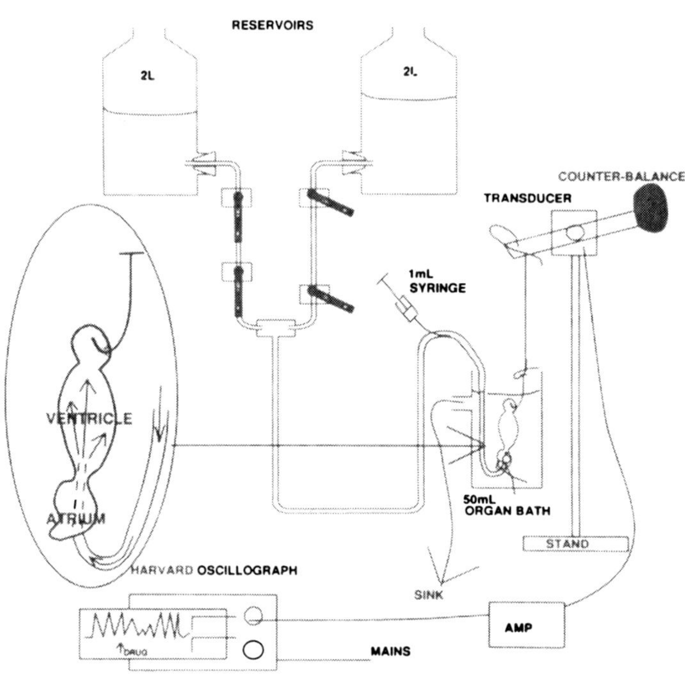

Figure 1. The set up for the registration of heart muscle contractility.

Responses on the application of NO donor SNAP were analyzed in three ways (Fig.2):

1. Recovery time: this was defined as the time taken, in seconds, for complete recovery.

2. Amplitude of response: the maximal deflection on the pen recorder was defined as 100%, responses were calculated as a proportion of this.

3. Percentage inhibition: this was defined as that inhibition caused by the highest dose of NO donor under normal conditions.

4. The Students t-test was used for statistical analysis.

86Rb uptake assay

^{86}Rb uptake assay was used for Na-K pump activity measurement. It is well known that Rb ions successfully replace K ions and Na-K pump transports Rb instead K. Removed hearts were incubated in physiological Ringer solution containing ^{86}Rb isotope (about 0,01 uCi per heart) with or without 10^{-4} M ouabain during the time indicated. Then hearts were washed three times per 5 min by cold K-free solution to remove isotope from extracellular spaces. Radioactivity was measured in liquid scintillate spectrometer and calculated in dpm/mg of wet weight. Each point is the mean of five simultaneous experiments.

cGMP level assay

Removed hearts were incubated in normal or K-free physiological solution with or without SNAP during 30 min. Then they were immediately frozen in dry ice in high EGTA containing solution. cGMP level was measured in alcohol extracts of hearts by radioimmunoassay by using ^{3}H-cGMP kits ("Amersham").

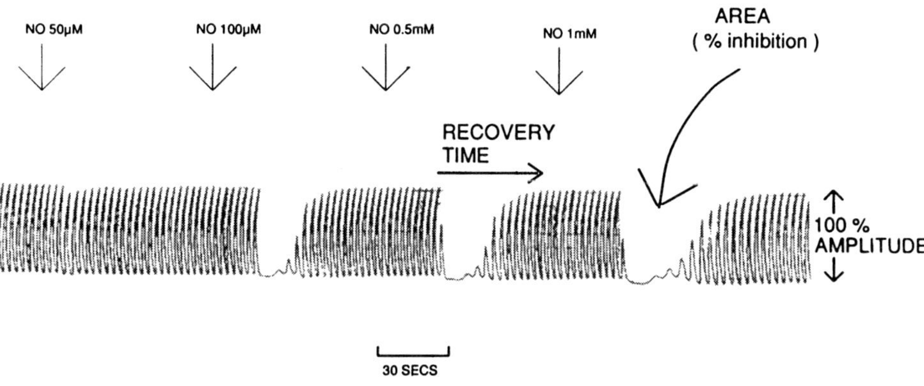

Figure 2. Dose response effect of SNAP on heart activity. Some characteristics used for data analysis are represented: recovery time, amplitude of response and percentage inhibition.

Results and discussion

First of all the role of Na-K pump in heart muscle contractility was investigated. It's well known that the removal of K ions from external medium leads to the inactivation of Na-K pump and restoration of K ions causes reactivation of pump. As can be seen such reactivation of pump causes transient inhibitory effect on heartbeat and relaxation of heart muscle (Fig.3, A, B). Long-lasting incubation in K-free (about 1hour) leads to the gradually inhibition of twitches and at last their stop in heart contracted state (Fig.3, B). While reincubation in normal Ringer solution produces dramatic relaxation of heart muscle which is followed by heart stop now in the relaxed state (Fig.3, B). About 10-15 min. wash in normal solution is needed to start heart beating activity. Ouabain which is known as Na-K-ATPase (the working molecule of Na-K pump) blocker has similar inhibitory effect on the heart contractility as K-free solution (Fig.3, C).

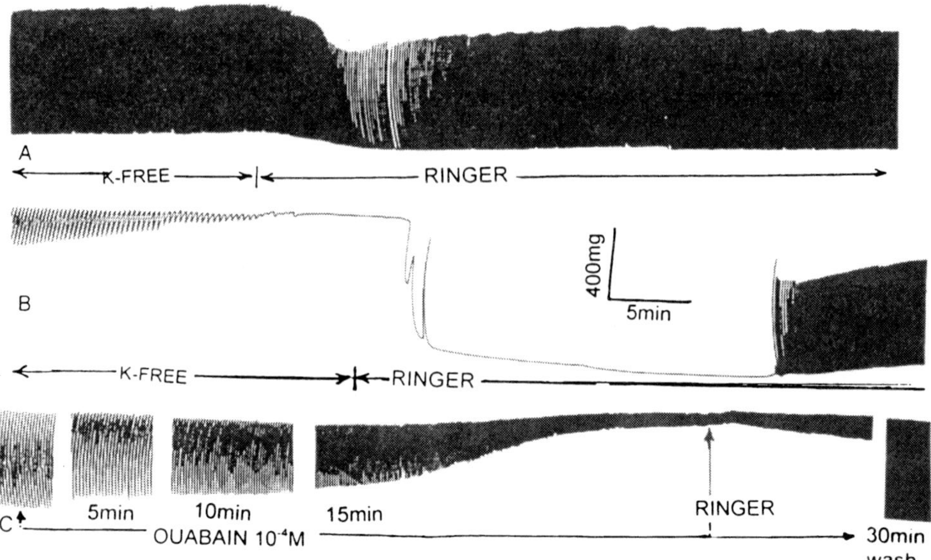

Figure 3. Effect of Na-K pump inactivation on heart activity.
A.Preincubation in K-free solution leading to Na-K pump inactivation followed by wash with normal Ringer solution;
B. prolonged perfusion with K-free solution and wash with normal Ringer;
C. perfusion with 0.1 mM ouabain followed by wash.

Thus, K-free and ouabain, both Na-K pump inactivating factors cause heart contraction and stop of beat after long incubation while the reincubation in normal physiological solution restores heartbeat following the powerful and long relaxation. How can be explained the effect of Na-K pump activity changes on heart contractility? Earlier in our work it has been shown that there is a close correlation between Na-K pump activity and Na:Ca exchange: inactivation of pump leads to the activation of cAMP dependent reverse of Na:Ca exchange, leading to the increase of Ca ions concentration in the cells (Saghian, 1991; Ayrapetyan et al, 1992). So, ouabain and K-free induced inhibition of heart activity by the increase of contraction of muscle can be explained by the elevation of intracellular Ca ions concentration which reaches its abnormal value as a result of long incubation in Na-K pump inactivating conditions. It is suggested that abundance of Ca causes stop of heart pacemaker activity likely through the sustained contraction of myosin. Recently the similar suggestion on the involvement of Na:Ca exchange in the support of twitch contraction of mouse diaphragm under the inhibition of Na-K-ATPase activity was made by Nishimura and coworkers (1996).

Thus Na-K pump induced heart muscle relaxation can be explained by the activation of Na:Ca exchange in forward mode while the inactivation of Na-K pump induces muscle contraction via the activation of Na:Ca exchange in reversed mode.

Previously Walker and coworkers have shown that SNAP has inhibitory effect on Helix aspersa heart activity (White et al., 1996). It was interesting to investigate this effect of SNAP, depending on Na-K pump activity. As it is shown on Fig. 4, inhibitory effect of SNAP on heart activity is accompanied by heart muscle relaxation also as in the case of Na-K pump activation.

So, both Na-K pump activation and SNAP cause heart muscle relaxation. The question arises whether SNAP induced effects could be explained through the activation of Na-K pump? Therefore in the next series of experiments the effect of SNAP on heart muscle contractility dependent on Na-K pump activity was studied.

In general, the application of K-free solution to the preparation result in a reduction in the magnitude of inhibition caused by the NO donor (n=15), this reduction being completely reversible (Fig.4). The analysis of data of 5 experiments are represented. Recovery time was also substantially decreased in K-free solution. The amplitude of the response was slightly increased under K-free conditions, again showing the depression of NO mediated inhibition.

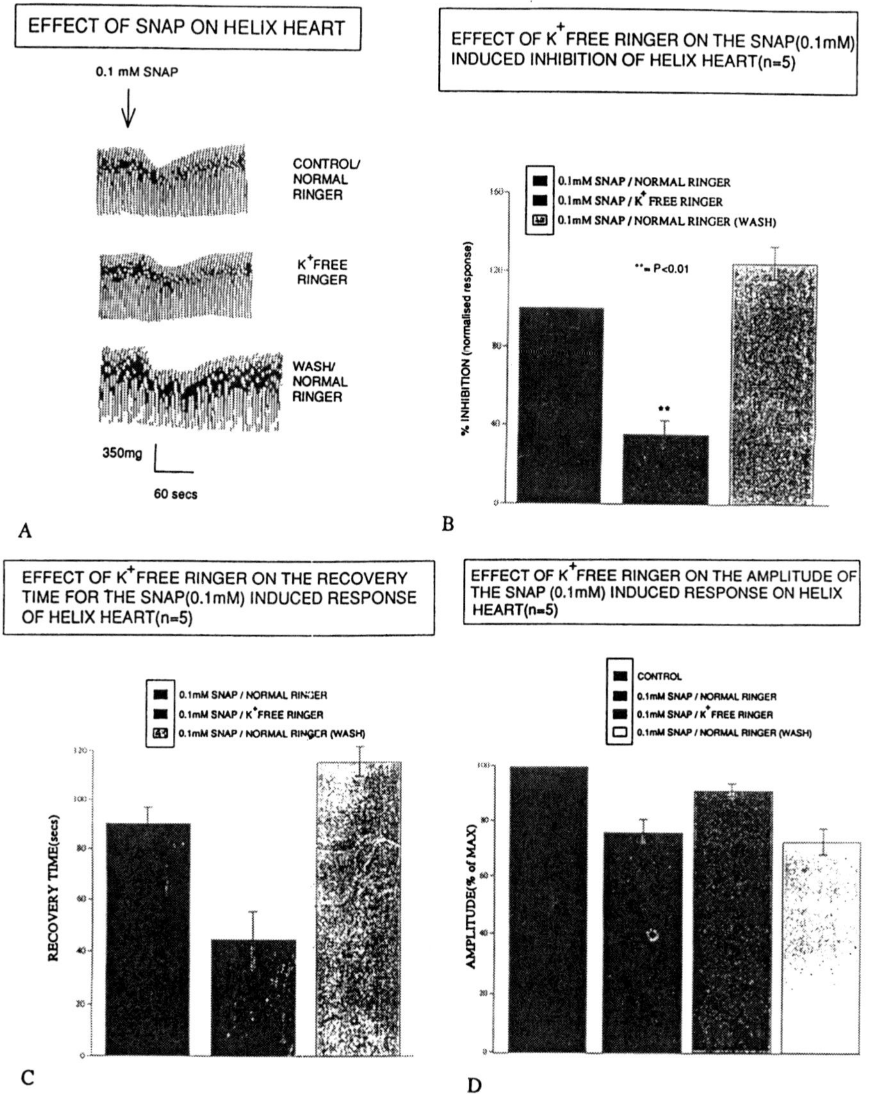

Figure 4. Effect of K-free solution on 0.1 mM SNAP induced heart muscle relaxation.
A. Effect of SNAP in normal Ringer, K- free and after wash. B. Effect of K-free on SNAP induced inhibition of Helix heart (n=5). C. Effect of SNAP on the recovery time for the SNAP induced responses of Helix heart (n=5). D. Effect of K-free on the amplitude of the SNAP induced response of heart (n=5).

Dose - dependent effect of SNAP on heart contractility in normal, K-free and after the wash in normal solution is shown on Fig. 5. K-free has depressing effect on SNAP caused relaxation and inhibition of heart activity. Dose response effects for SNAP on Helix heart in norm and K-free are represented on Fig.6. Thus, SNAP especially in large doses induces heart muscle relaxation which is very similar to Na-K pump activation induced one.

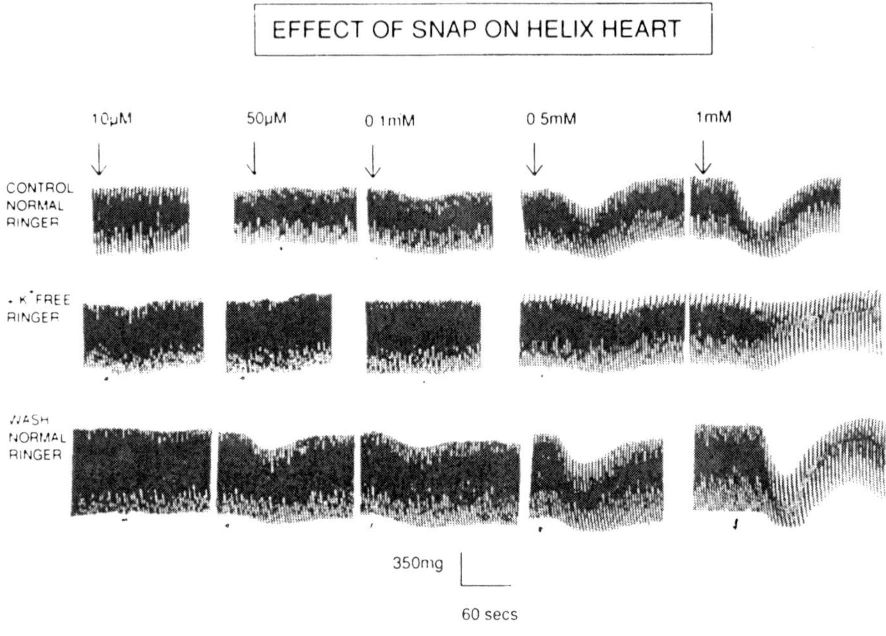

Figure 5. Dose dependent effect of SNAP on Helix heart activity in normal Ringer, K-free solutions and after wash. K-free depresses SNAP effect on these preparations (n=15).

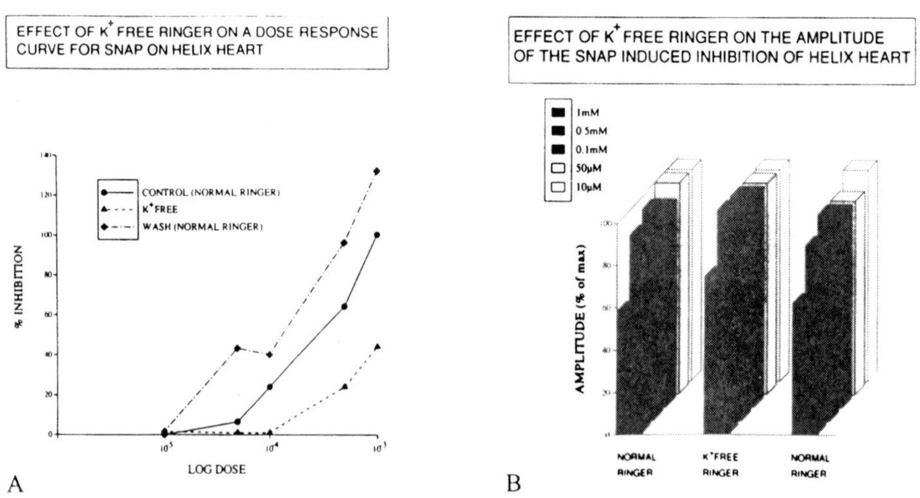

Figure 6. Analysis of data from Fig.5. Effect of K-free on SNAP induced dose dependent inhibition of heart activity (A) and on the amplitude of this inhibition (B).

However in few experiments (n=3) K-free showed a potentiation of SNAP effect (Fig. 7). Dose response effect of SNAP in normal and K-free solutions on inhibition and amplitude of twitches is represented on Fig.8.

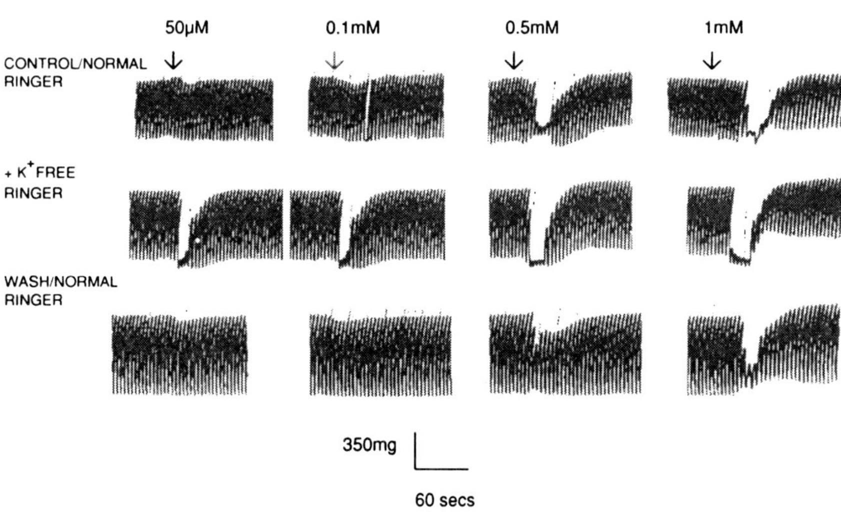

Figure 7. Dose dependent effect of SNAP on Helix heart activity in normal Ringer, K-free solutions and after wash. K-free potentiates SNAP effect on these preparations (n=3).

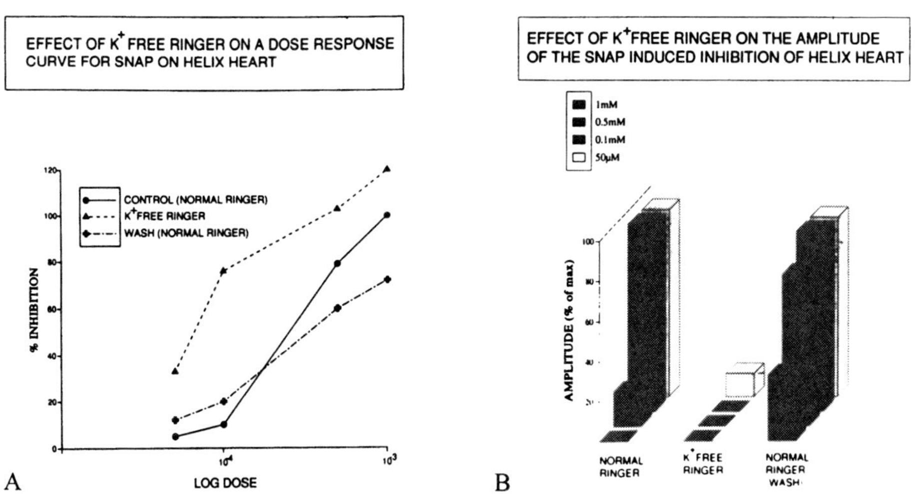

Figure 8. Analysis of data from Fig.7. Effect of K-free on SNAP induced dose dependent inhibition of heart activity (A) and on the amplitude of this inhibition (B).

Effect of ouabain on SNAP induced heart muscle relaxation was investigated. As in the case of K-free solution the effect of ouabain was differed on different preparations. On Fig. 9 it is shown that SNAP induced heart muscle relaxation is not influenced by ouabain while in some other preparations SNAP effect disappears in the presence of ouabain (Fig. 10).

The fact that on the group of preparations SNAP induced relaxation doesn't disappear under Na-K pump inactivating conditions (K-free solution or ouabain) allow us to suggest that SNAP effect could not be the result of Na-K pump activation.

How can be explained data on the disappearance of SNAP effect on heart muscle contractility in the presence of ouabain or K-free in some preparations? (Fig. 5,10). Earlier it was shown that Na-K pump blockers (K-free, ouabain) depress membrane receptors affinity to their ligands (Ayrapetyan et al., 1985) and this effect depends on initial level of membrane phosphorylation (Dadalian et al., 1988). Therefore it can be suggested that the same mechanisms may be involved in the Na-K pump induced inhibition of SNAP caused heart muscle relaxation.

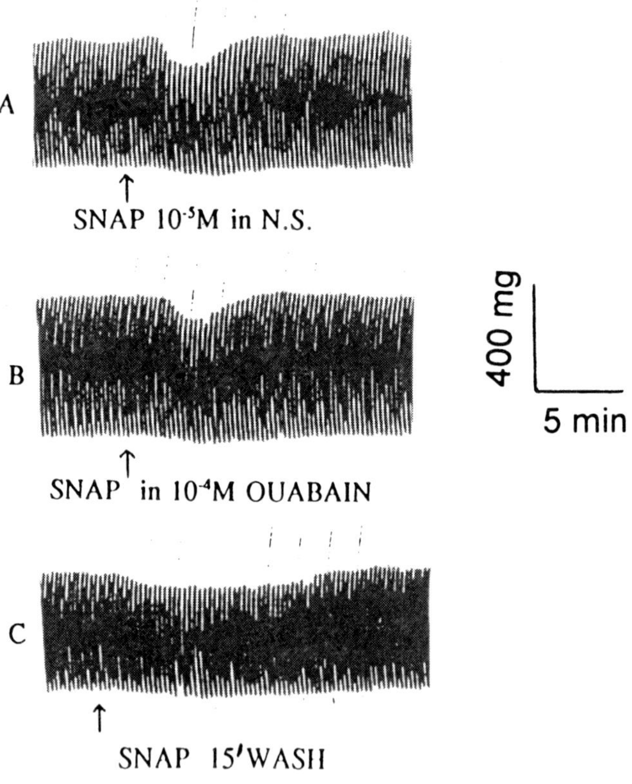

Figure 9. Effect of 0.1mM ouabain on SNAP induced heart muscle relaxation. Ouabain doesn't affect SNAP effect on this preparation.

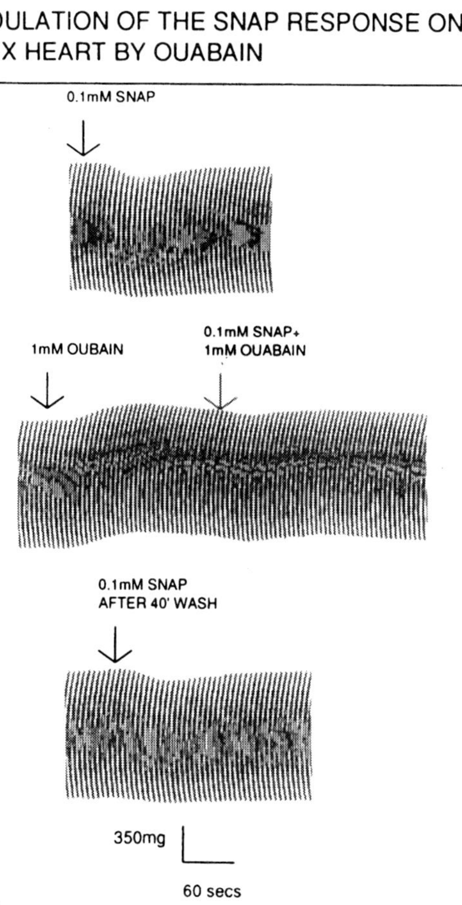

Figure 10. Effect of 0.1mM ouabain on SNAP induced heart muscle relaxation. SNAP effect on this preparation disappears in the presence of ouabain.

The difference in the effect of Na-K pump inactivation on SNAP induced relaxation can be explained also by initial level of membrane phosphorylation of different preparations. However more detailed investigations are needed for the final conclusion.

The following experiments also proved the conclusion that SNAP relaxing effect is not due to the activation of Na-K pump. It's well known that pump can be activated by preliminary incubation in K-free medium in result of cells' enrichment by Na ions. On Fig. 11 has shown that the magnitude of Na-K pump activation induced relaxation depends on duration of preincubation in K-free solution, while SNAP effect is independent on it.

These results allowed us to conclude that although both Na-K pump activation and SNAP cause muscle relaxation likely through the decrease of intracellular Ca concentration, but they apparently implicate different cellular mechanisms.

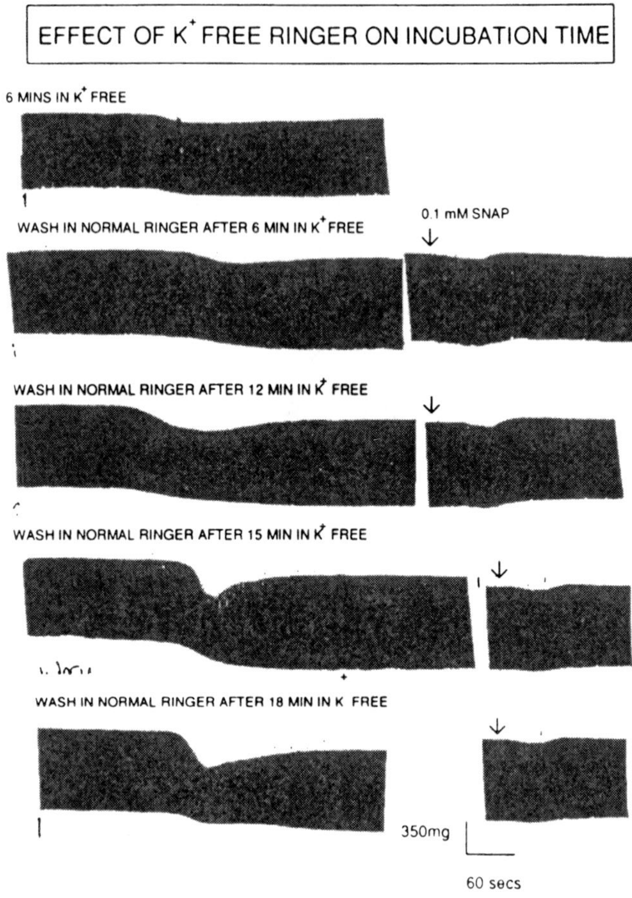

Figure 11. Effect of Na-K pump activation and 0.1 mM SNAP on heart activity dependent on the duration of preincubation in K-free solution.

In the next series of experiments the effect of SNAP on Na-K pump activation induced heart muscle relaxation was investigated. On Fig. 12 it is shown that SNAP in 0,1 M concentration has slight relaxing effect on this preparation. Reinclusion of K ions following about 10 min perfusion by K-free solution leads to the pronounced relaxation of heart muscle as a result of Na-K pump activation. SNAP applied in the beginning of Na-K pump activation induced relaxation potentiates this likely via causing additional efflux of Ca from the cells. These data confirm the suggestion made above that different mechanisms are involved in the Ca extrusion from the cells stimulated by Na-K pump activation and SNAP.

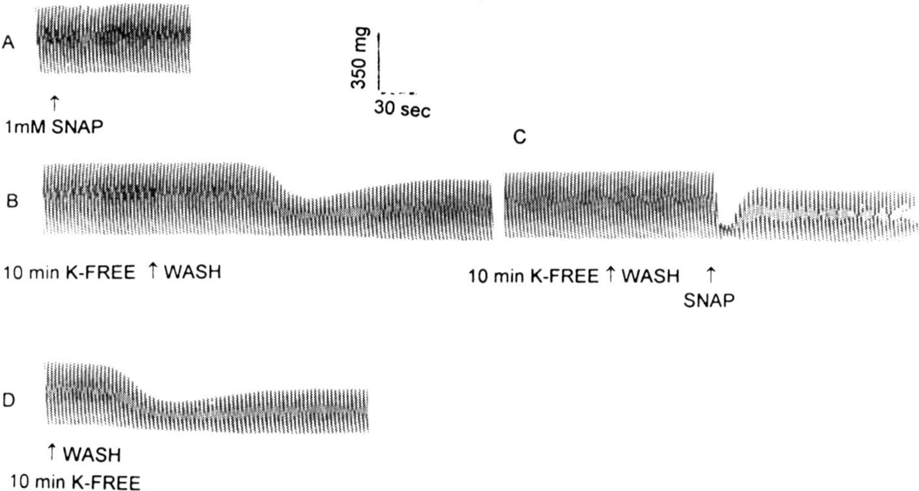

Figure 12. Effect of SNAP on Na-K pump activation caused Helix heart muscle relaxation. A. SNAP caused heart muscle relaxation; B. Heart was perfused by K-free solution 10 min and then washed with normal Ringer. C. SNAP was applied under the same procedure in the beginning of Na-K pump activation induced heart muscle relaxation. D. The restoration of Na-K pump induced effect after the wash.

For the final conclusion, direct measurements of SNAP effect on Na-K pump activity were performed. Fig.13 shows that SNAP decreases ^{86}Rb uptake at all measured periods of time. Ouabain inhibits ^{86}Rb uptake by about 70% confirming that the main part of Rb uptake composes Na-K pump dependent component. In the presence of ouabain depressing effect of SNAP on ^{86}Rb uptake is disappeared.

Therefore SNAP induced heart muscle relaxation is not due to the activation of Na-K pump.

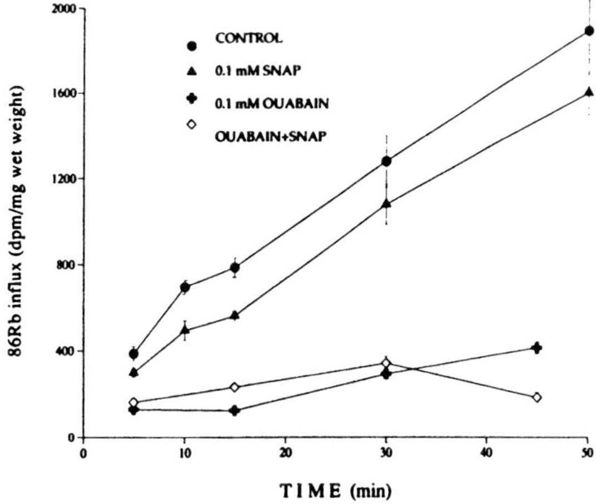

Figure 13. Effect of 0.1 mM SNAP on ^{86}Rb uptake by Helix aspersa cardiac muscle cells in normal physiological conditions and in the presence of 0.1 mM ouabain.

Some literature data show that protein kinase C and phosphatidylinositol pathways can be involved in NO effect on the cell (Bredt et al., 1992; Urushihara et al., 1992). On the other hand, results obtained in our lab show that protein kinase C is involved in neurotransmitters effect on Na:Ca exchange (Arvanov et al., 1992; Azatian et al., 1996). That's why it was interesting to investigate the effect of phosphatidylinositol specific phospholipase C (PL C) on SNAP induced alteration of Na-K pump activity. Hearts were preincubated with PL C (2 mg/ml) during 5 min and then tested on ^{86}Rb uptake. Although PL C in itself it doesn't influence ^{86}Rb uptake but SNAP decreasing effect on it becomes more pronounced (Fig.14). It means that phosphatidylinositol pathways implicate in the SNAP induced Na-K pump inactivation.

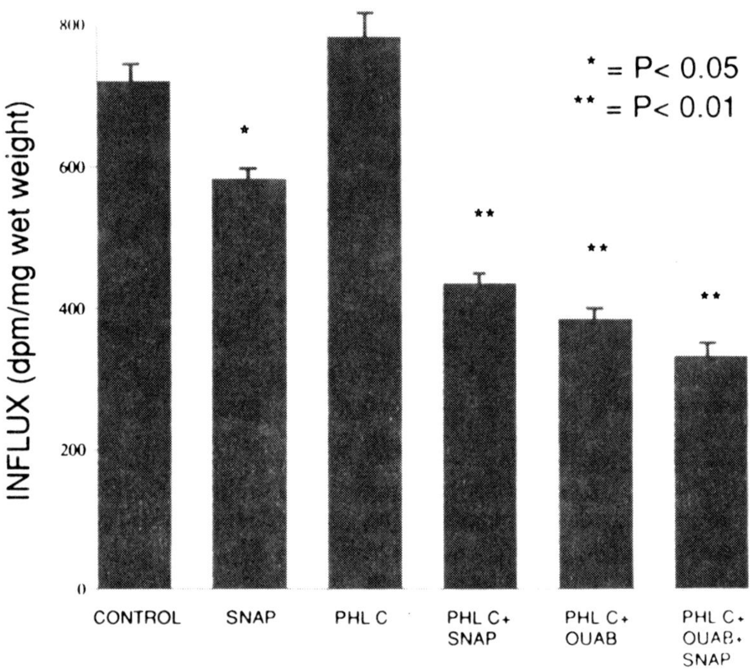

Figure 14. Effect of phosphatidylinositol specific phospholipase C (PhL C) on 0.1 mM SNAP induced inhibition of ^{86}Rb uptake by cardiac cells in normal and 0.1 mM ouabain containing solutions. Hearts were pretreated with PhL C (2mg/ml) 5 min and then tested for ^{86}Rb uptake.

To find out whether SNAP induced relaxation of heart muscle is due to the decrease of intracellular Ca concentration as a result of the activation of Na:Ca exchange, the dependence of SNAP effect on Na:Ca exchange activity was investigated. As the driving forces for Na:Ca exchange appear to be Na and Ca ionic gradients on the membrane (Baker&Blaustain, 1968), SNAP effect on heart muscle contractility dependent on Na and Ca concentrations was investigated. Fig. 15 shows that decrease of Na gradient by 50% removal of Na leads to the heart muscle contraction which evidence that Ca is accumulated in the cells. Under this conditions SNAP relaxing effect on heart muscle becomes more pronounced.

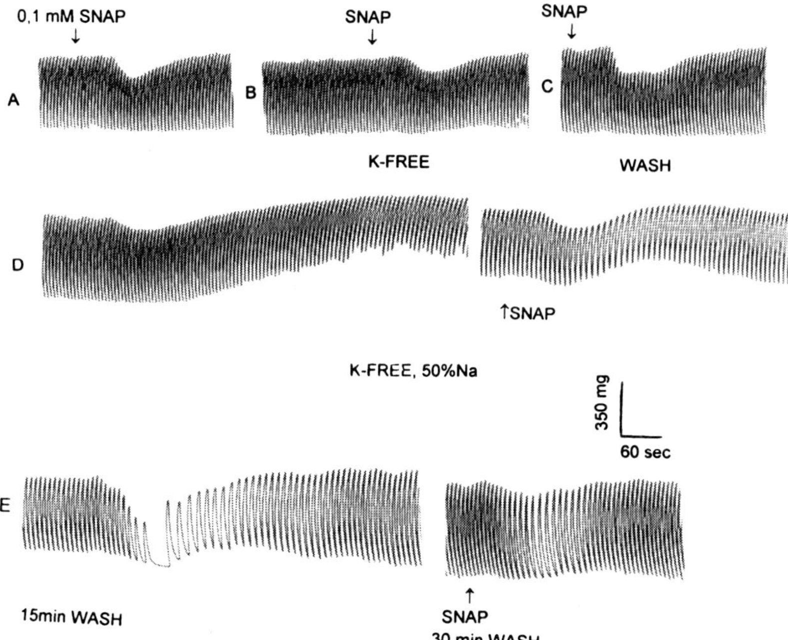

Figure 15. Effect of 50% removal of Na⁺ (it was replaced by equimolar concentration of tris) from K-free physiological solution on 0.1 mM SNAP induced heart muscle relaxation.
Effect of SNAP on heart activity in normal (A), K-free (B) solutions and after wash (C); D - effect of 50% Na⁺ containing K-free solution and SNAP effect in it; E - wash by normal physiological solution and SNAP effect in it.

The next mode of modulating Na:Ca exchange activity is to change external Ca concentration. As can be seen on Fig.16, in lower Ca containing solution SNAP effect decreases and in higher Ca - increases. Thus, this data show that any activation of reversed Na:Ca exchange leading to the elevation of intracellular Ca content, potentiates SNAP induced relaxation, while the depletion of intracellular Ca via the activation of forward Na:Ca exchange, decreases SNAP effect.

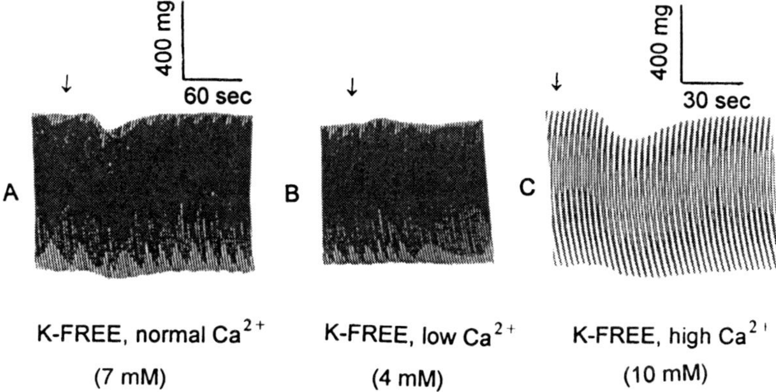

Figure 16. Effect of 0.1 mM SNAP on heart activity dependent on Ca^{2+} concentration in physiological solution. A - in normal Ca^{2+} (7mM); B - low Ca^{2+} (4mM) and C - high Ca^{2+} (10mM) containing solutions.

It's well known that high K-containing solution elevates intracellular Ca by the activation of both reversed Na:Ca exchange and voltage-dependent Ca-channels (Baker&Blaustein, 1968). Fig.17 shows that 10mM K leads to the increase of heart contraction and stop of heart activity. It's interesting to note that in heart contracted state SNAP produces relaxation and starting of heartbeat. This effect depends on preincubation time in 10 mM K: longer incubation leads to the decrease of relaxing effect of SNAP but increases its heart activity stimulating effect. This decrease of relaxing effect of SNAP along with increase of incubation time in 10mM K solution likely could be explained by abnormal abundance of Ca uptake when SNAP induced Ca removal is not enough to relax the muscle in the same extent as in norm. Washing by normal solution leads to the relaxation of heart muscle but about 15 min heart activity is still inhibited and application of SNAP leads to the significant relaxation likely due to additional extrusion of abundance of Ca followed by gradually starting of heart activity.

Thus, the present data strongly confirm that SNAP induced relaxation is due to decrease in intracellular Ca concentration in consequence of the activation of Na:Ca exchange through the membrane. If as a motive force for Na-K pump induced Na:Ca exchange activity changes serves ionic gradients through the membrane, what could be the driving force of SNAP induced Na:Ca exchange activation?

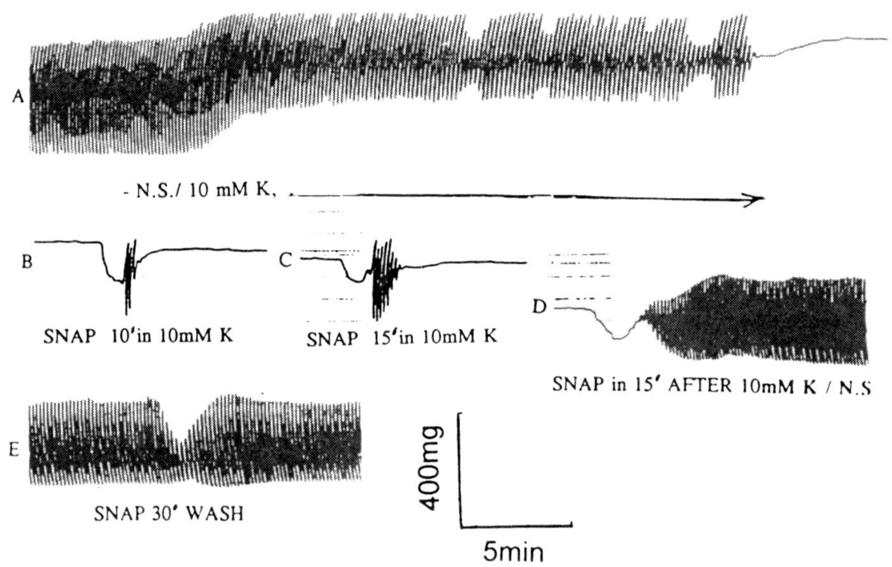

Figure 17. Effect of 10 mM KCl containing physiological solution on 0.1 mM SNAP induced heart muscle relaxation. A. Effect of 10mM KCl containing solution; B. Effect of SNAP applied after 10 min in 10mM KCl; C. SNAP applied after 15 min in 10mM KCl; D. Wash by normal physiological solution and SNAP effect after 15 min wash. E. Restoration of heart activity and SNAP effect after 30 min wash.

It's well known that the main mode of NO effect is the activation of guanylate cyclase and the elevation of intracellular cGMP (Garthwaite, 1993). Fig.18 shows that in Helix aspersa heart SNAP also causes about 70% elevation of cGMP level. It's interesting to note that in K-free solution this effect is disappeared. This is quite new phenomena which likely can be explained by K-free induced regulation of receptor-ligand affinity (Ayrapetyan et al.,1985) as have been mentioned above. Probably K-free induced phosphorylation mechanism is involved in the regulation of affinity of guanylatecyclase to NO as well. This is the question to be investigated in future.

EFFECT OF SNAP ON cGMP LEVEL

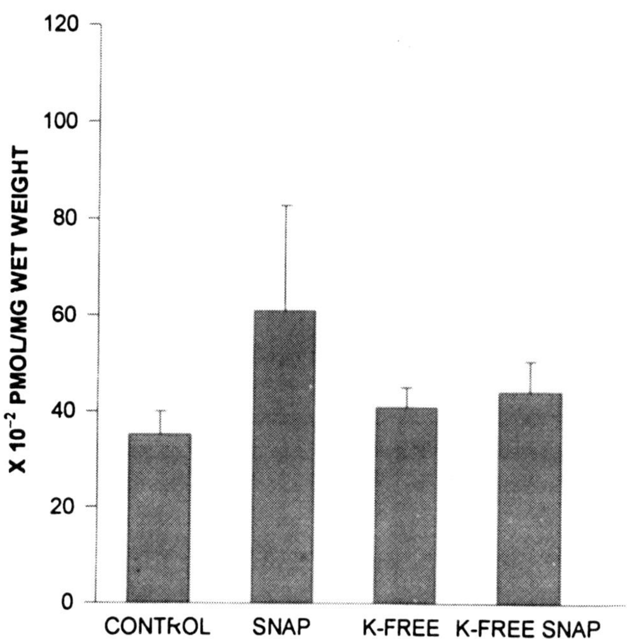

Figure 18. Effect of 0.1 mM SNAP on cGMP level in Helix aspersa heart in normal physiological and K-free solutions.

Our earlier works show that elevation of cAMP level results in the activation of reversed Na:Ca exchange (Dadalian et al., 1988; Saghian, 1991). Present results allow us to suggest that cGMP may activate forward Na:Ca exchange leading to the decrease in intracellular Ca concentration. If this speculation is correct then it will give the key for the explanation of NO-cGMP intracellular pathways.
All these data allow us to consider NO production as a powerful metabolic protective reaction to the abnormal excitation of cell.

Therefore, by this mechanism NO being retrograde messenger could depress transmitter release from presynaptic terminals as a result of decrease of intracellular Ca in presynaptic endings.

In conclusion, our results show that NO has inhibiting effect on Na-K pump activity in heart muscle cells. NO induced heart muscle relaxation is secondary to rises in cGMP level and as a result of it, the activation of Na:Ca exchange leading to the decrease of intracellular Ca^{2+} concentration.

Acknowledgements

This work was supported by grants from Royal Society (UK) and K. Gulbenkian Foundation (Portugie) (ARM-B/BUR/AG/96-0295 N3353).

References

Arvanov VL, Ovakimyan KS, Stepanyan AS, Ayrapetyan SN (1992) The effects of cAMP, Ca^{+2} and phorbol ester TPA on ouabain induced depression of neuron responses induced by rapid acetylcholine application. Cell Molec Neurobiol 12, 153-161.

Ayrapetyan SN, Arvanov VL (1979) On the mechanism of the electrogenic sodium pump dependence of membrane chemosensitivity. Comp Biochem Physiol 64A, 601-604.

Ayrapetyan SN, Arvanov VL, Maginyan SB, Azatyan KV (1985) Further study of the correlation between Na-pump activity and membrane chemosensitivity. Cell Molec Neurobiol 5, 231-243.

Ayrapetyan SN (1995) Cellular Mechanism of pain. In "Pain - Clinical Aspects and Therapeutical Issues" (B Kepplinger ed) Edition Selva Verlag Linz (in press).

Ayrapetyan SN (1996) The application of the theory of metabolic regulation to pain. Abstr. of Internat. Symposium "On the Application of the Theory of Metabolic Regulation to Pain", Stepanakert-Yerevan Armenia 11.

Ayrapetyan SN and Carpenter DO (1991) Very low concentration of acetylcholine and GABA modulate transmitter responses. Membrane and Cellular Biophysics and Biochemistry NeuroReport 2, 563-565.

Ayrapetyan SN, Carpenter DO, Azatian KV, Dadalian SS, Martyrosian DM, Saghian AA, Mndalian VG (1992) Extralow neurotransmitter dozes-induced triggering of neuronal intracellular messenger systems. In: Cellular Signallization (PG Kostyuk and MA Ostrovskii eds) "Nauka" Moscow 89-96.

Ayrapetyan SN and Suleymanyan MA (1979) On the pump-induced cell volume changes. Comp Biochem Physiol 64A, 571-575.

Azatian KV, Karapetian ITz, Ayrapetyan SN (1994) Effect of acetylcholine at low doses on ^{45}Ca influx into the Helix pomatia neurons. Biol Membranes (English) 7, 301-304.

Azatian KV, Ayrapetyan SN, Carpenter DO (1996) The metabotropic effect of low doses of GABA. Gen Physiol, (in press).

Baker PF and Blaustein MP (1968) Sodium-dependent uptake of calcium by crab nerve. Biochem Biophys Acta 150, 167-170.

Bialecki RA, Stinson-Fisher C (1995) Kca channel antagonists reduce NO donor-mediated relaxation of vascular and tracheal smooth muscle. Am J Physiol 268, 152-159.

Bredt DS, Ferris CD, Snyder SH (1992) Nitric oxide synthase regulatory sites. J Biol Chem 267,10976-10981.

Dadalian SS, Azatian KV, Ayrapetyan SN (1988) On the effect of low concentrations of neurotransmitters on sodium efflux and cyclic nucleotides level in snail neurons. Neurochem 7, 18-25.

Garthwaite J (1993) Nitric oxide signalling in the nervous system. Seminars in the Neurosci 5, issue 3, 171-180.

Mayer B (1993) Molecular characteristics and enzymology of nitric oxide synthase and soluble guanylyl cyclase in the CNS. Seminars in the Neurosci 5, issue 3, 197-206.

Nishimura M, Hasegawa T, Ito K (1996) Twitch responses dependent on external calcium ions in the mouse diaphragm in a potassium-free bathing solution. Gen Pharmac 27, 459-461.

Rand MJ (1992) Nitrergic transmission: nitric oxide as a mediator of non-adrenergic non-cholinergic neuro-effector transmission. Clin Exp Pharmacol Physiol 19, 147-169.

Saghyan AA (1991) The Ouabain-insensitive Fraction of Sodium Efflux from Helix Pomatia Neurons. Biol Membranes (Russ) 8, 711-718.

Schuman E M and Madison DV (1993) Nitric oxide: a multi-functional messenger substance in cerebellar synaptic plasticity. Seminars in the Neurosci 5, issue 3, 207-216.

Urushihara H, Tohda M, Nomura Y (1992) Selective potentiation of N-methyl-D-aspartate induced current by protein kinase C in Xenopus oocytes injected with rat brain RNA. J Biol Chem 267, 11697-11700.

White AR, Bascal Z, Holden-Dye L, Walker RJ (1996) Evidence for a possible role for nitric oxide in the modulation of heart activity of Achatina and Helix hearts. J Physiol 491, 108.

Williams JN, Errington ML, Li Y-G, Lynch MA, Bliss TVP (1993) The search for retrograde messengers in long-term potentiation. Seminars in the Neurosci 5, issue 3, 149-158.

Pain Management
(Social Issues)

Pain Mechanisms and Management
S.N. Ayrapetyan and A.V. Apkarian (Eds.)
IOS Press, 1998

The Tropho-Defensive System (T-DS) as Target to Prevent Chronic Pain in Orthopedics, Traumatology and Rheumatology

C. V. Morpurgo
Istituto Ortopedico G. Pini, Milano, Italy

... l'immagination se lassera plus tot de concevoir que la nature de fournir.
B. Pascal, Pensee, p. 118, Charpentier, Paris 1896.

The history of the Pio Istituto dei Rachitici di Milano, now Istituto Ortopedico G. Pini, is in many ways related to the development of the research on the connections between pain and metabolism in the last 120 years in Italy.

The Institution was founded in 1850 by A. Visconti d'Aragona as an "Orthopedic hospital to treat the children with rickets." It was first realized in 1874 by Gaetano Pini, to ensure proper care to the children of the lower social classes: hygienic and therapeutic support, adequate food, education, training and then a suitable job.

Under the direction of R. Galeazzi (1900-1937) the hospital became Clinica Ortopedica of the University of Milano with more than 300 beds. During this period the better life conditions and the preventive therapy of rickets with vitamin D, as well as the application of ultraviolet rays and gymnastics provided the end of this disease. Attention was then directed to the surgical therapy of the consequences of muscular paralysis caused by polio and to the large number of congenital diseases pertinent to Orthopedics.

After the damages of the 2nd World War the Institute was rebuilt to have 600 beds for orthopedics, traumatology, rheumatology and sport medicine. In the last few years it was reduced to 500 beds to provide more comfort for the patients and more space for the scientific activity and the laboratories.

The Service of Anaesthesia was started in 1951 and transformed into a Department in 1963. It has been a very efficient observatorium to study the prevention of pain, the plastic changes that can occur to the mechanisms of pain perception, the influences of the metabolism on pain and the outcome of therapeutics, from birth to the oldest age in patients with orthopedic, traumatic and, rheumatic diseases.

This paper has been prepared on data collected when the Service of Anesthesia was also responsible for the intensive, postoperative, and general medical cares, for pain therapy, and for the supervision of the clinical laboratories in the hospital.

The experimental researches were done in collaboration with the Ist. di Istologia e Anatomia Umana Normale (prof. Bruni), Ist. di Istologia e Anatomia Patologica (prof. Redaelli), Ist. di Fisiologia Umana (prof. Margaria), Clinica di Ortopedia e Traumatologia (prof. Poli), Clinica di Reumatologia (prof. Ballabio), Cattedra di Medicina Sportiva (prof. Lanzetta), Cattedra di Psicologia (prof. Cesa Bianchi) dell'Univ. degli Studi di Milano, Lab.

of Neuro-and psycho-physiology of the GRES of the Univ. of Massachusetts, Lab. de Neurophysiologie of the Univ. P. et M. Curie of Paris.

At the beginning of the 50's the research in our Institute was on the effects of corticosteroids on the T-DS in order to evaluate the possible applications on our patients. The possibility of modulating the response of the tissues with intraarticular injections of hydrocortisone after arthroplasties was studied. This technique gave optimal results as far as pain control and mobility of the joint were concerned. It was adopted until the advent of the arthroprostheses and contributed to the diffusion of the intraarticular use of corticoids in many orthopedic and rheumatic diseases.

In 1957 the Ist. di Fisiologia Umana of the University of Milano developed a project to study some elementary activity of the spinal cord, for NASA. The project was directed towards studying:

a) motor conduction speed of nerve fibers;
b) sensory conduction speed of nerve fibers;
c) central reflex time of H-reflex;
d) end plate delay;
e) the antidromic inhibition of the Renshaw reverberating circuit on the motoneurons.

These five parameters are constant in normal condition, but peculiar changes were observed in stress states and during the effect of some neurotropic drugs. The most important changes were observed on the Renshaw inhibition during mild hypoglycemia, hypoxia, sleep deprivation, muscular fatigue and after the use of alcoholics, tea, coffee, Ritalin, etc.

In Orthopedics the method was applied to test the integrity of the spinal cord during the surgical correction of scoliosis and then for pain researches while trying to act on pain through the inhibitory mechanisms. This study demonstrated that, in our patients, metabolic changes, as well as stress states and neurotropic drugs (when not used with great attention) can dramatically influence the functions of the CNS.

From 1960 to 1965 research concentrated on neuroleptoanalgesia and "vigil" anaesthesia in children, on the treatment of patients with multiple injuries and lesions of the spinal cord, and on the action of curari, sympathomimetic and parasympathomimetic drugs, and autonomic blocking agents. Rickets and polio in Italy were under control at the time, and the congenital deformities were treated in time to prevent a surgical therapy.

During 1964-74 most of the attention was directed to pediatric anaesthesia and to the treatment of spinal shock and its consequences on the survival of the patients. Beds were reduced to 400 to give more space to labs, radiology, immunohematology, and one-day surgery.

After 1975 all the research concentrated on the plasticty of the mechanisms of pain perception.

The exciting progress of the neurosciences in the last fifty years has diverted interest from the T-DS, although the entire organism is dependent, in physiological and pathological events, on this system derived from the mesenchyme. The plasticity and the higher functions of the central nervous system are also dependent on it.

Local, and general modulation of the T-DS with ice therapy, antiinflammatory drugs, corticoids, antihistaminics, etc. is always useful to prevent chronic pain. Examples in patients and in animal models will be presented.

A recent meeting has pointed out that 75% of the people in the world use only Traditional Medicine and that most of the immigrants cannot afford the expensive medical care of the western countries. In the meantime, many of the local inhabitants often have a personal magic ritual or prescription for emergencies, and in particular for pain.

Nowadays, everybody claims a multidisciplinary approach in doing research. In the meantime, most of the researchers in fact treat with suspicion or disregard Traditional Medicine without explaining whether they consider more important the outcome for the patients, or the modern culture of the empirism of some magicians, chamans, sorcerers faithhealers, and--why not?--medical doctors.

Formalism has been officially recognized: hyperspecializations with a modest content; and some papers with a noble signature are so thin and restrictive that is difficult to imagine any practical use for them.

The continuous increase of initiatives (departments, chairs, pain clinics, congresses, meetings, medical associations, scientific and popular writings, books, researches etc.), with pain as subject, suggests some questions:

a) How many patients and doctors are—and not because of negligence or mistakes--unsatisfied with the results?
b) What is the ratio cost/benefits of all these activities?
c) Which is the prevailing cause: altruism, professionality, profit, reputation--or what else?

While a physician still pursues a panacea (or has only adopted a single way to treat his patients), others discover new imaginative hyperspecializations or connections with other sciences. In this Babel a consistent number of patients are still in trouble and do not find any solution for their pain.

This meeting at last calls for attention on metabolism, T-DS and on Traditional Medicine.

In the last 100 years lots of researches, time, and money were invested in rationalizing all aspects of pain in humans. However, we still do not know how to prevent some difficulties that still can arise in patients with chronic pain.

Pain, as well as pleasure, is a paradigm of the peculiarity of life: an unstable disequilibrium in contrast with the static equilibrium of death. Therefore it is difficult to agree with the banal simplicity and the rigidity of the mechanisms of pain perception as it was expressed on the basis of the law of the neuron.

Pain indeed is a random experience, influenced by an incredibly large number of variables produced by metabolic, nervous, cultural and accidental events. It can affect, more than other mechanisms, the whole behavior of the patients and is influenced by the metabolism and vice-versa.

We are all aware of the irreversible changes that deafferentation can cause on the mechanisms of pain perception, but also of the damage produced by neurotropic drugs and destructive procedures. But there are few opportunities for the physician to find anything to prevent intractable chronic pain.

My teachers influenced me to follow a different approach. Therefore, I hope that my use of the term "somatic pain," which implies a more rational manageable meaning, when compared to "visceral" or to "neuropathic pain," will emphasize how determinant are the influences of the T-DS system on the mechanisms of pain perception, and how relevant the functions of this system are in producing plastic changes in the Nervous System.

This meeting is a good opportunity to verify these researches. I hope not to end as Stent (1972) when writing: "to be ahead of one's time deserves only the sympathy into oblivion."

The analysis of the data derived from the activity of the Dept. of Anaesthesia from 1950 up to 1995 suggests some considerations, and some critical remarks on the interactions between metabolism and pain.

While dealing with somatic pain, it is very important:

1) to keep normal the physiological parameters (temperature, glycemia, oxygenation, uricemia, etc.) and functions (circulatory, respiratory, urinary, digestive, motion, sleep alternated with alertness, etc.);

2) to take care as soon as possible and constantly of all the tissues injured by the trauma, surgery or disease (positioning to facilitate blood circulation, accurate hemostasis, evacuation of hematomas and debridement of pus, etc.);

3) to control pain where it originates by using ice treatment as soon and as long as possible (at best, immediately and at the place of the accident) to keep low the local temperature, with the application of antiinflammatory gels or spray, nerve blocks, TENS, etc.;

4) to ensure adequate social support and a decent environment to all patients.

The problem of cancer pain has been adequately emphasized, but a real project has not yet been proposed on the "prevention" of pain for the large population of subjects with congenital or post-traumatic affections of the apparatus of movement. Pain can debilitate these subjects physically and psychically. The problem was important in Italy until the 60's in children with rickets or with paralytic consequences of polio, or of Little's disease. It is still a problem for babies with hip dysplasia, club foot, torticollis, and other similar diseases (in certain areas of North Italy these congenital diseases have an incidence of 16% on the population). They need successive surgical operation through the period of growth, then at the end of the adolescence, and later when old.

The daily example of the connection between metabolism and pain is the ice treatment, which is used in sport-competitions to prevent and to decrease any kind of accidental pain. In this case, the effect of reducing the mesenchymal reactions is more important than the effect of decreasing the sensibility of the peripheral receptors and the conduction speed of the sensory and motor nerves.

The term "reticuloendothelial system," as opposed to the gross "tropho-defensive system," proposed by A.C. Bruni, does not remind us of the trophic functions (the physiological aspects) nor the defense mechanisms (the pathologic aspects) of the system. As a consequence, most of the dramatic contributions of the mesenchyme in the development of the evolutionary brain of the *Homo sapiens* has been underestimated.

In fact, the neurostructures of the neopallium, of the neocerebellum and all the small and very fragile interneurons modulating the activity of the large, resistent and highly specific motor-and sensory neurons, are more strictly dependent on the blood supply than any other cell.

The interneurons are also protected by specialized endotelial cells with the task of an "active" transport of all the metabolites in both senses across the capillary walls to and from these neurons. In the same years, the theory of the neuron was hyperemphasized in its rigid statement by Cajal, while Golgi and his direct heirs Fusari and Bruni, with a small group of colleagues were always considering the nervous system as more flexible and complicated, that is as influenced also by non-neuronal mechanisms.

In the summer 1975, during some experiments on the inhibitory circuits of the spinal cord, a hypothesis became consistent: the inhibition can spread out from an area of normally committed neurons to influence neurons committed to another task. More recently (1993) with L. Rossi we observed the influence of inhibitory neurons of the respiratory center on the pain-sensory nuclei of the trigeminal nerve.

During the sabbatical in 1976-77 in the Laboratory of neuro- and psychophysiology of the Graduate Research Center at University of Massachusettes, the persistent changes caused by a sensory training on the primary somatosensory cortex were studied on animal models. The research was supported by a grant by the Sloan-Kettering Foundation.

For this phenomenon, we used the term "plasticity" adopted by Sperry, Hirsch, and others, for new "physiological" commitments of pathways and neurons in "memorizing" experiences. For this reason, great care was adopted to use, for the training, stimuli not inducing damages to the tissues. We would never consider "plastic" the irreversible changes caused by surgery or drugs.

Our aim was to prevent chronic pain by protecting the inhibitory circuits from death from fatigue; this can be obtained by avoiding the damages produced by hyperergic reactions to pathological events. When the tropho-defensive system is guided in both the metabolic and the aggressive/protective aspects, it is possible to ameliorate the repairing and the destructive functions of the cells produced by the mesenchyme.

Pain Mechanisms and Management
S.N. Ayrapetyan and A.V. Apkarian (Eds.)
IOS Press, 1998

Pain Management in the Republic of Nagorno-Karabagh

V.R. Aghabalian[#] and E.I. Ghukasian[*]
[#] *Minister of Health of NKR,*
[*] *Chief Surgeon of Ministry of Health of NKR*

Pain is an inseparable part of human life, and it is not accidental that the problem of pain has become the subject of study by many leading scientists. It is accepted that pain is a protection mechanism of the organism in response to certain external stimuli. Among these stimuli, gunshot wounds are of great importance. The majority of wounded people first complain of pain, which is one of the main symptoms of wounds. The character of pain (acute, dull, etc.), and its duration are of clinical importance.

In surgery generally, and in field surgery in particular, one of main aims of each surgeon and medical worker is the treatment of pain since timely pain relief interrupts the stream of pain stimuli coming from the wound and helps to prevent such dangerous after-effects as traumatic shock. The latter is also a protection mechanism of the organism in response to pain itself.

The science which deals with pain relief, anesthesiology, is fairly successful, and uses effective pharmaceutical means with the help of which it is possible not only to "turn off" patient's conscious awareness, but also to remove pain reflexes. The types, ways and means of anesthesia are different, the detailed study of which we leave to the specialists. It is only necessary to mention that the anesthesiologist and the surgeon must work together to address the problems of pain relief, given that modern anesthetic means (general, local or complex) must be used taking into account the age, sex, body built and nervous system peculiarities of each separate patient, as well as the conditions where anesthetic means are used (hospital, first-aid station, village medical room, etc.). This approach, especially in battlefield conditions, will provide not only complete pain relief, but also unobtrusive conditions for surgical intervention, ensuring its success.

However, especially in battlefield conditions, one must bear in mind that bullet and shrapnel wounds do not always cause pain from the start. Sometimes, bleeding has to occur before the patient feels pain. This is because the force of the blow and the break inside the tissue causes stroke of nerve endings, so that they temporarily lose their excitability. The type and the force of pain which appears later depends on the type and anatomic position of the wound, the type of fire-arm, and other related factors.

Pain can be completely or partially absent in the case of nervous system trauma. When medical help and rescue are organized in time, pain abates and in 10-12 hours turns into the so-called "painfulness," which can be caused by repositioning or incorrect positioning of the wounded part of the body. We were convinced of this fact during the national liberation war of the people of Artsakh. Pain showed all of its "faces" in Artsakh. However, out of the whole range of all types of pain we would like to concentrate on pain caused by mechanical reasons.

We do not have access to the data of field surgery for the wars of the last 50 years, and especially of the Afghan war. In the beginning of the Artsakh war, we did not have a regular army and military medical service either, and one can imagine what difficulties we came across, and why we had to turn our medical service into a martial one. We hope that our medical officers and especially the surgeons will analyze in detail their experience, which will provide useful information.

Bringing ambulances as near the front line as possible played an important role in gaining success in this sphere. War raged throughout Karabagh, and there was no rear for the military medical service. That is why very often special qualified operations were performed at the battle field, with no special preparation. The importance of anesthesiology carried out under these circumstances becomes even greater when making allowance for the fact that there were very few specialists.

One of the most important problems of pre-hospital period is the organization of anesthesiology treatment. Through proper first aid and rescue measures (pain relief, temporary stop of bleeding, temporary bandaging of the wounded part of the body, etc.) it became possible to subdue pain syndrome and pathological reactions connected with it.
In first and pre-medical aid, the role of rescue groups was of utmost importance. Since during the war of Artsakh the entire country was a battlefield, there were many civilians - children and women - as well as soldiers in the hospitals.

We examined the records of 7,698 wounded people who had been at republican hospital and the central hospital of Stepanakert (operating since September 1991) between 1991-1993 (see table 1).

Table 1. Number of wounded people listed accoding to gender and age.

Number of wounded people	Men	Women	under 15	16-20 years old	21-30 years old	31-40 years old	41-50 years old	51-60 years old	61 and older
7,698	694 89.5%	753 10.5 %	324 4.2%	1,085 14.2%	2,644 34.5%	2,139 27.9%	832 10.5%	381 5%	288 3.7%

As can be seen from table 1, the number of wounded people under 15 and above 41 was 1,444 (23.4%), and those from 16-40 years old make up 76.6%. The rate of casualties is also high. These figures show a significant loss of genofond and a depletion of the work force.
According to the type of wound and the intensity of pain, the results are the following:

Table 2.

Severely and moderately wounded people (in-patients)	Slightly wounded people (out-patients)
4,185 (54%)	3,508 (46%)

People of both groups underwent anesthesia and first surgical treatment. Slightly wounded persons were exposed to local anesthesia and took analgesic drugs, and 2,409 (57%) severely wounded people who underwent operation in front-line military hospitals were exposed to local anesthesia. Severely wounded people who were brought to hospitals were exposed not only to first-aid treatment but also underwent qualified operations under some kind of anesthesia (see table 3):

Table 3.

Number of people who underwent the operation	Types of anesthetic means used				
	Intratracheal combined narcosis	Intravenous narcosis	Epidural anesthesia	Spinal cord anesthesia	Local anesthesia
1,772	1,056 59.2%	159 8.4%	79 5.3%	139 7.5%	339 19.5%

As can be seen from this table, less than half of 4,185 wounded people, that is only 1,772 persons, underwent operation at ordinary hospitals, the other part (more than half) underwent operation at battle field military hospitals.

The location of the wounds on the organism were:

Table 4. Classification of wounded people according to anatomic position of wounds.

Number of wounded people	wounded on the head (jaw, eye, nose, ear, neck)	wounded on the chest	wounded on the stomach and the hip	wounded on the lower and upper limbs	wounded on the spinal cord	burns	comb. wounds
7,698	1,865	951	688	3,874	109	211	757

As can be seen from table 4, the majority of the people (3,816 persons or 49.4%) were wounded on the upper part of the body. The numbers of these injuries could have been fewer if they wore helmets and protective vests.

The classification of gunshot wounds is shown in table 5.

Table 5. Classification of wounded people according to the types of wounds.

Number of wounded people	Gunshot wounds	Shrapnel wounds
7,693	1,334	6,359

As can be seen from this table, the number of shrapnel wounds is 4.8 times greater than that of gunshot wounds. This number could also have been lower if the population had access to refuges. It becomes clear that there are a number of non-medical and non-medicinal means, which could not only relieve pain but also reduce the number of causes of mechanical pain.

Thus:

1. In the case of armed conflicts as well as natural disasters, anesthesia must be carried out in time in all medical facilities, and especially in first-aid stations, according to number of victims and the strength of the pain syndrome. This is one of the most important conditions for shock prevention.

2. The general population and above all rescue groups must be involved in the activities of pain prevention and pain treatment organization.

3. Non-surgical medical workers must be familiar with the principles of pre-medical, first-aid and pain relieving help.

4. There must be a sufficient number of anesthesiologists and other specialists involved in the above mentioned activities.

5. There must also be sufficient technical and medicinal reserves to be used in case of emergencies.

6. When the Ministry of Health and the military medical service of NKR analyze their experience gained during war, it will have useful results.

Pain Mechanisms and Management
S.N. Ayrapetyan and A.V. Apkarian (Eds.)
IOS Press, 1998

Pain Management in Armenia

A. Minasyan, A. Virabyan and A. Boshyan
Emergency Medical Scientific Center, Emergency School
Yerevan, Armenia

Abstract. Pain is universally understood as a signal of disease, it is the most common symptom that brings the patient to a physician's attention. Numerous approaches to pain management prove that the problem is very urgent, and that it is to be studied and investigated thoroughly. The research carried out show the importance of pain management standards determination, especially when disasters and catastrophes occur. Our elaboration results in following principles:
I. Proper development of emergency services according to the modern standards building on the material and technical base of the Health Care system. In the pre-hospital stage, foundation of corresponding structures for pain management.
II. Constant development of educational programs for different specializations, aiming towards pain control and pain management study.

Introduction

Pain is universally understood as a signal of disease, it is the most common symptom that brings the patient to a physician's attention. Pain, especially acute pain, should be controlled immediately because long-term pain irritation may bring about shock. The function of the pain sensory system is to detect, localize, and identify tissue-damaging process. Since different disasters produce characteristic patterns of tissue damage, the quality, time, course and location of a patient's pain complaint, and the location of tenderness provide important diagnostic clues, which are used to evaluate the response to treatment. Medical care cost for patients with pain increases annually. That is why it is considered not only a medical problem but a social one as well. Our efforts with respect to pain are usually directed towards restraining pain seansations. However, the patient's interpretation of the pain, emotional reaction, and behavior are equally considered to be important factors and deserve the physician's attention.

Materials and methods

At present, there is no generally accepted pain classification, however, the work of many authors may result in following:

1. Classification according to anatomic and topographic features

head pain
face pain
chest pain
abdominal pain

pelvic pain
extremity pain

2. Classification according to the grades

Grade 0 No pain
Grade 1 Mild pain: patient calm, complains only when asked, no other signs
Grade 2 Moderate pain: patient spontaneously complains of pain, no other signs
Grade 3 Severe pain: patient groans, complains bitterly, nausea, vomiting,
    disphoresis or pallor can occur
Grade 4 Very severe pain: patient groans, writhes, weeps, or screams from pain,
    nausea, vomiting, diaphoresis, or pallor is usually present.

Numerous classifications show that the problem is very urgent nowadays, and that its to be studied and investigated thoroughly.

We have done the following investigations on the population of the city of Yerevan brought to a physician's attention with pain during the year 1994-1995. During the indicated period 287,766 calls were registered. Out of the total number, 31,654 (11 %) calls referred to pain with 4 grade intensity, 63,309 (22 %) calls to 3 grade intensity, 74,819 (26 %) calls to 2 grade intensity, 69,064 (24 %) calls to 1 grade intensity, and 17% calls with 0 grade intensity. This indicates the high frequency of calls due to high intensity grade pain.

During the period of the Karabagh war, the number of patients with grade 4 intensity pain was also very high. In the Emergency Medical Scientific Center, emergency care was provided to 1,028 victims with gunshot wounds and multiple traumas. There we observed 453 victims with 4th grade intensity, 447 victims with 3rd grade intensity, and 28 victims with 2nd grade intensity pain. Emergency care should be provided to victims from the military zone taking into account the pain intensity grade.

After the Spitak earthquake, in 1988, 500 victims were brought to the Emergency Medical Scientific Center. 65% of this number had sustained multiple traumas and had severe pain. According to the pain intensity grade, the division is as follows: 193 victims with intensity grade 4, 100 victims with intensity grade 3, 73 victims with intensity grade 2, 33 victims with intensity grade1. It should be noted that 193 victims out of 500 were conveyed to the Emergency Medical Scientific Center by air, then they were transferred from the airport by ambulances. 107 victims were brought in by passing cars and special ambulance transportation, 100 victims were transferred from other hospitals. High quality emergency care was provided to 112 victims at the place of disaster, and to 98 victims on the way to the hospital. No care was provided to 22 victims.

To organize the pain management process in cases of disasters and catastrophes, medical services should be properly equipped, provided with necessary transportation and medication. Thus, the principle approach to pain management is important, especially for disasters and catastrophes.

Various classifications are noted for the different authors (T. Harrison 1993, P. Radge 1994 et al.) Pain can be divided into somatic and neuropathic, as well as into "post(operative," "ontological," "chronic" and "psychogenic."

The goals of the pain control in emergency medicine are threefold: (1) relieve the pain and suffering, (2) rule out life threatening causes of the pain, and (3) attempt to diagnose the origins of the pain. All three tasks may be undertaken simultaneously.

Several avenues of pain control emerge from this simplified schema of the etiology of pain just presented:

1. Removal of the painful stimulus. Draining a subungual hematoma or treating coronary artery spasm or blockage with vasodilators, thrombolic agents, or angioplasty are examples of removing the pain-provoking stimulus to relieve pain.

2. Blocking the transmission of the pain message. Non-steroidal anti-inflammatory agents block the production of prostoglands, which are pain mediators. Local anesthetics and nerve blocks interrupt the transmission of the nerve impulse.

3. Centrally acting agents. Narcotics bound to opiate receptors in CNS effect analgesia.

4. Modulating the patient's perception. Headphones and music, suggestion, and guided imagery have been used to "take the patient's mind somewhere else," refocusing his or her attention away from the pain. Modification of the patient's cognitive response to pain might be as simple as putting the patient in pain in a quiet, soothing environment.

The above-mentioned acquaintance with pain classification will promote the pain management process organization. Our elaboration results in the following principles:

I. a. The development of primary Health Care material and technical bases, which is very important for early evaluation and diagnosis especially for pain syndrome, thus preventing further complications.
b. Pre-hospital stage development of pain management organization, especially in cases of disasters and catastrophes.
c. Hospital stage development

The Emergency Medical system must always be in the process of improvement and specialization to solve the raised problems, which include:

- Ambulance arrival timeliness
- Pre-hospital care management
- Medical and technical problems solution

Ambulances, including resuscitative ones, are being equipped and provided with medications according to the condition of the material and technical base of the Health Care System of the Republic of Armenia. Additionally, all the resuscitative ambulance teams (for example, cardiological, pediatric, neurological, traumatological, reanimation) are also being properly equipped.
For the further development of pain management, it is very important to train the ambulance personnel to work in close collaboration with rescue teams.
In addition, emergency pharmacology is also in the process of development to modern Health Care standards. Here, we consider it very important to enlarge physician's pharmacological bucket with injections and tablets and express-diagnostic sets. The physician's pharmacological bucket includes: narcotics, nonsteroidal anti-inflammatory drugs, local anesthesia, nerve blocks, low-dose "general anesthetics."
The elaboration of high quality evaluation and treatment of the patients and victims favors the development of an Emergency Department in the Emergency Medical Scientific

Center. The Emergency Department is equipped with modern express diagnostic sets, and provided with all the medications for pain management organization. The department makes it possible to establish closer contacts between medical personnel and critical patients' relatives, which favors hospital management of the human aspects. All the victims are being examined and evaluated; if necessary consultations are done. This is very useful and important in cases of massive admissions of injured and wounded patients.

II. Pain control and pain management education programs development for students and physicians of different specialties.

World experience of emergency care shows that the most drastic factor in pain control in the hospital and pre-hospital stage is high quality medical personnel.

Certainly, one of the most important ways of increasing the effectiveness of emergency care is medical staff training.

To solve this problem it is necessary to have worked out programs for training, and certification of medical personnel. All this presupposes implementation of a differentiated approach to special programs and specific elaboration for physicians, nurses, paramedics, and non-medical personnel involved in the emergency care. In 1994, the Regional Training Center in the Emergency Medical Scientific Center was founded to train medical and non-medical personnel not only in Armenia, but in the whole Caucasus as well. The education process includes lectures, practical lessons, simulations of disaster emergencies, and others.

The following programs were designed in the Emergency School:

1. 100-hour curriculum designed to improve the initial assessment and treatment skills of medical and non-medical personnel in pre-hospital stage.
2. 400-hour curriculum was designed to improve the nurses' ability to assist doctors in the emergency department, operating room, and all the other spheres of medicine.
3. Residency program for nurses
4. Emergency Department curriculum for the physicians working there
5. Residency program for physicians.

All the above mentioned programs include pain management and pain control. For example, the 100-hour curriculum includes training in all the measures of pain control for different traumas, such as skull trauma, chest trauma, abdominal trauma, burns, as well as pain management in cases of disasters. The residency program for physicians reviews pain syndrome in internal organs.

Results

Pain management continues to be an urgent issue and demands further specialization and development. Our elaboration results in following:
I. The research carried out shows the importance of pain management standards determination, especially when disasters and catastrophes occur.
II. Pain intensity and grade evaluation generally reflects on the dynamic and process of the pathology at hand.
III. Medical personnel adequacy provides opportunities to organize the pain management process in emergency cases.

IV. In order to organize the pain management process in cases of disasters and catastrophes medical services should be properly equipped, provided with the necessary transportation and medication.

V. The development of primary Health Care on the material and technical bases is of great importance both in the pre-hospital stage and the hospital stage.

VI. The Emergency System should possess all necessary mechanisms to organize pain management.

VII. Pain control and pain management education programs development to increase the qualification of students and physicians of different specialties.

References

Alexander D (1994) Pharmocological aspects of pain treatment. 9th European congress of anesthesiologists.

Andersen C (1994) Basic concept of pain treatment. 9th European congress of anesthesiologists.

Harrison T (1993) Internal diseases. Moscow "Medicine" v 1.

May HL, Agababian RV, Fleisher GR (1992) Emergency Medicine. Volume I. Little brown and Company.

Minasyan AM (1995) Emergency System Reforms in Armenia. Dissertation for Doctor of Medicine degree. Yerevan.

Radge P (1994) Basic principles of pain treatment in USA. International congress of anesthesiologists.

Rosen P (1983) Emergency Medicine The CV Mostby Company Volume II.

Schwarts GR (1986) Principles and Practice of Emergency Medicine. WB Saunders Company.

Tailor R (1988) Difficult diagnose. Moscow "Medicine" v 1.

Pain Mechanisms and Management
S.N. Ayrapetyan and A.V. Apkarian (Eds.)
IOS Press, 1998

Pain Perception in War and Disease: An Epidemiologic Outlook

Haroutune K. Armenian
Department of Epidemiology, School of Public Health
Johns Hopkins University
Baltimore, MD, USA

Introduction

For an epidemiologist dealing with research about the determinants of disease incidence in human populations, pain is important for three reasons:

1. As the leading symptom for the diagnosis of a number of conditions, it affects our *measurement of the occurrence* of these diseases. Thus, pain *perception* will affect our estimates of the prevalence and incidence of arthritis as well as migraine and a number of other important public health problems. Depending on the threshold of pain perception, different levels of the iceberg of disease in human communities may be detected. Thus, pain perception will affect detection as well as measurement of disease load in human populations.

2. Epidemiology is also interested in *the effectiveness of health services*. A large component of the health services is dedicated to the management of pain; more effective processes of such management could provide economies in limited resources that are available to the health care sector. This is the framework for the evaluation of various interventions. Response variation to management creates major problems of analysis where the role of the epidemiologist may be very critical.

3. In a number of investigations, pain is a *determinant of disability*, and coping mechanisms with pain may play an important role in minimizing such disability.

This presentation will provide examples of research that were conducted in populations that were exposed to unusual situations and/or lived in an unusual environment. These examples will focus primarily on the relationship of pain perception to psychosocial stressors and mental and physical illness.

The effect of various psychosocial stressors on mental and physical illness is well documented by a number of clinical investigations but only a few population based epidemiological studies. Epidemiologists have to deal with a number of issues within the context of some of the complex relationships that exist between psychosocial stressors and mental and physical illness.

Our presentation of epidemiologic research done during the civil war in Lebanon and investigations following the 1988 earthquake in Armenia, illustrate the potential for learning about the role of massive environmental stressors on both physical and mental health from such research. Our current investigations from within the Epidemiologic Catchment Area Follow-up Study in Baltimore provides us with an opportunity to test these relationships using a more systematic approach.

At the conclusion of this paper, the need for an integrated approach in dealing with such complex situations will be highlighted.

Psychopathology in disaster situations

There is a rich literature of studies that have looked at the relationship of disasters to psychopathology. Whether it is following a hurricane, an earthquake or war, it is well established that, as a result of a major disaster, there is a high level of psychopathology in the exposed population (Bromet and Dew, 1995).

Psychopathology in wartime

A number of studies have reported increased psychiatric illness in persons exposed to war stress. These reports include high rates of psychiatric disorders among concentration camp survivors following the Second World War (Eitinger, 1962 and Eitinger, 1969), in East European refugees (Krupinski et al., 1973), and in Vietnamese evacuees (Murphy, 1977). Many of these studies have a clinical focus, and few are population based.

While the protracted war in Lebanon was in progress, we conducted a number of investigations that assessed the role of stressors on illness in the population. During the siege of Beirut, in the summer of 1982, we conducted an Emergency Health Surveillance Project that was designed to provide ongoing information on the health status of Beirut residents and to quickly identify health problems requiring assistance and intervention (Fac. Of Health Sciences, 1984). As part of this project, we conducted a population based household survey of about 1,345 families in Beirut and its suburbs. The analysis of data from this population survey revealed that, parallel to high rates of common infections, this population also reported high rates of psychological distress symptoms (Lockwood Hourani et al., 1986). The frequency of these symptoms in this population was related to worsening physical health and loss of home and income.

In another study, requirements for analgesics following appendectomy were used as a model to assess the impact of the civil war situation in Lebanon on patient reaction to pain. The records of 246 patients who had undergone appendectomy for acute appendicitis under general anesthesia with no complications or concurrent diagnoses were reviewed. 67 of these patients were operated in the pre-war years, 67 during the war, and 112 in a period of relative calm and peace. The total dose of analgesics in pethidine equivalents and number of injections was calculated for each patient. In addition, socioeconomic, demographic and clinical data were collected on all these patients. Patients operated during and after the war required significantly less postoperative analgesics compared to prewar patients. We explained these findings on the basis of changes of perception regarding intensity of pain by providers and patients during the war.

Physical illness and stressors in wartime

The role of psychosocial stressors in physical illness has been highlighted in a number of studies. The ongoing war in Lebanon provided an opportunity to assess the impact of war stressors on coronary artery disease (CAD) within a case-control study at the American University of Beirut. A total of 127 patients who underwent coronary angiography were individually matched with visitor controls free from any evidence of clinical CAD. Arteriographic cases were compared to two control groups: arteriographic controls with entirely normal coronaries, and visitor controls. Cases reported significantly higher number of exposures to acute war events compared to both control groups. Crossing the "green line" separating the two fighting factions in Beirut, considered as an attribute of war related chronic stress, was more frequent in cases compared to both control groups. Adjusting for the effect of well-established CAD risk factors did not alter the above reported findings (Sibai et al., 1989).

Psychopathology following an earthquake

Psychiatric morbidity, particularly post-traumatic stress disorders (PTSD) following disasters are a major public health problem. Estimates of PTSD following disasters vary between 2 and 60 percent (Saigh, 1992). Although measurement issues may explain some of the differences in these estimates, it is more probable that these could result from differences in the nature of the disaster and the sociocultural environment within which these disasters occur.

Following the earthquake of December 7, 1988, in Armenia, we embarked on a number of population based epidemiological studies of the determinants of death and injury during the earthquake as well as of the long term effects of the earthquake in a cohort of 33,000 survivors of the disaster. Within this population, a geographically stratified sample of 1,785 persons between the ages of 16 and 70 were interviewed using a special psychiatric questionnaire over a period of one year. Within two years following the earthquake, about 60 percent of this adult population had symptoms that could fulfill the diagnosis of either PTSD and/or depression. The risk of PTSD and depression was related to the amount of loss in the individual's family. Thus, the intensity of the ensuing loss from the disaster was related to the intensity of the psychiatric morbidity in this population (H. Armenian et al. Manuscript in preparation).

Psychopathology and physical illness

Although there is a wealth of clinical reports in the literature about psychopathology following physical illness, most of these are based on cross sectional studies and very few of these are population based. The role of psychopathology itself as a determinant of physical illness has been difficult to study. A major problem for such studies is the difficulty in establishing antecedence of diagnostic specific psychopathology to physical illness.

The Baltimore Epidemiologic Catchment Area (ECA) Follow-up project is a population based study of assessment of diagnostic specific psychopathology and other comorbidity in 1981, 1982 and 1993. From an original population-based cohort of 3,481 persons who were interviewed in 1981 for psychopathology, chronic physical illness, and disability, 1,862 were alive and reinterviewed in 1993. In this study, we were able to investigate psychiatric antecedents of a number of physical illnesses including arthritis, diabetes, migraine, and coronary heart disease.

A number of associations between antecedent psychopathology and these chronic illnesses have been demonstrated within the ECA study. In a recent analysis, the possible interaction between antecedent psychiatric illness and arthritis as determinants of incident disability was studied (H. Armenian et al. Submitted to publication.)

Conclusions

The review of these studies, in particular the ECA study, has highlighted the fact that the relationships between pain, psychosocial stressors, physical and mental illness are not simple. In order to understand these relationships, one has to use more complex models of etiology. As we were able to study within the ECA study population, psychopathology could be a determinant of, as well as a result of, physical illness. Similarly, the intensity of pain perception could be determined by physical illness as well as psychopathology. If we consider the role of social and demographic characteristics, in addition to factors affecting access and utilization of health services, within the framework of these relationships, the need for a more integrative approach to such research has to be underscored. Such an approach is dependent on the use of more complex models of etiology, like the web of causation of MacMahon and newer approaches of investigation and analysis.

One such approach that epidemiologists could learn from and could adapt to their needs, is systems analysis. Epidemiologists need to view disease and wellness within systems of interacting elements. Such systems have inputs, processes and outcomes, and are integrated within systems at higher levels. In addition, outcomes in one system are inputs to other systems. The relationship of psychopathology and physical illness that we discussed here is a good example where such an approach could possibly be more productive than existing approaches.

Epidemiologists have primarily focused on simple models of etiology where the direction between one primary independent variable is studied as it affects one outcome. Multivariate analyses in such a context are used to hold constant or adjust for other determinants of the primary relationship of interest. The underlying philosophical model for such an approach to etiology is essentially univariate and simple. Progress in epidemiology is contingent on adapting our powerful computing and statistical tools to study more complex models of interacting factors within identifiable systems.

We need to study how the whole web of causation works rather than just how a thread or a knot is held within the web.

Plenary discussion

Carpenter D.: Did you investigate the effects of age on post-traumatic separations such as depression or PTSS?
We have a separate study on a subsample of about 2,000 survivors of the earthquake in Armenia, looking at PTSD and depression. Our study population was made of adults who were individually interviewed. Age is introduced as a covariate in our analyses.

Berkley K.: What amongst your findings surprised you?
The strong effect of wartime stressors on physical illness, and the finding of a dose/response relationship between amount of loss as a a result of the earthquake and the intensity of subsequent PTSD and depression.

Apkarian V.: I noticed that the analgesic dose used decreased even further at the postwar period. How do you explain this?
What was called a post-war period in that study was essentially a lull period between two periods of fighting. Also, the effects may be longer term than we may expect.

References

Armenian HK (1986) In wartime: options for epidemiology. Am J Epidemiol 124:28-32.

Armenian HK (1989) Perceptions from epidemiologic research in an endemic war. Soc Sci Med 28:643-647.

Bromet E, Dew MA (1995) Review of psychiatric epidemiologic research on disasters. Epidemiol Rev 17:113-119.

Eitinger L (1962) Concentration camp survivors in the post-war world. Am J Psychother 26:191.

Eitinger L (1969) Psychosomatic problems in concentration camp survivors. J Psychosom Res 13:183.

Krupinski J, Stoller A, Wallace L (1973) Psychiatric disorders in East European refugees now in Australia. Soc Sci Med 7:31.

Murphy J (1977) War stress and civilian Vietnamese. A study of psychological effects. Acta psychiat scand 56:92.

Faculty of Health Sciences, American University of Beirut (1984) Emergency health surveillance project, July-November 1982. WHO Wkly Epidem Rec 58:7-8.

Lockwood Hourani L, Armenian H, Zurayk H, Afifi L (1986) A population-based survey of loss and psychological distress during war. Soc Sci Med 23:269-275.

Day RC (1986) Psychological study of children in Lebanon. In: In wartime: the state of children in Lebanon (JW Bryce and HK Armenian eds). American University of Beirut, Beirut, 105-116.

Saigh PA (1992) History, current nosology, and epidemiology. In: Posttraumatic stress disorders (PA Saigh ed). A behavioral approach to assessment and treatment. Allyn and Bacon, Boston, London, Toronto, Sydney, Tokyo, and Singapore 1-27.

Sibai AM, Armenian HK, Alam S (1989) Wartime determinants of arteriographically confirmed coronary artery disease in Beirut. Am J Epidemiol 130:623-631.

Pain Management
(Clinical Issues)

Pain Mechanisms and Management
S.N. Ayrapetyan and A.V. Apkarian (Eds.)
IOS Press, 1998

Percutaneous Radiofrequency Nucleotomy in Symptomatic Disc Protrusion

A. Witzmann[1], E. Mozes[1], B. Kepplinger[2], A. Popadic[1]
[1]*Landeskrankenhaus Feldkirch, Department of Neurosurgery*
[2]*Landesnervenklinik Mauer, Department of Neurology*
Austria

Introduction

Pain resulting from degenerative spinal diseases occurs with increasing frequency all over the world. Practicing neurosurgeons, neurologists, and orthopedists observe this phenomenon almost every day.

Local pain in the cervical region with variably associated pain radiating to the shoulder and the arm is suffered by 9% of all men and 12% of all women at some time of their lives (BLAND 1986).

In most cases, both lumbar and cervical pain syndromes may be alleviated by conservative treatment. Many treatment modalities like physiotherapeutic techniques, biofeedback, medical therapy, psychological strategies, and, increasingly, alternative methods like acupuncture, manual therapy, and so on are offered to the patients. All of these treatment modalities have their merits and lead to pain reduction in a great number of patients. However, pain recurrence is observed in a considerable percentage, and extensive diagnostic assessment takes place to reveal a disc prolapse, or other noxious pathological abnormalities that require surgical interventions.

But, such abnormalities are not found in all patients. For these cases, a set of targets for radiofrequency lesions has been developed. All of these lesions are located adjacent to the spine and were developed to alleviate pain (Sluijter And Mehta 1981, Sluijter 1990). Therefore, we would like to call these kinds of procedures *"percutaneous perispinal pain procedures"*. These techniques comprise facet denervation, radiofrequency lumbar sympathicotomy, radiofrequency rhizotomy (cervical, thoracic and lumbar), and radiofrequency nucleotomy (RF-NT). The latter technique is presented in this article.

Anatomical remarks

The highest density of nociceptors in the spine is found on the dorsal longitudinal ligament, the anulus fibrosus (mostly on its dorsal part), the dura, the facet joint and the spinal nerve root (Krämer 1994). There is some evidence that the dorsal root ganglion carries nociceptive cell bodies of both somatic and visceral afferent fibres from all potentially nociceptive spinal structures (Van Kleef et al. 1996). This implies the conclusion that the dorsal root ganglion is an important structure conducting nociceptive stimuli from various sites.

The spinal nerve root is divided into a ventral and a dorsal part. After division, the ventral part delivers the ramus meningeus, also called "recurrent nerve" or "Nerve of Luschka". This nerve runs back to the spinal canal via the intervertebral foramen. In the spinal canal it innervates the dura, the dorsal parts of the anulus fibrosus (the ventral parts are innervated by sympathetic fibres) and the inner part of the facet joint. The dorsal part of the spinal nerve root innervates the large outer part of the facet joint, and its capsule which are extremely densely packed with nociceptors.

Patients and previous treatment

23 patients were treated with RF-NT from January 1995 to December 1995. 12 of them were women, 11 male. The mean age was 40.9 years (27 to 72). In all patients extensive conservative treatment without success was performed prior to the RF-NT. No other perispinal pain treatment modality was performed before RF-NT.

Symptoms and signs

The clinical substrate of irritation of these structures is mostly local spinal pain in the lumbar level called "low back pain," and in the cervical level called "cervical syndrome." In most cases this local spinal pain is associated with some kind, and different degree, of irradiation into the leg and arm, respectively. This irradiation is also called "pseudoradicular pain." The compression of the spinal nerve root itself caused by a disc prolapse leads to the well-known lumbar radiculitis and cervical radiculitis, respectively.

Two of our patients suffered solely from low back pain. 21 patients showed irradiation in addition to the local pain. In 4 patients, the local pain was more disabling than the irradiation. Three patients felt more disabled by the irradiation, and 14 patients were disturbed equally by both the local pain and the irradiation. The 3 cervical patients were also found in this group.

Description of RF-NT

Disc protrusion creates pressure on the nociceptors of the dorsal part of the anulus fibrosus and is, therefore, one of the sources of local spinal pain. Alleviation of this type of pain by denervating the dorsal part of the anulus fibrosus by heat via an inserted electrode is the possible underlying mechanism of RF-NT.

First, a puncture of the interspace with a Sluijter-Mehta needle under fluoroscopic control is carried out. Then a discography is performed with 1 to 2 ml of a solution consisting of 2% lidocaine and contrast medium. The purpose is twofold: first, one can test the condition of the disc and detect leaks in the anulus and dorsal longitudinal ligament, and secondly, diagnostic blockade of the anulus receptors is achieved. The patient should be pain-free for at least 6 hours after discography. If there is no reduction of pain over this period of time, a RF-NT is not performed. Otherwise, a RF-NT will be performed in a second session one or two days later. In the lumbar region the needle is inserted 8 to 10 cm lateral from the midline. In the cervical region the interspaces C2/3 and C3/4 are approached laterally, and the cervical interspaces caudal from the C3/4 interspace are approached ventrally.

In the beginning of our work, we performed RF-NT with 72°C for 240 seconds. Later, after discussion with Sluijter we applied 75°C for 240 seconds with somewhat better results.

Treated levels

L4/5 was treated 13 times, L5/S1 once, a combination of treatment of L4/5 plus L5/S1 was performed twice, L4/5 plus L3/4 3 times and L2/3 plus L3/4 plus L4/5 was treated in one patient.

In the cervical region C4/5, C5/6, and C6/7 each was treated in one patient. In summary, we have treated 30 levels in 23 patients. All patients were carefully examined preoperatively, clinically and with CT scan or MRI. All patients revealed disc protrusion in the treated levels without the signs of disc prolapse.

Results

All 23 patients were evaluated before, and one day after the procedure, by means of the Visual Analog Scale (VAS). Three months later follow up examination was performed in 18 patients. 5 patients were lost for follow up because of various reasons. Out of these 5 lost patients, 4 were painfree after the procedure. One of them was treated without effect.

Patients were categorized as painfree (VAS 0 to 1), improved (difference between pre- and postoperative examination 3 or more points in VAS) and unchanged (difference only 2 or less between pre- and postoperative examination).

After the procedure, 14 patients were pain free, 5 had improved and 4 had no benefit from the treatment. Only 3 out of 18 patients at follow up were pain free, 9 had improved and 6 were unchanged. In 3 out of these 6 unchanged patients clinical reexamination and repeat CT scan revealed disc herniation, instead of the previous protrusion as the cause of their disability. These 3 patients underwent microsurgical disc removal and were pain free after this surgical procedure.

Discussion

In sum, it can be said that RF-NT has proved a safe method with no side-effects for the treatment of disc generated pain without spinal root compression. However, the results of our study strongly suggest that RF-NT is not a panacea, but only part of the treatment armamentarium for spinal pain. After three months only 3 out of 18 patients were pain free. One has to keep in mind that, perhaps, 3 patients who were later on operated for removal of a prolapsed disc should not have undergone RF-NT. Careful patient selection and careful clinical and radiological examination (CT or MRI) are essential for the outcome.

RF-NT should be the last point in the percutaneous perispinal procedures even when a disc protrusion is detected. Facet joint and spinal nerve root blockade and denervation should be done before insertion of an electrode into the interspace. We have changed our attitude during the last months. From January 1996 to August 1996 we performed 97 percutaneous perispinal pain treatment procedures in 49 patients. Out of these 97 procedures only 2 were RF-NTs. Both patients are pain free up till now.

Plenary discussion

Ayrapetyan S.: I am interested in what frequency was used in your treatment?

Witzmann A.: This is a thermal lesion with 75°C applied for 240 seconds. The heat is the critical factor in this kind of lesion (as compared to root lesions). Therefore, the frequency doesn't play an important role.

Ayrapetyan S.: Does it depend on age?

Witzmann A.: Older people show more frequent recurrence of pain than younger individuals. This is probably because of the progressive degenerative changes of the spine which involve more pain generating structures than in younger patients. Furthermore, in older patients pain is usually experienced for a long time and, therefore, contains a lot of chronic mechanisms which are very difficult to treat by invasive methods. Not to forget are also psychological and social mechanisms, which are known to play an important role in pain generation and pain assessment.

Knapp D.: What percent of patients with chronic back and neck pain have the origin of their pain in the spine and adjacent structures?

Witzmann A.: Low back pain and neck pain origin is a very complex problem. There are several structures like the dorsal part of the arilius fibrosus, the facet joint, the dura mater, and the posterior longitudinal ligament, all of which can contribute to the pain in various degrees. Because all of these structures belong to the spine, a high percentage of low back and neck pain is actually of spine origin. But, one should not forget that pain is a psychic event and comprises the entire human being, and can, therefore, originate elsewhere in the nervous system.

References

Band JH (1986) Cervical spine syndromes. J Muskuloskel Med 3: 23-41.

Krämer J (1994) Bandscheibenbedingte Erkrankungen. Stuttgart, New York, Thieme, 63 - 70.

Sluijter M and Mehta M (1981) Treatment of chronic neck and back pain by percutaneous thermal lesions, In: Persistant Pain, Modern Methods of Treatment. London (Lipton S., Miles J. eds), Academic Press, Vol. 3, 141 - 179.

Sluijter ME (1990) Percutaneous Thermal Lesions in the Treatment of Cervical Pain Syndromes. Radionics Procedure Technique Series. Burlington, Radionics Inc.

Van Kleef M, Liem L, Lousberg R, Barendse G, Kessels F and Sluijter ME (1996) Radiofrequency lesion adjacent to the dorsal root ganglion for cervicobrachial pain: a retrospective double blind randomized study. Neurosurgery 38: 1127 - 1132.

CT-Controlled Instillation of Tramadol, Cortison and Lidocaine - a Comparative Study

B. Kepplinger, H. Schmid, P. Kalina, J. Wallner and C. Derfler
Diagnostic and Therapy Center, Department of Neurology, NOE LNK
Mauer, Austria

Introduction

The pain controlling effect of nerve root blockades with local anesthetics in radicular pain is generally accepted. Nerve root blockades, especially in the cervical region are performed very restrictively because of quite often observed complications and hazards e.g. cardiovascular and/or cerebrovascular complications.

As the recent literature hints that perineural (and intraarticular) morphine is effective due to morphine receptors within the peripheral nerves, the question arises if and to what amount local anesthesics blockades can be substituted by nerve root blockades performed just with morphine. In this study we compared the therapeutical effect of periradicular applied Tramadol, periradicular applied Cortison and Lidocaine.

Method and patients

Three statistically independent probes of one population (each 15 patients with acute radicular pain due to disc herniation or stenosis of the neuroforamen L4/5 or L5/S1) were compared. Patients from the first group were treated with 50 mg Tramadol, the patients of the second group were treated with 50 mg Lidocaine, and the patients of the third group were treated with 10 mg Volon (cristall corticoid). The treatment was performed equally due to CT-guidance of the canulla and application of 2 ccm Jopamiro 300 (CT-contrast medium) for evaluation of the exact placement of the canulla. In case of exact placement (periradicular position of the cannula and the contrast medium) either Tramadol (50 mg), or Lidocaine (50 mg), or Volon (10 mg) was instilled.

Evaluation of pain intensity was performed using a visual analogue scale (VAS). VAS scores were performed before, 1, 6, 12, 24 and 48 hours after application of the agent. The statistical evaluation was performed with the Wilcoxon test for dependent probes and with the U-test for independent probes.

Results

Comparison of VAS-scores before the blockade did not show any difference between the three groups. One hour after CT-controlled application of the respective agent, statistically significant lower VAS-mean values (p<0.01 - 0.05) showed in all three groups. The analgesic effect for all three agents lasted on a statistically significant level (p<0.05) for 24 hours. The pain reduction after Volon application lasted at the 5 % level, also at the 48 hour measure point; whereas, the Tramadol and Lidocaine effect at this time did not show statistically significant differences to the base-level.

Discussion

Prior investigations (Stein, 1994) have already shown the analgesic effect of periradicular applied morphine. Our study shows, that in radicular pain (due to disc herniation) Tramadol, a morphine-like agent, when instilled to the nerve root, provides an almost equal analgesic effect compared with Lidocaine or Cortison within a 24 hour period.

Taking into consideration that the morphine effect can be antagonized by Naloxone, while no antidote can be kept ready for local anesthesics, the use of morphine-like agents for periradicular blockades might be less hazardous, and therefore recommendable for clinical praxis.

References

Kepplinger B, Schmid H, Derfler C (1995) Computertomographic controlled nerve root infiltration with Tramadol. In: Ilias W. K.: ZAK 95, Volume of free communications. Monduzzi Editore, 497-499.

Kepplinger B, Schmid H, Rettenstreiner G, Derfler C, Papst H, Erhart H, Wallner J (1995) Wirkungsvergleich zwischen intramuskulär und periradikulär verabreichtem Tramadol. Neuropsychiatrie, Band 9, Heft 4; 196-200.

Rettensteiner G, Schmid H, Derfler C, Kalina P, Papst H, Kepplinger B (1996) Computertomographisch kontrollierte periradikuläre Applikation von Tramadol versus Lidocain. Kongressband der 5. Jahrestagung der Österreichischen Schmerzgesellschaft, Hrsg.: Lanner G und Wessely P, Norea Verlag, Klagenfurt, 36-37.

Stein C (1994) Interactions of immune-competent cells and nociceptors. In: Gebhart G. F., Hammond D. I., Jensen T. S.: Progress in pain research and management on pain. Vol. 2, Proceedings of the 7th World Congress on Pain. IASP-Press, 285-297.

Computertomographic Guided Percutaneous Interventions for Chronic Pain Treatment

B. Kepplinger[1], C. Derfler[1], P. Kalina[1], J. Wallner[1], G. Vogl[2], V. Belan[3], B. Szalay[4], J. Reiss[5], J. Matejka[6] and P. Fencl[7]

[1]*Diagnostic & Therapy Center/Neurology/NOE LNK, Mauer, Austria*
[2]*Center for CT-controlled disc management, Innsbruck, Austria*
[3]*Radiologic Dept./L. Derer Hospital, Bratislava, Slovakia*
[4]*Pain Clinic/CT-Institute, OOE GKK, Linz, Austria*
[5]*Neurol. Dept./Bezirkskrankenhaus Haar, Munich, Germany*
[6]*Radiologic Dept./General Hospital, Dunajska Streda, Slovakia*
[7]*Radiologic Dept./General Hospital, Czeske Budejovice, Czech Republic*

Introduction

The advantages of computertomographic assisted pain therapeutic interventions in comparison to conventional (i.e. only anantomically oriented) and fluoroscopic guided blockades and ablative methods results are due to the exact positioning of the canulla tip, while vulnerable structures can be spared. Many physicians believed that this new technique we developed and proved would be an unnecessary "technical overkill" which would make the procedure only expensive and time consuming. But the technical developement of CT-devices moves towards "realtime imaging" with scan slices available within 0.75 seconds and towards "CT-fluoroscopic imaging" with "cinemode characteristics" (six to nine images per second), the semiconductor-detector technology lowering drastically the x-ray dosage which makes it possible to introduce and forward the probe without preplanning to the target point. This results in a higher efficiency of the treatment, and on the other hand to a greater safety for the patient, and, in times of "legal medicine," also to fewer risks for the physician.

The following CT-assisted methods for pain treatment are in use
A) Epidural scar tisssue infiltration,
B) Nerve root blockades and percutaneous thermoselective rhizotomy,
C) Cervical and lumbar sympathetic blockades and chemical/thermal
   "sympathectomies",
D) Percutaneous mechanical and thermal (radiofrequency) nucleotomy,
   sequestrectomy and chemonucleolysis.
E) Facet joint blockades and - radiofrequency denervation,
F) Blockade/chemical destruction of the coeliac ganglion.

The mentioned institutions are performing following indicated methods
Inst. (1): A, B, C, E,
Inst. (2): A, B, C, D, E,
Inst. (3): B, C, F,

Inst. (4): B, C, E,
Inst. (5): B, C,
Inst. (6): B, C,
Inst. (7): B, C, D,

Results

Within a time period from one up to seven years a total of 13,407 CT-controlled interventions were performed in mentioned institutions. The most often performed method was a CT-guided lumbar nerve root blockade, followed by CT-guided lumbar facet joint infiltration and lumbar nucleotomies. The longest time of experience, the broadest spectrum of CT-interventions, and the greatest number of interventions are revealed in institution 2, followed by the institution 1. Cervical nerve root blockades are performed in mentioned institutions, exclusively CT-controlled. No major complications occured under CT-guided interventions.

Discussion

The increasing importance of CT-interventions for pain treatment is due to the easier access to CT-devices nowadays, and also due to the new developments in CT-technology-- i.e. real time imaging, fluoro-CT, semiconductive detectors, subsecond scanning, greater gantry aperture. Important is the fact, that CT controlled interventions are safer, and generally less traumatic. There are less canulla positioning corrections necessary compared to fluoroscopic-controlled or "only anatomically" oriented infiltration techniques.

References

Dominkus M, Kepplinger B, Bauer W.and Dubsky E (1991) Percutaneous Radiofrequency Thermolesion of the Sympathetic Chain in the Treatment of peripheral Vascular Disease. AMA (Acta MedAustr), 18/ Sonderheft 1, 69 - 70.

Kepplinger B, Papst H, Dubsky E and Benischek B (1988) Lumbale perkutane Radiofrequenz Fasettdenervierung und Sympathektomie. Abstract Proceeding Jahreskongress der Gesellschaft zum Studium des Schmerzes (DÖS), 51 - 62.

Kepplinger B and Derfler C (1993) CT assisted percutaneous lumbar radiofrequency coagulation of the lumbar sympathetic chain. In: Pain - Clinical Aspects and Therapeutical Issues - Part II, Edition Selva, 75-78.

Kepplinger B and Defler C (1994) CT-gesteuerte Interventionen in der Neurologie. Neuropsychiatrie, 8, 36.

Kepplinger B (1995) Interventionelle neurologische Schmerztherapie. ÖKZ, 36:5, 4-8.

Kepplinger B, Rettensteiner G, Reiss J, Szalay B, Vogl G, Wallner J, Papst H, Derfler C, Ambros G and Fencl P (1996) Computertomographisch assistirte Interventionen in der Schmerztherapie. In: 5. Jahrestagung der Österr. Schmerzgesellschaft - Kongressband, Hrsg.: G. Lanner und P. Wessely, Norea Repro Druck & Verlag, Klagenfurt, 32 -35.

Vogl G and Kepplinger B (1992) CT-aided infiltration of cervical nerve roots. In: Pain - Clinical Aspects and Therapeutical Issues - Part I, Edition Selva, 75-79.

Vogl G and Mohseipour I (1993) CT assisted percutaneous treatment of lumbar and cervical herniated disc. In: Pain - Clinical Aspects and Therapeutical Issues - Part II, Edition Selva, 108-114.

Pain Mechanisms and Management
S.N. Ayrapetyan and A.V. Apkarian (Eds.)
IOS Press, 1998

Computertomographic Controlled Epidurography for Safe Epidural Blockades

B. Kepplinger[1], D. Embey-Isztin[2], C. Derfler[1], P. Kalina[1], A.E. Oygar[3] and H. Schmid[1]
[1]*Diagnostic & Therapy Center/Neurology, NOE LNK Mauer, Austria*
[2]*Pain Clinic, National Institute of Oncology, Budapest, Hungary*
[3]*Eisenhower Medical Center, Rancho Mirage, USA*

Introduction

In 1885, the first attempts for an epidural analgesia were performed by J. L. Corning. In 1933, this method was established by A. Gutierrez for surgical anesthesia. During the last 30 years epidural blockades are performed also for the treatment of subacute and chronic pain, especially in sciatica. To prolong the therapeutical effect, the local anesthetic agent is combined with a cristal corticoid suspension. Observing the effect of epidural blockades showed a vast difference in the short and long term outcome of this treatment. In this investigation, the clinical effectiviness of epidural blockades was compared to the definitive reached area, controlled by CT-imaging; in this way, the participating phycicians could assess their own aptitude.

Method and patients

Epidural blockades were performed at the level of L3/4 in sitting position using a 20 Gauge B-D Yale canulla. Reaching of the epidural space was indicated by loss of resistance, and then 2 ml Jopamiro 200 (x-ray contrast medium), 1 ml Volon A 10 and 4 ml Xylocaine 1 % were instilled. Afterwards, the canulla was retrieved and one (to three) CT scan(s) in prone position were performed at the level of puncture to detect and evaluate the distribution of the instilled contrast medium. Eleven physicians participated in this study on 145 patients, who suffered from low back pain, sciatica, lumbar radicular pain due to disc protrusion, epidural fibrosis, spondylarthrosis and spinal canal stenosis.

The following contrast medium distributions were found
Contrast medium paravertebral
Contrast medium paravertebral and epidural
Contrast medium epidural
Contrast medium epidural and intrathecal
Contrast medium intrathecal
Contrast medium not detectable

The clinical effect of the epidural blockade was estimated by the patient according to the following criteria during an observation period of three days:

Score 0: No effect.
Score 1: Moderate pain relief.
Score 2: Distinct pain relief.
Score 3: (Almost) pain free.

The average scores of pain relief from the first, second and third day were compared with the radiological findings.

Results

Epidural distribution was found in 78 % of all 121 patients, the clinical outcome being score 2.2 on the first day, 2.1 on the second day and 1.7 on the third day. Paravertebral distribution was found in 9.7 %, the clinical outcome being score 1.7 on the first day, and 1.0 on the second and third day.

Paravertebral and epidural distribution was found in 7 %, the clinical outcome being score 1.8 on the first day, 1.7 on the second and third day. Intrathecal distribution was found in 3,5 %, the clinical outcome being score 3.0 on the first and second day, 2.5 on the third day.

No contrast was detectable in 1.8 %, the clinical outcome being score 2.0 on the first day, 3.0 on the second, and 2.0 on the third day.

The idcal distribution was estimated to be the epidural space solely. The eleven different physicians who performed the procedure reached this desired contrast medium distribution in a widespreaded spectrum between 50 and 95 %. The patients in total reported an average pain reduction of 2.0 (according to the above mentioned scores) at the day of blockade, a pain reduction of 1.7 on the next day, and of 1.4 on the third day.

Discussion

According to the CT results, the participating physicians could assess their skill in performing an epidural blockade. The differences in reaching the ideal target point (i.e. the epidural space) varied from 50 to 95%.

The clinical outcome of epidural blockades was distinctly different when the different target points reached were evaluated with respect to contrast medium distributions. Best results were found when the contrast medium was detected only in the intrathecal space, followed by the results when contrast medium was found epidurally and intrathecally, an observation which has already been made by clinicians who used to give cortison intrathecally in severe cases of pain due to epidural fibrosis.

The results were poorest when the contrast medium was found only in the paravertebral space, better results were seen when the contrast medium was also found intrathecally.

One of the interesting results of this study was the fact that, in 1.8 % of all cases, no positive contrast was found in the epidural space, although there was air visible in the epidural space, which leads to the conclusion, that a technically perfect epidural blockade "per se" does not necessarily guarantee an optimal distribution of the therapeutic agent, and therefore a so-called diagnostic blockade should always be performed under CT control.

References

Kepplinger B, Kalina P, Derfler C and Allen C (1995) Epidural blockade in CT-epidurography - a preliminary study. In: 24th Central European Congress on Anesthesiology. Volume of free communications. Ed.: W. K. Ilias, Monduzzi Editore, Bologna, 493-495.

Kepplinger B, Kalina P and Derfler C. (1995) CT-kontrollierte epidurale Blockade. Anästhes. Jg 44, Suppl, 417.

Kepplinger B; Wallner J, Schmid H, Derfler C, Allen C, Kalina P, Rettensteiner G, Baaz A, Dubsky E and Erhart H (1996) Qualitätskontrolle bei epiduralen Blockaden. In: Kongressband / 5. Jahrestagung der Österrreichischen Schmerzgesellschaft, Hrsg.: G. Lanner und P. Wessely, Norea Verlag Klagenfurt, 58-60.

Kepplinger B, Embey-Isztin D and Schmid H (1996) The save method of epidural injection: The role of CT and X-ray image intensifier controls. Abstract book 7th International Symposium: The Pain Clinic, ed. by S. Erdine, 325.

Papst H, Derfler C and B Kepplinger (1994) Perkutane lumbale Sympathikusausschaltung - Sicherheitsaspekte. In: VASA, Suppl. 44, 13.

Author Index

Printed in the United Kingdom
by Lightning Source UK Ltd.
132499UK00001B/160-162/P